RESEARCH IN PHYSICAL THERAPY

RESEARCH IN PHYSICAL THERAPY

Edited by

CHRISTOPHER E. BORK, Ph.D., P.T.

Dean, School of Allied Health
Professor of Physical Therapy
Medical College of Ohio
Toledo, Ohio

With 12 additional contributors

J. B. LIPPINCOTT COMPANY   Philadelphia

Sponsoring Editor: Andrew Allen
Coordinating Editorial Assistant: Miriam Benert
Production Editor: Virginia Barishek
Indexer: Barbara Littlewood
Cover Designer: Susan Blaker
Production: Publishers' WorkGroup
Compositor: Bucks County Type & Design
Printer/Binder: R. R. Donnelley & Sons Company

6 5 4 3 2

Library of Congress Cataloging-in-Publication Data

Bork, Christopher E.
    Research in physical therapy / Christopher E. Bork ; with 12
additional contributors.
        p.   cm.
    Includes bibliographical references and index.
    ISBN 0-397-54803-6
    1. Physical Therapy—Research.   I. Title.
RM708.B67   1992
615.8'2'072—dc20   92-23674
                                                                              CIP

Any procedure or practice described in this book should be applied by the health care practitioner under appropriate supervision in accordance with professional standards of care used with regard to the unique circumstances that apply in each practice situation. Care has been taken to confirm the accuracy of information presented and to describe generally accepted practices. However, the authors, editors, and publisher cannot accept any responsibility for errors or omissions or for any consequences from application of the information in this book and make no warranty express or implied, with respect to the contents of the book.

Every effort has been made to ensure drug selections and dosages are in accordance with current recommendations and practice. Because of ongoing research, changes in government regulations and the constant flow of information on drug therapy, reactions and interactions, the reader is cautioned to check the package insert for each drug for indications, dosages, warnings, and precautions, particularly if the drug is new or infrequently used.

This book is dedicated to the memory of our colleague and friend,
STEVEN J. ROSE, P.T., Ph.D., F.A.P.T.A.

His keen insights, constructive criticism, support of colleagues,
and belief in the physical therapy profession
shall be missed but not forgotten.

CONTRIBUTORS

Christopher E. Bork, Ph.D., P.T.
Dean, School of Allied Health
Professor of Physical Therapy
Medical College of Ohio
Toledo, Ohio

Mark W. Cornwall, Ph.D., P.T.
Assistant Professor, Physical Therapy
Northern Arizona University
School of Health Professions
Department of Physical Therapy
Flagstaff, Arizona

David E. Krebs, Ph.D., P.T.
Associate Professor
MGH Institute for Health Professions
Boston, Massachusetts

Marilyn J. Lister, B.S., P.T.
Editorial Consultant
Berryville, Virginia
Former Editor, *Physical Therapy*, Journal
   of the American Physical Therapy
   Association

Paulette Murrell, M.Ed., P.T.
Assistant Dean and Associate Professor
School of Physical Therapy
Texas Woman's University
Dallas, Texas

Otto D. Payton, Ph.D., P.T.
Medical College of Virginia
Richmond, Virginia

Ernest D. Prentice, Ph.D.
Associate Dean for Research
University of Nebraska
Medical Center
Omaha, Nebraska

Ruth B. Purtilo, Ph.D.
Professor of Clinical Ethics
Center for Health Policy and Ethics
Creighton University
Omaha, Nebraska

Jules M. Rothstein, Ph.D., P.T.
Professor and Head
Department of Physical Therapy
University of Illinois at Chicago
Chief of Physical Therapy Services
University of Illinois Hospital
Editor, *Physical Therapy*
American Physical Therapy Association

Beverly J. Schmoll, Ph.D., P.T.
Associate Professor and Director
Physical Therapy Department
School of Health Professions and
  Studies
The University of Michigan—Flint
Flint, Michigan

Katherine F. Shepard, Ph.D., P.T.
Professor and Assistant Dean
Department of Physical Therapy
College of Allied Health Professions
Temple University
Philadelphia, Pennsylvania

Ann F. Van Sant, Ph.D., P.T.
Associate Professor and Chair
Department of Physical Therapy
College of Allied Health Professions
Temple University
Philadelphia, Pennsylvania

**Wanda C. Wilkes, M.S., M.T.
(ASCP), CLS (NCA)**
Professor
Department of Physical Therapy
College of Allied Health Professions
Temple University
Philadelphia, Pennsylvania

FOREWORD

The need for performing, directing, and comprehending research in physical therapy has been recognized and advocated by many. Authors have published manuscripts about the need for validating theory related to practice and the need to demonstrate the efficacy of treatments we apply as physical therapists. Journal and book editors have frequently attempted to facilitate proliferation of research activity. Esteemed lecturers and American Physical Therapy Association (APTA) activists have also been intensely involved in raising the level of attention and resources given to research within physical therapy. Because the lack of literature substantiating practice patterns will predictably continue, most practitioners and academicians would readily agree that there is a need to strengthen research efforts pertaining to both the theory and practice of physical therapy. Thus the publication of this volume is important and timely.

Encouragingly, there is evidence from a variety of sources that the number of physical therapists and their level of active involvement in research are increasing. Manuscript submissions to *Physical Therapy*, the flagship journal of the association, are increasing in number and improving in quality. New journals have also been established by sections within the APTA and by private vendors. Poster and paper presentations at the Annual Conference and the Combined Sections Meeting of the APTA have also dramatically increased over the last several years. Further, physical therapists have become more prestigiously involved in research presented at other meetings, for example, the Society for Neurosciences. Interest from the community of physical therapists is apparently driving the increase in oral and written presentations.

Within the APTA, the Section on Research has been particularly active in advocating the proliferation of research, both in quantity and quality. Growth of membership within this Section has been exceedingly strong and predicates further interest in research activities within the profession. Most recently the Section sponsored a Gordon-like retreat, the first of its kind offered by an APTA component. The topic, muscle function in normal and pathological states, brought together approximately 125 of the leading researchers in and those associated with physical therapy. Subsequent retreats now being planned will foster the continuation of this scientific process which facilitates development of our knowledge base.

The efforts of the Foundation for Physical Therapy have also had an important impact on research within the profession. Awards for advanced degree students have been given since 1986, and requests for grants to other physical therapist researchers usually exceed the amount available from the Foundation by a factor of two or three. The precedent set by the designation of the first Clinical Research Center in Physical Therapy in 1991 should also stimulate external private and governmental agencies to recognize physical therapy research.

However, the profession still faces dilemmas. The first is time. Despite recognizing the need for research, many clinicians must manage patient care first. Completing and presenting research is not usually a performance criteria within most practice arenas. The shortage of physical therapists provides some explanation as to why investigative work is not done—"I'm too busy treating patients in order to be able to do research." Despite the time dilemma, research within the clinic remains important because it is in this setting that many of the studies related to theory and patient assessment and treatment protocols can best be performed. A second dilemma relates to the shortage of faculty serving in academic centers. This concern is confounded by the fact that existing faculty often do not assign a high-enough priority to their own participation in scholarly activities. In addition, many institutions of higher education that offer physical therapy curricula neither hold nor hold fast to a philosophy that requires physical therapy faculty to participate in research activities. Physical therapy faculty even debate the role of introducing entry-level students to research in the curriculum, asking, "Do we train consumers or individuals who can actually perform research?" The resulting contribution to the body of knowledge associated with physical therapy is thus less than we could achieve.

Completion of the research effort required for continued growth of the profession may remain problematic because physical therapists need better training and/or a time allotment and ability to perform studies of this nature. Physical therapists who serve either as clinicians or academicians can make an impact by facilitating their research productivity. Toward that end, this volume will serve to facilitate the goals of physical therapists, the profession, and, ultimately, the clients that we serve.

Gary L. Soderberg, Ph.D., P.T., F.A.P.T.A.
President, Section on Research, 1992–94

PREFACE

Most people who teach research courses will, at some time or another, tell their students that research begins with a problem. It seems fitting, then, that this book is a result of a problem. A number of years ago, when I began to teach research design and statistics, I looked without success for a text that covered both research design and statistics in a straightforward manner. At that time most of the statistics texts were highly mathematical and the research design texts contained little, if any, integration of statistics into the fabric of research design. In addition, qualitative research was largely ignored. This text is designed to provide an understanding of the fundamentals of research design and common statistical tests used in clinical research by physical therapists.

The topics of research design and statistics evoke fear in many people, including many physical therapists and physical therapy students. Because each of you has undoubtedly "survived" (and probably actually enjoyed) anatomy and neuroanatomy, you certainly can learn research design and statistics! The authors of this volume have consciously worked to demystify research and statistics. It was my intention to produce a book that was sufficiently detailed yet not bogged down in unnecessary detail. As our late colleague, Steve Rose, used to say, "Tell the students what they *need* to know; save the 'nice to know' information for advanced classes." This book contains *essential* information. Readers who desire more detail are encouraged to seek other resources, many of which are referred to by the contributing authors.

Over the years it has become clear that students, in particular physical therapy students, have a staggering amount of information to learn in a very short time. As a result, they tend to read sparingly; they simply do not have the time. Similarly, professionals in the discipline find themselves busier every year and must carefully choose what they read. Thus, while it is to be hoped that each reader reads this entire book, that may not be realistic. Recognizing these facts, each chapter here can stand on its own. Optimally, the book can be used as a reference or, better still, as a tool by the student and clinician alike.

The underlying focus here is on eliminating or controlling bias. Reliability and validity are central themes. Optimally the reader will understand that statistics are a tool, just like a goniometer, and, similarly, must be applied appropriately and interpreted with care and caution. Just as using a goniometer to measure range of motion at a given joint does not explain why movement may be limited, statistical tests do not explain a phenomenon. Both are tools; it is the application of human wisdom that provides the explanation.

This book will not make you a researcher, no matter how diligently you read it. To become a researcher you must engage in research, and this is best learned under the tutelage of an experienced researcher. This book will not provide everything you need to know about research design and statistics; it *will* provide fundamentals. In a sense, this is an introduction to an interesting way of looking at the world. I hope that you will become fascinated by this "new" way of looking at the world and will continue to study these topics.

I would like to acknowledge each of the authors and thank them for their contributions. They are all very busy, and much of this work represents burning the midnight oil. I would also like to thank my friends, colleagues, and family for their encouragement and support during this process. Last, and certainly not least, I wish to thank all the people at the J.B. Lippincott Company, and especially Andrew Allen and Miriam Benert. I would also like to recognize and thank Stephanie Egnotovich of Publishers' WorkGroup for her help. Their patience, persistence, and encouragement were exemplary.

Christopher E. Bork, P.T., Ph.D.

CONTENTS

8. Questionnaire Design and Use   176
Katherine F. Shepard

PART III: DATA ANALYSIS

9. Populations, Samples, and Statistical Significance   207
Christopher E. Bork

10. Nonparametric Statistics   223
Ann F. Van Sant

INTRODUCTION: AN INVITATION

Christopher E. Bork

THE IMPORTANCE OF RESEARCH

THE PHYSICAL THERAPIST AS CRITICAL CONSUMER OF INFORMATION

THE PHYSICAL THERAPIST AS CONTRIBUTOR TO RESEARCH

SURVIVAL AND GROWTH THROUGH RESEARCH

THE NEED FOR PROFESSIONAL RECOGNITION AND CREDIBILITY

SUMMARY

If research is to remove physical therapy procedure from the realm of empiricism, it can only be accomplished through the presentation of resulting facts and principles in the literature of the physical therapy and related professions.
—Catherine Worthingham (1959)

THE IMPORTANCE OF RESEARCH

Learning research methods is similar to learning a foreign language. First, there is a vocabulary to master, just as there is when one studies French or, for that matter, anatomy. Understanding research methods will also broaden your knowledge, provide insights, and allow you to view your profession in a different way.

1

Some readers of this book may be graduate physical therapists who wish to refresh their memory or who are taking the first step toward learning a rather intimidating subject. Others may be students for whom this is a reading assignment. In my experience, it is the rare physical therapy student who is excited about a research or statistics course. Most believe it is better to take a course in a clinically relevant area and view such courses as more important for physical therapy practice.

That attitude is mistaken. The skills learned in research can be the basis for continued improvement in clinical practice in a number of ways. First, research skills enable a physical therapist to become a critical consumer of information. Second, they provide the clinician with a basis for contributing new knowledge. And third, these skills are essential for the survival and growth of physical therapy as a profession. The ultimate result will be a contribution to improved health care for the clients and patients who receive physical therapy.

THE PHYSICAL THERAPIST AS CRITICAL CONSUMER OF INFORMATION

More than half of what I learned in my entry-level physical therapy education has been modified by new findings, and some of what I was taught has been rejected.* For example, when I was a student in the 1960s, patterning was included as a form of advanced therapeutic exercise. Although patterning was an accepted form of exercise in the mid-1960s, it was later believed to be a fad and not of therapeutic value. As a result, it is no longer included in the curriculum. Given such advancements in knowledge, it would be tragic if one had to function in clinical practice with only half of the knowledge necessary. It is, moreover, a professional responsibility to decide when "new" knowledge should be incorporated into one's existing knowledge base.

Understanding research methods gives a clinician the ability to analyze critically the literature and new approaches to clinical practice. Skill in critical thinking allows clinicians to add regularly to their professional knowledge and to recognize fads and theories that are not supported by sound evidence. These skills are fundamental to continuing one's education.

The physical therapy profession has its share of what can be best referred to as "gurus," who profess to know wondrous techniques and approaches for improving treatment success. A glance at the periodicals for health professionals reveals a plethora of continuing education seminars for clinicians. It is incumbent upon the clinician to demand evidence based on rigorous studies that support new approaches to patient care. Too often, treatment approaches are supported only by anecdote or the personal experience of the instructor. By balancing an openness to new ideas with a healthy amount of skepticism, the clinician will continually learn and improve patient care. In a practical sense, research skills help a clinician determine what is useful and what is not.

*For a sense of the state of therapeutic exercise knowledge during the 1960s, see the Northwestern University Symposium on Therapeutic Exercise Project (NUSTEP).[1]

THE PHYSICAL THERAPIST
AS CONTRIBUTOR TO RESEARCH

Becoming familiar with research methods gives the physical therapist the opportunity to contribute to the knowledge base of physical therapy. The notion of the physical therapist as a contributor is not new. As early as 1959 Worthingham stated:

> To be professional, members of a group must possess a body of knowledge that is both identifiable and different from that of other professions. They must also assume responsibility for adding to that body of knowledge.[1]

The responsibility to contribute does not obligate every physical therapist to be a competent clinical researcher. That objective is generally unattainable in an entry-level program and often difficult to attain even in an advanced master's degree program. Rather, each physical therapy clinician should be conversant enough with research methods to know from whom to seek help when initiating a research project. Through participation in such clinical research the physical therapist can improve patient care.

In clinical practice, physical therapists are keen observers. When a patient demonstrates even a subtle change, the physical therapist is usually aware of it. In fact, much of physical therapy practice unfortunately appears to have been based upon physical therapists' repeated observations of patients' responses to specific treatment procedures. Two examples will help to clarify my statement. Brunnstrom's classifications of recovery following stroke and her treatment approach were based upon her observations of the return of function in her patients.[2] Additionally, theorists such as the Bobaths noted that when patients were placed in certain postures, specific movements were either facilitated or inhibited.[3] These revered clinicians then went on to explain *why the observed changes in their patients occurred without first establishing that the changes were related to, if not caused by, the treatment administered.* Such flawed methodology is the basis of some of the theory in which physical therapy practice is rooted.

Clearly, to improve the practice of physical therapy, we must combine clinical and research skills. A clinician who has studied research methods knows rigorous investigation is required before any conclusions about the effect of a treatment can be drawn. The clinician knows how to administer treatment and measure changes in the patient's function and can contribute to the body of knowledge by seeking to determine whether the observed changes occur randomly or are related to treatment. By being conversant in research methods and seeking advice, the clinician can assist in a study of the treatment phenomenon. The researcher, while perhaps not familiar with the treatment or the measurement of change, is competent in designing studies and analyzing data. Through combined skills, communication, and a shared interest in studying a treatment's effects, the clinician and the researcher become a team whose objective is determining whether a treatment results in changes in patients' function.

Conclusions about the treatment's effect(s) will be based upon an analysis of data obtained in an unbiased manner. This approach is the very essence of research design: to allow observed changes to be due to the result of a treatment rather than biases or beliefs. The clinician who has an understanding of research methods can potentially contribute to the profession through collaboration on a research project.

SURVIVAL AND GROWTH THROUGH RESEARCH

Health care costs have become a concern for individuals, the business community, and government. Over the last four decades the cost of health care has risen at a faster rate than the gross national product or rate of inflation. Increasingly, health care professions are being asked to justify their contributions to the consumer's return to health. Consumers want and deserve to know what they are receiving for their health care dollar. Health care professions unable to prove that they prevent disease, improve health, or restore function will not be reimbursed for their services. When individuals cannot earn a living as practitioners of a specific health care profession, that profession will eventually disappear. Thus, if physical therapy cannot justify its existence on the basis of what it does for patients, it will cease to be a profession in all too short a time.

The possibility of the demise of physical therapy as a profession is unconscionable to those of us who have witnessed the benefits our patients have derived from physical therapy. We must prove its value. Instead of viewing increased accountability as a problem or threat, we must view it as an opportunity to document the positive contributions physical therapy makes to the public it serves. By accepting the challenge to validate through research what we do clinically, we can educate the public about what physical therapy has to offer.

The bridge between what physical therapists believe they contribute to improving patient function and the documentation of those improvements is clinical research. As more is known about the effects of physical therapy on various conditions, opportunities develop to explore the contribution physical therapy can make in treating other conditions that result in movement dysfunctions. By examining and documenting the value of physical therapy, the professional body of knowledge grows and so does the profession.

THE NEED FOR PROFESSIONAL RECOGNITION AND CREDIBILITY

Even though we might like to believe otherwise, the physical therapy profession is neither well known nor understood. By and large, the public does not know what the physical therapist does. Those people who are aware of the profession learned about it when they or a relative needed physical therapy. When individuals suffer from a movement dysfunction, they do not generally seek physical therapy. When we are able to prove our effectiveness in treating certain conditions, more people may request our services directly.

For the most part, physicians and other health care professionals do not know what physical therapy clinical practice encompasses. Typically, physicians are relatively aware that physical therapy exists, but, for the most part, they do not understand it is useful for conditions other than severe rehabilitation problems. For example, if you experienced low back pain, where would *you* go? Some individuals will seek a chiropractor, while others will go to their family physician (who will "treat" the *symptoms*, as opposed to the cause, with drugs), and other people will just ignore the problem and live in pain until it goes away or gets worse. Many physicians do not even know the education required to practice physical therapy. Their knowledge tends to be limited to and a result of their contact and experience with a physical therapist. Unfortunately, professional credibility may be adversely affected by the way in which we present ourselves to physicians.

We must consider the kind of relationship we want with physicians and other members of the health care team. Most physical therapists want to be recognized as valuable members of that team, respected for their knowledge, and therefore able to exercise their professional judgment, including recommending, if not deciding upon the best physical therapy treatment for their patients. Physical therapists are often unaware of the importance physicians place upon the literature in clinical decision making. Problems sometimes arise when the physical therapist attempts to justify a treatment approach whose efficacy is not established in the literature.

Michael Crichton, a physician and writer, provides interesting insights in his book *Five Patients*.[4] He describes the physician's clinical education as a socialization process that is very different from the clinical education of physical therapists. To an outside observer, the physician's clinical education may appear to be an intellectual game whose equipment is knowledge and the research literature. Imagine a hypothetical senior resident and junior resident who are engaged in a discussion about a patient in or outside of a patient's room. The junior resident examines the patient, and the senior resident asks for a diagnosis. A questioning process follows wherein the junior resident has to defend her or his diagnosis and treatment plans. The defense must not be based strictly upon classroom lectures but also upon the most recent literature. In many cases, the senior resident will play the devil's advocate and quote literature that does not support the junior member's defense. The debate continues until one is unable to rebut the other's evidence. The winner quotes not only the most but the more recent literature in defense of the diagnosis and treatment plan.

To be successful one must be aware of the most current literature, well read in the literature, able to recall the literature, and able to apply it to clinical practice. Although the clinical education is an often uncomfortable process for the junior resident, its result is a physician who is adept at explaining and defending diagnosis and treatment based upon literature and research.

Physical therapists face disadvantages in their dealings with physicians. First, they are not similarly trained. Physical therapy students are not expected to quote the literature in defense of their diagnosis, assessment, or treatment plan, and thus do not even know the rules of the game. Another disadvantage is our profession's relatively small body of knowledge. A substantial amount of physical therapy treatment is either not well documented in the research literature or is anecdotal; the referring physician remains unconvinced of its effectiveness. In an attempt to convince the physician, the therapist may quote theory that is conjectural and has not been tested. One does not establish credibility by citing support based on speculation. Difficulty arises when a therapist believes in a given treatment approach or philosophy to such an extent that she or he ignores the fact that there is no documentation of its efficacy through research. Often the rationale for such a belief is that to deprive the patient of the treatment (which is sincerely believed to be helpful) is unethical. Interestingly, a scientist, or perhaps even a reasonable person, would inquire how the clinician could be so certain of the effect in the absence of rigorous investigation.

The physical therapist, in my experience, makes recommendations based upon what she or he "knows," which tends to be based upon what has been taught, or experienced, but not necessarily based upon physical therapy research litera-ture. Rarely is a therapist prepared to quote a particular journal or able to produce an article supporting a recommendation.* Even when the recommendation is actually based upon literature, that literature is generally not familiar to physicians.

What we now know about how physicians value research literature also allows us to begin to understand why they may look askance at treatments we recommend for the patient. Fortunately this awareness provides insight as to how we can enhance our professional recognition and respect: expand our body of profes-sional literature through research and publication.

SUMMARY

Clinical research in physical therapy is necessary for the survival and contin-ued growth of the profession. Physical therapists must be prepared to examine and justify what they contribute to health care on the basis of rigorous investigations. One major theme in this book (and of research itself) is ascertaining that what we do is responsible for the changes we observe in the people we treat. What we must do is assess the likelihood that the observed differences in our patients and clients are due to chance or other extraneous factors. Optimally our investigations will validate that what we do for and with our patients is responsible for the improve-ments in their movement and that those successes that occur in our clinics are due not to chance but to the care we provide.

REFERENCES

1. Worthingham, C. The development of physical therapy as a profession through research and publication. *Physical Therapy Review* 40:573–577, 1960.
2. Sawner, K. and Lavigne, J.M. *Brunnstrom's movement therapy in hemiplegia.* Philadel-phia: J.B. Lippincott Co., 1992.
3. Bobath, K. A neurophysiological basis for the treatment of cerebral palsy. *Clinics in Developmental Medicine No. 75.* Philadelphia, PA 1980.
4. Crichton, M. *Five patients.* New York: Random House, 1989.

*I have a strong suspicion that one of the reasons physical therapists are concerned with credentials and honorifics (and have "alphabet soup" after their names) is related to the inability to support what we do via the literature. In essence the message we try to convey is, "Trust me, I know what I'm doing!"

PART I

BASIC
CONCEPTS
OF RESEARCH

1

TRUTH AND THEORY

Christopher E. Bork

> Science is nothing else than the search to discover unity in the wild variety of nature—
> or more exactly, in the variety of our experience.
> > Jacob Bronowski, "Science and Human Values"

A profession must have a way of knowing in order to establish, add to, and modify its body of knowledge. But what are the ways we come to know? The purposes of this chapter are to present first the typical approaches to discovering knowledge and then ways in which to apply these approaches directly to physical therapy. The chapter begins with philosophical constructs and then discusses inquiry, theory, approaches to research, hypotheses, variables, and, finally, levels of measurement.

WAYS OF KNOWING

What is truth? What is reality? Ultimately, those are topics for philosophers. Some philosophers maintain that human beings cannot know truth—or even reality. Nonetheless, we want to know about our world and to be able to make sense and order out of the chaos that is characteristic of life. Knowledge is liberating. Understanding events and phenomena gives a person a certain sense of confidence. Perhaps one cannot control the onset of night, but to the primitive the knowledge that light will return can provide comfort.

We acquire knowledge in two ways: by faith and by inquiry.

Faith

Knowledge gained through faith rests upon the foundation that all knowledge was revealed by a deity or deities through sacred writings. This deity is responsible for the universe as we see it and for revealing all truths to humankind. With faith, one believes that explanations of the creation of the universe and of the condition of the world are contained in sacred religious documents. Greek and Roman mythology, the Talmud, the Bible, chronicles in Sanskrit, and other sacred writings explain to the faithful why the world is the way it is. The interrelationships and constructs of the explanations and beliefs form the dogma of religions.

The method for obtaining knowledge is the scholastic method, that is, studying and interpreting the sacred writings. The scholastic approach to the discovery of knowledge is based upon the belief that everything that needs to be known is already available and accessible because it has been revealed to humankind. To seek the answer to a question, religious scholars go to their great books and read them, interpret them, and try to explain different phenomena. If the explanation, the new knowledge, is widely accepted, it becomes a belief. It is, however, difficult to assess the verity of most scholastic knowledge for beliefs are not testable.

Inquiry

Inquiry is based upon observation. The central tenets of this approach are that not everything is known and that new knowledge can be discovered through observation, explanation, and verification. The focus of inquiry is on understanding, explaining, and predicting a phenomenon. The inquiry approach develops explanations, or theories, of phenomena.[1]

THEORY

Inquiry and research help us to explain and predict phenomena. This statement of prediction of the relationship between elements within a given phenomenon is loosely called a *theory*. The role of theory is to give structure to and make sense out of the world. Theory, however, is not truth. It is an explanation or a speculation about a given phenomenon.

Sometimes, theories have components that appear incompatible. Consider, for example, explanations of radiant energy. Physical therapists study about light in terms of wavelength. We use the wave theory of light transmission and are well acquainted with the energy spectrum. We study ultraviolet and infrared light and their properties. However, we are also acquainted with photons and the particle theory of light. Photons are useful to explain other qualities of light. Is light particles or is it waves? We do not know. And to most of us, it does not matter. Both theories of radiant energy are convenient for explaining different qualities and phenomena associated with light.

A useful theory allows the development of hypotheses with which to test its applicability to specific situations or conditions. As hypotheses are tested, the results verify, modify, and refine the theory. Through the process of theory development and testing, knowledge is enhanced and refined. The method associated with inquiry as the way to discover and verify knowledge is termed *research*.

RESEARCH

According to the Merriam-Webster dictionary, research is a "studious and critical inquiry and examination aimed at the discovery and interpretation of new knowledge."[2] Let us dissect this definition. One key point is that the inquiry is critical; evidence is weighed and decisions are made. Discovery is another key point. Discovery implies that research will reveal knowledge—but that the investigator must be willing to seek it. Interpretation suggests that the investigator must decide what the results mean. The ultimate result is new knowledge. Even though this definition is a good start, let us consider one that is narrower in scope.

I define research as a premeditated, reproducible process for gathering and analyzing data in order to answer a question. First, research is premeditated. One does not do research spontaneously, waking up one bright morning and saying, "Look at that sunshine! I think I'll do research today!" Research requires planning and preparation. Research must be reproducible. Findings are useless if someone else follows the same steps and produces contradictory results, for there will be no basis for prediction. Data must be gathered and analyzed. The analysis of data requires the application of human intelligence to understand or explain the phenomena being studied. Research cannot take place without thinking; the data cannot speak for themselves. It is the interpretation of the findings, in light of extant theory, that advances knowledge.

There are two major approaches to addressing a research question—the qualitative and the quantitative.

Qualitative Research

Qualitative research[3] has its roots in phenomenology. It looks at the entire phenomenon being investigated, the perspective of the researcher, and the variables involved in the phenomenon. The focus of qualitative research is understanding. The qualitative researcher describes, explains, and interprets events and phenomena because this research does not yield quantitative results. Thus, qualitative research is often theory-generating rather than strictly testing.

Qualitative research activities are unobtrusive and uncontrolling. The key element of data gathering is the researcher rather than instruments. The researcher's goal is to understand the phenomenon from multiple perspectives. Data is analyzed through a constant comparative process wherein themes are identified, tested, and verified.

The principal approaches to qualitative research include ethnography, grounded theory, and the case study. Let us take one example, ethnography. Ethnography is practiced by the cultural anthropologist like Margaret Mead, or even a more biologically oriented anthropologist like Diane Fossey. These researchers go into and among a population to be studied and try to develop a theory to explain what is going on. For a further discussion of qualitative research, see chapter 5.

Quantitative Research

The approach that most people tend to associate with the word *research* is quantitative research, which contends that there is a single objective reality. The quantitative approach tries to break a particular theory into many constituent elements and tests each element separately. The quantitative researcher believes that once all the elements have been examined, one can use them—like building blocks—to build theories and eventually to understand the phenomenon. The most common research approaches are experimental, correlational, and descriptive.

The key concept in quantitative research is objectivity: the phenomenon under investigation must be observable and verifiable. Quantitative researchers try to validate or test a hypothesis by setting up a controlled experimental situation in which they can be assured that only the item that is being manipulated can cause observable, objective changes. The data gathered tend to be quantitative and to be analyzed by statistical analysis.

Both the quantitative and the qualitative approaches are useful. The strength of the qualitative approach is the understanding that comes from seeing interrelationships. The strength in the quantitative approach lies in the fact that one can usually be sure that for a given situation the intervention is causing the observed differences. The result of both quantitative and qualitative research is the confirmation, expansion, refutation, or refinement of a given theory. Theory is confirmed, expanded, refuted, or refined by virtue of hypothesis testing.

HYPOTHESES

A hypothesis is a statement of the relationship between dependent and independent variables in order to test a construct and questions derived from a theory. Hypotheses can be classified into two categories: the research, or guiding, hypothesis, and the statistical, or test, hypothesis.

The Research Hypothesis

The research hypothesis can be thought of as the hunch, the speculation, or the expectation the investigator has when embarking upon an investigation. Very rarely does a quantitative researcher embark upon a research project with absolutely no idea of what the results or outcome will be. Since the researcher does have an idea of what the results will be or expects certain findings, one of his or her objectives is to minimize the bias that is inherent in those expectations. That, in fact, is the reason that a careful research design is chosen. A research design minimizes or eliminates bias so that any changes are due to manipulation of the experimental conditions rather than the biases or prejudices of the individuals associated with the experiment or study.

The Statistical Hypothesis

The statistical, or test, hypothesis is a statement of the relationship between the dependent and independent variables that allows a mathematical test to ascertain the probability of obtaining a result similar to that obtained in the study but strictly due to happenstance or chance. That is the function of any statistical test. The three main types of statistical hypotheses are (1) the null hypothesis, (2) the alternative hypothesis, and (3) the directional hypothesis.

The *null hypothesis* (H_o) states that there will be no specifically significant difference between the conditions compared (that is, between the variables). As Cornwall and Murrell discuss in chapter 7, on research design, the null hypothesis is based upon the principle of falsification. If one is unable to falsify a particular hypothesis or theory, then one must accept it as being true. The *alternative hypothesis* (H_a) is a statistical hypothesis which generally states that there will be a statistically significant difference between the dependent and independent variables, but does not state the magnitude or direction of the differences. The *directional hypothesis* (H_d) not only states that there will be a statistically significant difference but, in fact, identifies where or under what conditions the difference will occur.

Let us consider a physical therapist who wants to examine the effect of exercise versus no exercise on a particular condition:

The null hypothesis: There will be no statistically significant difference between subjects who exercise and subjects who do not.

An alternative hypothesis: There will be a statistically significant difference between subjects who exercise and who do not.

The directional hypothesis: Subjects who exercise will show a statistically significant increase in strength when compared to subjects who do not.

VARIABLES

In order to pose a hypothesis you must know something about variables. Variables can be classified as independent, dependent, or intervening. An *independent variable* is the condition that the experimenter or investigator is able to manipulate for purposes of comparison. Independent variables have levels, that is, different conditions, categories, or classifications. For example, an investigator who wishes to manipulate the independent variable "mode of exercise" can assign people to treatment groups and nontreatment groups or to the exercise or nonexercise group. The independent variable is "mode of exercise." The levels or subcategories are "exercise" and "no exercise."

The *dependent variable,* on the other hand, is the *outcome* the investigator measures. The dependent variable is expected to change in response to manipulation of the independent variable. Using the previous example, a dependent variable that would change in response to manipulating the mode of exercise might be "subjects' strength."

Intervening, or confounding, variables are *those factors other than the independent variable* that can cause differences in the dependent variable. Intervening variables are those factors and conditions (e.g., a biased sample) that the investigator wants to account for and control. In our example, if two individuals measure strength but they do not measure the same way, either the method used to measure strength or the difference between the way the people measure could account for differences in subjects' strength and would represent an intervening variable. The way in which the intervening variable is controlled in the example ensures that people measure strength the same way.

A nontechnical example summarizes variables quite well: we're going to make a cake. The independent variable is "ingredients." It has levels, or subcategories, of A, B, and C. Level A is flour, eggs, sugar, and milk. Level B is sawdust, glue, sugar, and monosodium glutamate. Level C is sand, gravel, water, and limestone.

The *intervening variables* are "directions," "baking temperature," "amount of each ingredient," and "baking time." The intervening variables are those factors that must be controlled or stabilized in order to be sure differences in the dependent variable are associated with, if not caused by, manipulating the independent variable. In this example, the proportions of ingredients, the temperature, and the directions are all intervening variables. If the "cakes" are not baked at the same temperature, for example, one cannot assume that the changes were due to the "ingredients"—it might be temperature that is causing differences.

The dependent variable is chosen by an investigator and is critical to the outcome. It is driven by the theory and by the hypothesis. To illustrate its importance, consider the outcomes of this example. If one is concerned with color, the best cake may be the one that is comprised of Level B ingredients. If taste is the dependent variable, Level A would probably be chosen. If weight were the dependent variable, the choice would probably be Level C, which includes gravel and limestone.

Thus, the choice of dependent variable is critical. If one is going to measure a dependent or independent variable—a patient, for example—one needs to know the common levels of measurement of the variable.

LEVELS OF MEASUREMENT

Levels of measurement are categories for measuring variables. The levels are generally accepted by researchers, statisticians, and people who deal with measurement. From the least to the most sensitive, they are: nominal, ordinal, interval, and ratio. The nominal and ordinal levels of measurement are *discrete variables*. Discrete variables have a finite number of values or categories. *Continuous variables* have an almost infinite number of categories or values. The interval and ratio levels of measurement are continuous variables.

Nominal level measurements are used to classify or categorize data. Nominal levels of measurement do not imply any type of magnitude, simply category. A clinical example would be arthritis. One could categorize patients into patients with osteoarthritis, rheumatoid arthritis, psoriatic arthritis, or traumatic arthritis. The differentiation is simply according to the type of disease.

Ordinal level measurements add magnitude to the categorization. One example is a ranking: normal, good, fair, poor, trace, zero. These categories may be recognized by the readers as the manual muscle test, which is an example of an ordinal level of measurement. A manual muscle test grade or range of normal can be thought of as indicating strength that is greater than that of a muscle measured in the good range. There is no assumption that the categories are the same in terms of the quantity that they represent. For example, the amount of strength that one must have to move from a zero to a trace is not the same amount of strength needed to move from a fair to a good rating.

The values of ordinal and nominal measurements can be summarized by frequency of occurrence, by percentage of the whole, or by counting the members in a category. Nominal and ordinal level data is not generally appropriate for arithmetical computations.

Interval level measurements include all the qualities of the ordinal level measurement and also include units that are equal in size. Therefore, the distance between levels is equal. This permits the use of arithmetical operations. In the interval level of measurement, the zero point is arbitrary. An example of an interval level of measurement is the centigrade temperature measurement, where zero does not indicate the absence of heat but rather is an arbitrary point.

The *ratio level of measurement* includes all the qualities of the interval level of measurement and also includes a zero point that is absolute. Using the example of temperature, the Kelvin scale would be a ratio level measurement because zero degrees Kelvin is absolute zero and indicates the absence of heat.

Be careful that you do not misuse levels of measurements. For example, a qualitative measure is sometimes used to try to quantify change in patients. Some misuses of functional indices are very good examples of this. Consider a 5-level scale where 0 represents no function and 5 represents full independence. Level 1 denotes maximum assistance of two staff members. Level 2 requires maximum assistance of one staff member. Level 3 requires moderate assistance. For level 4, the patient requires only verbal assistance. It might seem that one could ascertain the success of a treatment by subtracting the patient's functional score on admission from the functional score at some later time or when they leave, then dividing by 5 and multiplying by 100. One might think this would yield the percentage of increase in function so that a patient who came in functioning at a 1 and left at a 4 had a 3/5 or 60% increase in function.

This seems logical until one examines the underlying assumptions. Is the change from complete dependence to maximal assistance the same as from verbal assistance to independence? Most therapists would say no. With ordinal level measurements one cannot perform mathematical functions. Thus, if you see individuals, for example, adding manual muscle test scores, be critical. If you construct scales without proving that the increments between the scales or classifications are equal, the increments cannot be added or subtracted. Such basic mistakes still occur once in a while in the literature.

SENSITIVITY TO CHANGES

The choice of a level of measurement is the decision of the investigator. In each case the investigator is encouraged to use the most sensitive level of measurement available because subtle changes will become more apparent. Concerns about our ability to validate what we do in clinical physical therapy are, I believe, a result of the lack of sensitivity of the measurements that we use in typical physical therapy patient evaluations. In assessments of strength, sensation, and pain, the level of measurement typically used is ordinal; sometimes it is purely descriptive and nominal. Is it any surprise that as the patient makes progress we are often unable to document the change? The question is not whether change is taking place or not; the question is whether the tool we are using to measure the patient's sensation, pain, or strength is sensitive enough to detect subtle changes.

It is not uncommon for a physical therapist to notice an improvement or a decline in a patient's functional ability, even though there has not been enough change to move from one level in the ranking to the next. To one who would just be looking at the measurement, the patient demonstrates no change and seems to be receiving very little benefit from physical therapy. However, within that ranking the patient *has* made some progress, although the progress is not clear to anyone but the physical therapist. A physical therapist's ability to document change may be limited by the sensitivity of the measurements conventionally used in physical therapy practice.

In the late 1980s and early 1990s, the professional journal *Physical Therapy* focused on issues of validity and reliability in measurement. Some physical therapists were not pleased with this emphasis and wanted research and articles that focused on clinically relevant material. There were other individuals who saw the journal's focus as a very exciting and positive change. While the focus on measurement may not appear to be clinically relevant, it is what will ultimately not only enable physical therapy to validate what the profession contributes to health care but also serve as a launching pad for future clinical applications. In other words, when physical therapists use measurements that can accurately document change in their patients' function and keep accurate records, eventually researchers will have access to a database that will enable them to determine the most effective procedures for a given movement dysfunction. The choice of treatment will be supported by theory and evidence as well as the therapist's judgment and experience.

REFERENCES

1. Tammivaara, J. and Shepard, K.F. Theory: The guide to clinical practice and research. *Physical Therapy* 70:577–582, 1990.

2. *Merriam Webster New Collegiate Dictionary.* Springfield, MA: G. & C. Merriam Co.

3. Jensen, G.M. Qualitative methods in physical therapy research: A form of disciplined inquiry. *Physical Therapy* 64:492–500, 1989.

2

RELIABILITY AND VALIDITY: IMPLICATIONS FOR RESEARCH

Jules M. Rothstein

Newcomers to the research process are often overwhelmed by the jargon of the researcher. We use terms that are arcane and often intimidating. Novices fear that they will violate some sacred law of research and forever shame themselves in the eyes of the seasoned veteran. Novices are unaware of the reason the seasoned researcher knows so much about making mistakes. We know because we have made the mistakes, and those of us who actively conduct research make many mistakes. Learning by doing and learning from your mistakes are essential parts of the research process. The purpose of this chapter is to deal with some of the more important terms used in research, specifically, reliability and validity, and, perhaps, to make the learning process a little easier.

There are no sacred laws in research that should be blindly followed; rather, there are logical rules that should be understood. These logical rules are derived from knowledge in four different disciplines. First and foremost, researchers must have *content knowledge* in the area in which they are working. As a reviewer for several journals and as the editor of *Physical Therapy*, I can attest that the need for content knowledge appears to have been forgotten by many physical therapists. Later in this chapter we will see why no one should ever attempt research without thorough knowledge of the topic.

The other three disciplines relate to the process rather than the content of research. They are *measurement science, research methodology,* and *statistics.* Many researchers, including authors of other chapters in this text, may disagree with my classification scheme. I believe, however, that all three areas represent unique, though related, bodies of knowledge. In this chapter we will consider aspects of two of these disciplines, measurement science and research methodology. And, most importantly, we will consider how content knowledge relates to both.

MEASUREMENT SCIENCE: ISSUES FOR THE RESEARCHER

Operational Definitions

During the process of measurement, we assign numbers to things or we categorize things.[1-3] In a real sense this is a human trait. When we awake in the morning and determine that the weather outside is good or bad, we are categorizing, and that is a form of measurement.* When we count change we are assigning a number to represent each coin. In clinical practice we measure the angle formed by two limb segments, and we categorize muscle performance by assigning manual muscle test grades. Because measurement is a ubiquitous part of our lives, it seems reasonable to question the need for measurement science, the need to study this process that we normally take for granted.

The categorization of the state of the weather that we make before leaving home is usually not very consequential—unless, of course, we forget an umbrella or leave a convertible top down. Therefore, we make such judgments casually. However, classifying a patient according to some administrative scheme could result in that patient being transferred to another, perhaps less desirable, facility. We need to approach such measurements with more sophistication so that we may use the measurements with greater certainty.

---

*Some authors insist that measurement occurs only when numerals are assigned to a variable. Fortunately that view is becoming increasingly rare, and for the purposes of this chapter, the broader definition, one that includes categorization, will be used.

The first prerequisite for meaningful measurement is an *operational definition*.[4] In order to assign numbers to a variable or to classify someone or something based on a variable, terms must be defined. However, a definition that is purely conceptual will not assist in the process of measurement. *Operational definitions must specify the procedure used in making the measurement.* They must guide the measurer through the process of assigning a numeral or a classification. My idiosyncratic definition for classifying the weather in the morning is that a good day is one in which the National Weather Service has predicted that the temperature will not exceed 70 degrees and there is less than a 20% chance of precipitation. A bad day is one in which either of these two conditions is not met.

There are two criteria for evaluating the quality of an operational definition.[5] The first is *universality*, whether the operational definition can be used by all those who are likely to apply it. I suggest that my definition for weather classification can be used by anyone who knows how to phone the National Weather Service, read a morning newspaper, or listen to a television or radio weather forecast. The second quality for an operational definition is *theoretical soundness.* Judging this is more difficult and in most cases requires content knowledge. You cannot judge the theoretical soundness of an operational definition without considering the purpose of a measurement and the underlying theory associated with that purpose.

In our simple example, the purpose of the measurement was to know whether or not I would be happy with the weather, and from that standpoint you can hardly argue with the definition. However, you could argue that my definition does not relate to how *you* would classify the weather. That is true, but the purpose of my classification scheme was to judge how *I* would view the weather. Operational definitions cannot be considered in a vacuum; rather, they can only be judged when the purpose of the measurement is clearly understood.

Validity deals with the purpose of a measurement. The purpose of my weather classification scheme was to judge whether I would like the weather. Therefore, it was a good operational definition because it had theoretical soundness relative to the stated use for the measurement.

In physical therapy school, we were all taught how to measure passive range of motion (PROM). The description of the process of how to apply the goniometer to known anatomical landmarks was an operational definition for the measurement of the angle formed at the joint. Before using these operational definitions in clinical practice, we should have asked whether these were good operational definitions. Apparently the operational definitions for measuring some types of motion are universal. Several recent studies have demonstrated that although for many joints two different therapists can measure the same patient and get the same numbers, for other joints their measurements do not agree.[6-8] Replicating deals with reliability, but reliability is often a function of the universality of an operational definition.

We can still question the theoretical soundness of the definitions. But before we can do that, we have to ask about the purpose of goniometry. As Miller has noted, the purpose of goniometry is to measure the angular relationship between adjoining limb segments.[9] When multiple measurements are taken, the excursion of the segments can be calculated and noted as PROM. Therefore, it appears that there is some theoretical soundness to goniometric measurements if we use them to describe angles. Nothing in the process of goniometric measurement tells us why PROM may be limited. That is not an inference that we can base on the measurement, because that was not part of the theoretical basis for the measurement. If we want to know why someone has a PROM deficit, we must use other tests. The theory behind an operational definition should clearly support the use of the measurement. In the case of goniometry, the theory allows us to describe angular relationships of limb segments but not to explain why those relationships exist.

We have discussed PROM, but it should be clear that use of the goniometer to measure active range of motion (AROM) represents a different construct and would have a different operational definition, as well as a different inferential use. PROM measurements reflect distensibility of tissues and the integrity of joint structures. AROM measurements reflect many of the same factors as do passive PROM measurements, but in addition they test the function of the neuromuscular system.

All measurements must be based on operational definitions. In our daily lives and in clinical practice most operational definitions are implicit, while in research reports they must be explicit.* Operational definitions must be described in the methods section of a research report. If they are not described, the credibility of the research cannot be evaluated and the research cannot be replicated.

Any research that uses inappropriate operational definitions is not useful research. Therefore, the quality of the operational definition must be defended in the research report. The justification for an operational definition can be found in the demonstration of the reliability and validity of the measurements used. This is because reliability relates to the universality of the measurement, and validity deals with the theoretical soundness of a measurement approach.

Validity

Validity of a measurement is a quality that all measurements must have if they are to have any use. I use the term *validity* in this chapter to describe two things. This section will deal with the use of the term *validity* in describing a measurement (*measurement validity*). Later in the chapter we will consider *experimental validity*, a term that deals with whether research is credible and, to some extent, what conclusions and generalizations can be made from a research report.

There is no more misunderstood and misused term in measurement science than validity. Physical therapists have done more than their fair share to contribute to the confusion. One dictionary defines valid as "well grounded or justifiable; being at once relevant and meaningful . . . ; having such force as to compel serious attention and usually acceptance . . . ; valid implies being supported by objective truth or generally accepted authority."[10] The definition magnificently captures the essential ideas that must be considered in measurement.

---

*Elsewhere I have made a strong argument that one of the major problems facing physical therapy is the absence of operational definitions for clinical measurements (see reference 5). Because this chapter is about research and not clinical practice, that argument will not be repeated. In observing that most clinical measurements are made without specific operational definitions, I am not endorsing this practice.

For a measurement to be valid it must, therefore, be relevant and meaningful based on the preponderance of available evidence. Relevancy and meaningfulness are deceptively simple terms and can be misapplied. Clinicians may manual muscle test (MMT) the quadriceps femoris muscles. As a result of this, they may classify a muscle contraction as normal, good, fair, poor, trace, or absent. They have classified, which is a form of measurement. As Lamb has noted, the MMT appears to be a logical method of assessing the ability of a muscle to create forces.[11] However, that does not mean that the MMT is valid. According to the dictionary, valid relates to something being relevant and meaningful. Therefore, in order to judge the validity of a measurement we must first know what the measurement is supposed to reflect.

It is ridiculous simply to say that a measurement is valid. *A measurement is only valid for some specific purpose.* My weather scale was designed to predict whether *I* would like the weather. If it did so, it was valid. The scale was valid for a specific and identified use. The weather scale is not necessarily valid for predicting whether you or anyone else would like the weather. Measurements can only be valid for specified purposes. A ruler may be used to obtain valid measurements of the length and height of a table, but those measurements can only be used to infer something about the linear dimensions of the table. When people say that a device has been shown to be valid, they are revealing how little they know about validity. A device cannot be shown to be valid; a measurement can, and that measurement can only be valid for a specified inferential purpose.

For most measurements, there are obvious limitations to the inferences that can be made. However, sometimes tradition, bias, or sloppiness causes us to assume that measurements tell us more than they really do. For example, Kendall and McCreary contend that the MMT grades can be used to predict the presence of postural deviations (e.g., weak abdominal muscles mean that a person will have lordosis).[12] And for many years therapists have assumed that this is true. In essence, Kendall and McCreary were saying that MMT grades had the inferential capacity to predict the existence of postural defects. Research by Walker in our laboratory demonstrated that this assumption may be incorrect.[13] Therefore, we question whether MMT grades can predict postural deviations.

We believe we have provided evidence that the MMT of the abdominal muscles is not a valid predictor of lordosis. We have not examined the validity of MMT for judging innervation or for predicting whether a patient can perform activities of daily living (ADL). Unfortunately, no one else has examined these assumptions either—yet some therapists use MMT grades as a predictive measurement of ADL performance. Evidence for validity must be specific to the inferential use of a measurement.

Because of the complex nature of validity, some people have tried to simplify the concept by saying that validity deals with whether a measurement measures what it is supposed to measure. Moffroid et al. took this view in their often-quoted study of the Cybex dynamometer.[14] In that study they said that they validated the Cybex by testing whether it accurately measured loads applied by placing weights on the machine's lever arm. If this was a validity study, then what use of the measurement did it validate? The authors showed that the Cybex could be used to measure weights. They did not show that the Cybex could meaningfully measure torques derived from muscular activity, and they did not demonstrate the correctness of any inference made from torque readings.[15-18] They did examine some of the mechanical characteristics of the Cybex.*

Studies such as that conducted by Moffroid et al. are sometimes referred to as *bench studies* because they are the type conducted in laboratories without regard to the application of a measurement instrument. Bench studies describe the mechanical properties of a measurement device. Such studies are often a vital prerequisite to use of an instrument, but they do not take the place of reliability and validity studies.

A measurement should have some valid use, and that is true whether the measurement is used for clinical practice or to quantify a variable (independent or dependent) in a research report. In that sense, measurement validity is no different in the context of research than it should be in the context of clinical practice. In clinical practice we should not say that a measurement demonstrates something unless we have data (i.e., evidence of validity) to support that claim.

In a research report we should use measurement appropriate to the question and should carefully draw conclusions based on the demonstrated validity of these measurements. For example, it would be inappropriate to conduct a study that demonstrated that MMT grades improve through treatment and then to conclude that this meant the patient was more functional. The measurement is not valid for that inference. In such a study the authors could hypothesize that function will be improved, but they should only base their conclusions on their results—and in this case the results related only to MMT grades.

Types of Validity

In view of the ease with which one can misuse the term *validity*, it is fortunate that experts in the field of measurement have developed a logical scheme for categorizing types of validity.[19] The terms and categories are quite useful, but too often the novice researcher will consider them part of the arcane and intimidating terminology that was promised at the beginning of this chapter. If you want to do research or, for that matter, if you want to understand clinical measurement, these terms must be understood.

Face Validity

When you assume that a measurement is valid for an inference, you are saying that it has face validity.[20] Many of the measurements we use in physical therapy clinical practice appear to be based on the assumption of face validity. Face validity for a measurement is a lot like the shine on a new car. It's a nice thing to have, but if that is all you have you cannot get very far. Face validity is the appearance of a justifiable use for a measurement—but this does not mean there are any data or

---

*Because of the widespread use of isokinetic dynamometers, the study by Moffroid et al. is one of the most often-cited references in physical therapy research. This is unfortunate because of the conceptual errors in the article. It is even more unfortunate because many authors misrepresent the study in an effort to justify their own use of isokinetic measurements. More complete discussions of the problems associated with this article can be found elsewhere (see references 5, 14–18).

theory to support the use. Not surprisingly, many experts on measurement do not include face validity in their discussions of validity.

Construct Validity

Measurement must proceed from a logical understanding of the phenomena being measured. Here, knowledge of content is paramount. Construct validity is the conceptual (theoretical) argument that supports the use of a measurement for a specific inference. If we want to measure the ADL potential of a patient, we must first have an idea of what defines ADL. To do this, we need a construct. The construct guides the development of the measurement procedure and will ultimately determine the persons who can be measured and the inferences that can be made from the measurement.

The MMT was developed with a clear construct in mind, one that is often forgotten by those who use the MMT. When polio was widespread, Lovett developed the MMT to characterize the weakness caused by the effect of the virus on anterior horn cells.[21] The construct was simple: fully innervated muscles can generate more tension than partially innervated muscles, and totally denervated muscles can generate no tension. The construct behind the test meant that it could be used to localize not just the effects of the lesions due to polio but also any lesion leading to complete or partial denervation.

A case for construct validity is made through the logical use of existing knowledge. Construct validity is a *theoretical form of validity.* A conceptual argument must be made. Therefore, construct validity may be based on arguments cited from research literature, but there can be no direct test of construct validity. There is no absolute way of knowing when measurement has construct validity. In my experience, however, unless there is a reasonable construct, poor operational definitions will be developed, and the deficits will become apparent when other forms of validity are considered. We need to remember that part of a good operational definition is theoretical soundness, and in practice it is hard to develop a logical operational definition unless there is thorough understanding of the construct being measured.

Content Validity

Once there is a construct for the variable to be measured, there is a need to consider what will be measured. Content validity deals with how measurement schemes relate to their constructs. The classic test of content validity asks whether we have chosen an adequate constellation of items to measure from the universe of items defined by our construct. But then again, we might say that such a definition represents the kind of arcane intimidating jargon that turns people off to research. An ADL example can help cut through the jargon.

To examine the functional capacity of a patient with hemiplegia we had a construct. ADL deals with our ability to carry out the demands we face in a day. For the patient, ADL could consist of the patient's ability to dress, feed, toilet, and ambulate without assistance. A measurement would have to reflect all relevant elements before we could consider the measurement content valid. Therefore, if an ADL test measured only a patient's ability to put on his pants, it would not be content valid relative to the item "dressing" and possibly only for men. In our society a man also needs to be able to put on shoes, socks, underwear, and a shirt. The manual skills required to slip into pants seem sufficiently different from putting on a shirt so that one could not predict the ability to do one from an ability to do the other.

I have made a judgment call in suggesting that an ADL dressing scale limited to putting on pants was not content valid. Content validity, like construct validity, is based on theory and logical argument. The argument may be supported by research. For example, if a study showed a high correlation between putting on pants and putting on a shirt and underwear, that would be evidence that one could infer one skill from the other. In that case, not all of these skills would need to be tested.

In an effort to have content validity, a test developer could go overboard. To assess eating capability, does a patient have to eat every imaginable food item in the world? If that were so, then most of us would fail because most Americans cannot keep a taco from extruding its contents into our laps. The test of the ability to eat should include items that test important elements, for example, the ability to use eating implements for a representative variety of foods that the person will really eat. Therefore, for some Asians, a meaningful test might require the use of chopsticks. Content validity requires adherence to the construct and an understanding of the measurement, the type of variable being measured, and the type of subject being measured.

When we developed our construct, we attempted to define the variable being measured. In our ADL example, the content would be different for an athlete than for the patient with hemiplegia. Therefore, the content of tests of ADL should reflect these differences. ADL for an athlete includes far more than personal care.

At the present time, we have no criteria for judging whether muscularly generated forces or torques can predict ADL or athletic performance.[14] There is often the assumption of face validity for such measurements, but unfortunately the data do not exist. As a researcher in the field of muscle biology, I am not surprised. Measuring muscle performance for the purpose of predicting some type of functional capacity makes sense. But what makes us think that we can do so by measuring torque at one angular position of a limb? Will measuring the forces generated during one contraction type (e.g., isokinetic, isometric, concentric, or eccentric) really predict the others and allow for functional inferences?

To infer function from muscle performance measurements requires more sophisticated constructs than we appear presently capable of generating. Someday, perhaps, we will develop the construct, but my guess is that such a construct will require the measurement of muscle performance under a variety of contractile and mechanical conditions. To be true to such a construct, a test battery must sample all the meaningfully different conditions to be content valid. This is in direct contrast to the MMT. Lovett's original construct dealt with innervation. To grossly judge if a muscle is contracting and whether it appears significantly weak does not require a great diversity of test conditions.

Criterion-Related Validity

Construct validity dealt with the theoretical basis for a measurement. Content validity dealt with implementation of theory. Both construct and content validity are based on theory and can never be directly tested. This is in contrast to criterion-related validity, which can be directly tested. There are two major types of criterion-related validity, *predictive validity* and *concurrent validity*. A third type of criterion-related validity, *prescriptive validity*, may also be included in this category.

Since validity deals with whether we can legitimately make an inference from a measurement, we could say that criterion-related validity represents the ultimate test of validity. To demonstrate criterion-related validity, a measurement is compared to a criterion to determine whether or not the inference was appropriate. We test a measurement by comparing it to something else, the criterion.

There is widespread belief that isokinetic torque values can be used to determine whether an athlete can safely return to competition. Malone et al. and Davies have suggested that, following knee injuries, athletes may be returned to activity when the quadriceps femoris muscles of their injured lower extremities are capable of producing a given percentage of the isokinetic torque of their noninjured extremities.[22,23] They are contending that peak torque is a valid predictor of whether an athlete can increase activity levels.

Malone et al. and Davies appear to be basing this contention on clinical experience because to date they have published no data to support this inferential use of peak torque measurements. Clinical experience is invaluable, but objective research would be a lot better—especially where patient safety is concerned. Because they are making a case for the predictive use of a measurement, they should test predictive validity. Such a test would be relatively easy.

To examine predictive validity, a researcher would need to collect and report data that show that when patients attain the necessary percentage of torque, the patient can safely return to competition. The researcher could obtain torque measurement on a number of patients and count the number of patients who were reinjured when they returned to activity. Here the researcher would be testing the measurement (a percentage of peak torque) versus a criterion (the frequency of reinjury). Because the researcher would be contending that the measurement could be used to predict future occurrences, the type of criterion-based validity he or she would demonstrate is *predictive validity*. Only through such a study could we know whether the measurement of peak torque has the inferential capacity claimed by some clinicians.

A second example of isokinetic measurements can also be used to illustrate concurrent validity. Davies contends that by examining the shape of the torque curve you can tell whether a person has a lax anterior cruciate ligament (ACL).[23] Davies supplies hand-drawn torque tracings in his text to make his point. His argument is one of *concurrent validity*, because he contends that, using his protocol, the torque curve can be used to show the presence of a pathology at the time of the measurement. He says a dip in the torque curve means an ACL deficiency is present. A study to test this hypothesis would take very little time and effort.

A sizable number of patients with ACL injuries, patients with other injuries, and persons with normal knees need to be tested using a described protocol. The strip-chart recordings of the torque curves can then be uniformly cut and coded. A record can be kept of the known diagnoses. The strip-chart recordings can then be shown to a whole series of therapists who know Davies' rules for judging the presence of the dip in the curve. These therapists would see only the curves, not the patient and not the patient's chart. This would test the argument that the judgment of ACL integrity is based only on the torque tracing and not on other factors.

Therapists' determinations of ACL injury can then be compared to the criterion— the known status of the ACL as determined at the time of either surgery or arthroscopy. A less convincing study could compare the judgments from the torque curves with those made by an expert's use of the anterior draw test or, better yet, the Lachman test.[24]

The study I have suggested would examine the concurrent validity for determining ACL injuries through isokinetic measurements. The generalizability of the study would depend on the patients and the therapists. If the study found that only Davies could determine ACL status by examining the curve, then only he could claim this inferential capacity for the measurement. If only experts (based on some criteria) were found capable of determining ACL injuries, then concurrent validity would be limited to that skilled group. A really useful test, however, is one in which anyone with reasonable training can follow a set of rules (operational definitions) to obtain a measurement to make correct inferences.

After seeing how criteria are used to validate the inferential uses of a measurement, we begin to see the specificity required for validity. Because we had two different inferences that people were making from isokinetic torque measurements, each needs to be tested and each needs to be tested on appropriate patients by the people who would really use the test. There is little to be gained from knowing that an expert can use a measurement—unless, of course, we expect that expert to be the only one ever to use the measurement. The reader should now see why a device cannot be valid or why a measurement such as peak torque cannot be valid. *Measurements can only be valid for specific purposes; therefore, each specific use of a measurement must be validated.*

Predictive and concurrent validity are considered forms of criterion-related validity. The literature in the behavioral sciences suggests that a third type, *prescriptive validity,* may also be useful.[19] If a measurement indicates a course of patient management, then the measurement is being used for prescriptive purposes. Some people hypothesize that some foot pain is due to a positional deformity of varus or valgus at the subtalar joint.[25] They say that the subtalar neutral position (STNP) for a person may be in either valgus or varus.

Many persons with foot pain, especially active people treated by physical therapists, podiatrists, and orthopedic surgeons, are given orthotic devices to adjust or to correct for their STNP. Therefore, the measurement of the position of subtalar neutral is used for prescriptive purposes. Based on the measurement, a specific type of orthosis is constructed. The prescriptive use of this measurement could be tested by examining whether treatment based on the measurement really does alleviate pain. The criterion would be some measurement of pain. My own bias suggests that the data would indicate that the measurement could not be used for prescriptive purposes. Elveru's research in our laboratory indicates that measurement of the STNP is not reliable. A measurement that is not reliable cannot be valid. Therefore, it is unlikely that there could be prescriptive validity for STNP measurements.[8,26] My rationale will be clearer after the discussion on reliability. I am not suggesting that orthoses are bad or that they do not work. I am suggesting that, based on the available data, the use or construction of an orthosis should not be based on the measurement of the STNP.

Another potential research project examining prescriptive validity could examine the treatment methods suggested by McKenzie.[27] In the McKenzie approach to low-back-pain patients, a classification scheme guides treatment. The measurement (evaluation) protocol McKenzie suggests is designed to have inferences as to the best type of treatment. Does use of his measurement scheme lead to effective treatment? The question is one of prescriptive validity.

Measurement Validity and Research

The use of a measurement for any purpose is questionable unless there is evidence for the validity of that use. Should there be a special standard for research and another for clinical practice? I think not. My patients deserve quality care based on scientific evidence, not on anecdotal conjecture. I care as much about my patients as I do about my research.

Based on the discussion of validity presented here, it should be clear that validity cannot be proven with absolute certainty. A careful case can be made for the valid use of a measurement, but acceptance of the case is up to the user of a measurement or the reader of a research report. Intelligent decisions about whether validity has been demonstrated can only be made when someone understands the phenomena being measured and the related issues. For example, without an understanding of muscle physiology, related bioelectric phenomena, and biological amplifiers, you cannot judge whether an electromyographic signal can be used to infer the extent of muscle activity. While the terms and process for judging the validity of a measurement may be derived from measurement science, the ability to evaluate validity is dependent on content knowledge.

There are some special issues that relate to research. No research report can be considered worthwhile unless it uses valid measurements. But even when valid measurements are used, researchers must be careful to limit what they infer from changes in dependent variables to those inferences that are supported by evidence for validity. When reading research reports, the critical consumer of research should be wary of making excessive generalizations that exceed the capacity of the measurements. Most good research is very focused, while the needs of our profession require broad generalizations. Attention to measurement validity, like a taste for nonalcoholic beverages, may lead us from temptation.

Reliability

Reliability deals with whether a measurement consistently reflects the variable of interest. In electronics the term *signal-to-noise ratio* is used to reflect how much extraneous information is carried as part of a signal.[28] Good amplifiers and recorders have very little noise per unit of signal. If there is a predictable amount of noise the signal can be interpreted. However, if there is too much noise then the signal can be totally obscured.

The concept of signal to noise can help in understanding reliability. In order to allow readers without expertise in electronics to follow my example, I have taken some liberty with terms. Let us imagine that we were recording an electronic signal and obtained a value of 6 volts. Based on previous studies of the signal-to-noise characteristics of our measurement system, we know that there is about a 2-volt error seen in measurements of this magnitude. Therefore, we really do not know the *true voltage* but, rather, a range. We can be relatively certain that the measured voltage was between 4 and 8 volts.

Reliability tells us something about the error associated with a measurement. Estimates of reliability, like those of signal-to-noise ratio, help us find not true measurements but ranges in which the true measurement falls. Reliability estimates make measurements interpretable because they indicate the amount of error associated with the measurement. Using the example of measuring a voltage, even though our measurement was 6 volts we certainly would not want that signal going into a device that could safely handle only a maximum of 7 volts. Based on our assessment of error, the true value could be as high as 8 volts, and we do not want to see our device going up in smoke.

Measurements, based on operational definitions, are supposed to reflect the quantity of some variable or the classification of something. If the measurement has some valid use, we make a judgment based on the assessment of the quantity or on the classification. Often we look for changes in classification or changes in quantity to tell us whether treatments are working or diseases are getting worse. We use the term *variable* to describe things we are measuring because *measured phenomena are expected to vary*, either within or between people (or groups).

If we measure flexion AROM at the glenohumeral joint, we do so for a reason. Perhaps we are afraid that someone may be losing motion and developing a frozen shoulder. In order to determine whether the patient is losing AROM, we may use *serial measurements*. These are measurements repeated over time to determine changes. In our discussion of validity we made the case that most PROM measurements appear to have some construct validity for inferring angular relationships between adjoining limb segments. How different is the construct for AROM? It seems that we could use goniometric measurements to determine AROM, and through serial measurements we could then calculate whether there was a loss of motion. However, AROM is based not just on the passive properties of tissues, but also on the ability of a patient to try to move, on muscular activity, and presumably on the presence of normal joint mechanics. AROM measurements can be used to infer whether neuromuscular and joint structures are functioning.

With this is in mind we could use AROM to determine angular relationships obtained by the patient, and then use other tests and, finally, our clinical judgment to decide if a frozen shoulder was developing.

In using a measurement of ROM to infer a loss of active motion over time, we implicitly accepted the assumption that changes in the measured variable (AROM) were real and actually represented a change in the ability to move limb segments. We call change in a variable that is understood to represent the phenomenon of interest *true variance*.[29] In our example, the phenomenon is the angular relationship between limb segments as obtained through active motion.

To illustrate true variance we need to contrast it to error variance. Using the same AROM example, let us imagine that we planned to measure AROM in this patient once a week for ten weeks. During the measurement session of the fifth week, we found severely decreased motion. We could conclude that joint and neuromuscular structures no longer allowed the patient to move the limb. But that would only be true if the AROM measurements represented only true variance. Perhaps on that day the patient had been told of a death in his family. During therapy he had little interest in his shoulder and made little effort to move. Our simple AROM measurements would then have become a reflection of the affective state of the patient, rather than of joint and muscle capabilities. The measurements obtained on that day would have been error-ridden because the obtained numbers would have been affected by a variable other than the one we were measuring. The variability that was not due to a change in the phenomenon of interest is called *error variance.*

When we measure, we usually obtain a number that characterizes our variable along a measurement continuum. This number, which is our total variance, really consists of two distinct components. *Total variance is the sum of the error variance and the true variance.* Every measurement has error associated with it, and in practice we can rarely know the causes of error. We can, however, make estimates of the error that will be present. We do this through determining the reliability of a measurement.

Types of Reliability

There are many types of reliability in measurement that are especially important when measurement techniques are developed. A full discussion of these is beyond the scope of this chapter, and these forms of reliability have been described elsewhere in general terms and specifically as they relate to physical therapy.[5,19] In practice, few of these forms of reliability relate to the research process. In conducting research it is imperative that reliability for measurements be evaluated—but only the type of reliability relevant to the study.

Two major types of reliability in measurement are intratester and intertester. The degree to which one person can replicate the measurements he or she obtains is *intratester (or intrarater) reliability.* The degree to which multiple testers can obtain measurements that agree is *intertester (or interrater) reliability.* A research report needs to show reliability that relates to the method of the research. If, in a study, all measurements are taken by one person, then, either as part of the method or by use of evidence from other sources, intratester reliability should be reported. Normally it is a good idea to have a reliability component of a study so that researchers can demonstrate the degree of reliability (amount of error) associated with their measurements as they take them from the population they are studying.

In studies where many people take the measurements, it is essential that intertester reliability be assessed. Once again that assessment is best made as part of the study. When reliability of any kind is not assessed as part of a study, researchers need to make a case as to why they did not examine reliability.

When there is considerable evidence (i.e., research literature) to support the idea that under the conditions of the study reliability is known, the researcher can argue that a reliability study is not necessary. Articles cited to demonstrate reliability must have examined a similar type of reliability using similarly trained examiners and similar types of subjects. For example, the dependent measure in a study examining the effects of a treatment on rheumatoid arthritis (RA) patients might be the distance the patient can walk in 15 seconds. In such a study we would need to know the normal variability (or reliability) seen between repeated measurements of distance. But that normal variability must be assessed for the kind of subject in the study—in this use, rheumatoid arthritis patients. Healthy persons would certainly demonstrate a different variability between repeated measurements than would persons with RA.

Normal subjects, especially physical therapy students, are relatively easy to measure and are often available for research projects. In fact, some study "volunteers" are required by their instructors to be subjects in studies. All too often the data generated from this rather atypical group is used in research, both for assessments of reliability and for experimental effects. This is contrary to all logic and to minimal scientific standards—unless of course you want to know the reliability and experimental effects on physical therapy students.

ASSESSING MEASUREMENT RELIABILITY AND VALIDITY FOR RESEARCH

Novice researchers, particularly graduate students, often go through an evolutionary process that sees them first as excessively quiescent and then uncritically overcritical. With knowledge of reliability and validity fresh in their minds, they read articles and act like members of the Spanish Inquisition. They decry studies where reliability estimates predict up to 30% error associated with repeated measurements. They forget that there is no absolute rule for essential values of reliability and validity estimates. The "goodness" of these estimates is relative, not absolute.

If, in an experiment, you have 30% error associated with repeated measurements but show statistically significant changes in excess of 70%, then I suspect there really was a change. There may not have been a 70% change, but the change is probably real, and there are statistical techniques for assessing the size of the change.[30] Similarly if a criterion-related validity study shows that a new measurement can only predict 50% of the variability of a well-proven measurement, I would prefer to use the tried-and-tested method. However, if for some reason I could not use the older and better method, then I might need to use the measurement that has 50% error associated with predictions. Before proceeding with my experiment, I had better be sure that I was conducting a study where the expected changes were large enough so that the error would not obscure my results.

In conducting research you need to know reliability and validity estimates so you can interpret your own data. Sometimes when dealing with studies that are looking at very small changes, even reliability estimates of 97% may not be good enough. The desired reliability and validity is a function of the study being conducted.

Only researchers with thorough knowledge of their content areas can anticipate a proper strategy to conduct their research. Student research is often guided by faculty members who have not worked in an area and, as a result, proper attention to nuances of measurement as applied to the specific topic is missed in the research design. I believe that this results in frustration for novice researchers. Students should only attempt research in areas in which their advisors have some expertise, regardless of the topic the student wants to examine. I can assure students that they will suffer less frustration and learn more.

Researchers are obligated to discuss their results in the context of their estimates of reliability and validity. In a study we conducted with Walker and colleagues, we did not have the level of reliability we desired for MMT grades of the abdominal muscles.[13] When we analyzed our results, we had to ask whether the results were real or just a function of measurement error. We concluded that, because of the magnitude of our results, we had a real finding rather than one based on measurement error. We also discussed this issue in the research report so that the reader could independently agree or disagree with our interpretation.

RESEARCH METHODOLOGY: VALIDITY

Elsewhere in this book, research designs are discussed and the strengths and weaknesses of these designs are examined. We frequently assess designs in terms of whether they will lead to valid research. The logic behind experimental validity is similar to that applied to measurement validity. By briefly discussing both types in this chapter, the two can be contrasted and each better understood.

Campbell and Stanley first described experimental validity in an article in a book.[31] Their ideas were so powerful and their logic so clear that their chapter has now become a classic book of its own.[32] Although they offer criteria that are now the standards used to judge many forms of research, they made it clear that they appreciated how painful it was to be judged. They wrote:

> For the experimenters, a personal avoidance-conditioning to experimentation can be noted. For the usual highly motivated researcher the nonconfirmation of a cherished hypothesis is actively painful. . . . This can lead, perhaps unconsciously to the avoidance or rejection of the experimental process. . . . We must somehow inoculate young experimenters against this effect, and in general must justify experimentation on more pessimistic grounds—not as a panacea, but rather as the only route to cumulative progress. (p. 3)

Campbell and Stanley appeared to realize that much published research is of poor quality and that they were offering new tools for critical readers. Therefore, they were suggesting that researchers need to be ready for criticism and show not just a "willingness to accept a poverty of finances, but also a poverty of experimental results."

Experimental Validity

An experiment or a descriptive study is conducted so that some knowledge may be gained or some inference made about the world. In experimental studies, the inference is the effect of the independent variable on the dependent variable. In descriptive studies, the inference deals with relationships. In the case of both forms of research, the term *validity* is used much like it is in measurement.

The major difference between measurement validity and experimental validity concerns the supporting arguments. In measurement validity, we need to justify the use of a measurement. In experimental validity, we need to justify the use of a research method.

Experimental validity has two subcategories, internal validity and external validity. Campbell and Stanley only relate these to experimental and quasi-experimental designs; however, their terms can also be cautiously applied to descriptive research. In experimental research, *internal validity* deals with whether an independent variable (a treatment) causes a change in the dependent variable. I suggest that internal validity for descriptive studies is present when demonstrated relationships are real, that is, when they are not an artifact of some methodological flaw. *A study without internal validity has no meaning and is not worth discussing.*

A study examined the effects of two different diathermy treatments on a host of variables in patients with recent ankle sprains. The day after injury, the researchers measured, among other things, the force the patient could generate in holding the foot either in an inverted or everted position. Not surprisingly to those of us who have lived through ankle injuries, the forces were negligible. After a week of either diathermy treatment, the patients' forces increased many hundred-fold. Did the diathermy improve the force-generating capability of the muscles? Fortunately there was also a placebo group that showed similar force improvements. If there had been no placebo group, the researchers might have falsely concluded there was an effect from the diathermy.

The researchers saved their study from being internally invalid by using a control. They could have done even better, however, if they had used a little common sense and realized that the day after an ankle injury they should not have assessed muscle performance around an injured joint. They apparently thought they were testing muscle performance, but in reality they were probably testing pain—or perhaps masochism. I make this point to emphasize that knowledge about internal and external validity is nice but useless without a common-sense approach and a knowledge of the phenomena and the subjects being measured. Only by knowing about the content of research can someone know when there are factors that threaten the internal validity of a study.

External validity deals with whether the results of a study are generalizable. The reliability and validity studies of clinical measurements that use healthy persons for subjects have little or no external validity. Even the best studies usually have limited external validity. You can generalize only so far. The author of a research report must be aware of this, and because researchers are sometimes intoxicated by their own results, the reader also had better be wary of excessive generalizations.

The practical world sometimes limits the type of research we conduct. Some friends were once interested in seeing whether rheumatoid arthritis patients could generate less torque isokinetically than could healthy persons. My friends had a colleague at the local Veterans Administration hospital who had a large number of willing patients. There was, however, one gigantic limit on their external validity. At the VA hospital they measured typical patients—and all of them were men. Unfortunately, my friends were characterizing muscle performance deficits in patients with a disease that is approximately three times more common in females than males.[33] Their study described an atypical group of patients with RA. The study, therefore, had limited generalizability. My friends were experts on research methods and are generally good scientists but they had limited experience with rheumatic diseases and were not aware of this limitation.

My friends never published the study. If they had, then they should have discussed the limitation to external validity. In the draft of a paper I reviewed, they had not. Their failure to develop content expertise about their subjects could have been embarrassing.

Assessment of experimental validity, like that of measurement validity, is based on logical application of rules to specific situations. Elsewhere in this book, the threats to experimental validity described by Campbell and Stanley are described, but for anyone who plans to conduct research, a review of the original will be a worthwhile experience.

SUMMARY

This chapter is meant to be a primer on some important issues for beginning researchers. Novices may be students or clinicians. If you are choosing to do research for the first time, I urge you to read on and read carefully. But I also urge you to seek the assistance of someone with experience before you start a project. You can no more learn how to do research by reading a book than you can learn how to sculpt from reading a book. The written word may give you some insight into process and technique, but that is not the same as application and implementation. Too many of our enthusiastic clinical colleagues have been turned off to research because their first projects were frustrating failures. That is a shame because we need their zeal and their insights.

Many who read this chapter will be students who were required (forced) to do so for a course. Many of them will then be forced to do research. Such students remind me of children forced to take castor oil. In both cases, observation of the results is not aesthetically pleasing. I hope that students who are being coerced into research will think carefully about the words of Campbell and Stanley. Nobel laureates usually have more humble expectations for the research than do students. Knowledge grows slowly and in a cumulative fashion—and only for those with the patience to wait while it does.

I hope that as a result of this chapter students will realize that research involves logical processes. Almost all of my graduate students who return to clinical practice admit that their new knowledge is helpful. However, they say that, more importantly, they are better clinicians because they have learned to think more critically. To new physical therapists and to seasoned veterans I say that if you can think clearly in order to conduct research, then you will be a better physical therapist. If you can stand the frustration of research, then you will be better at dealing with the frustration that comes from never being able to do enough for your patients.

REFERENCES

1. Stevens, S.S. Measurement psychophysics and utility. In Churchman, C.W. and Ratoosh, P., eds., *Measurement: definitions and themes.* New York: Wiley, 1959.

2. Hays, W.L. *Quantification in psychology.* Belmont, CA: Brooks Cole, 1967.

3. Lyle, V.J. *The nature of measurement in educational measurement,* 2nd ed. Washington DC: American Council of Education, 1971, p. 8.

4. Wilks, S.S. Some aspects of quantification in science. In H. Woolf, ed. *Quantification.* New York: Bobbs Merrill, 1961, p. 5.

5. Rothstein, J.M. Measurement and clinical practice: Theory and application. In Rothstein, J.M., ed., *Measurement in physical therapy.* New York: Churchill Livingstone, 1985, p. 1.

6. Rothstein, J.M., Miller, P.J., and Roettger, R.F. Goniometric reliability in a clinical setting: Elbow and knee measurements. *Physical Therapy* 63:1611, 1983.

7. Riddle, D.L., Rothstein, J.M., and Lamb, R.L. Goniometric reliability in a clinical setting: Shoulder measurements. *Physical Therapy* 67:668, 1987.

8. Elveru, R., Rothstein, J.M., Lamb, R.L., and Riddle, D. A clinical method for determining the position of subtalar neutral. *Physical Therapy* 68:678–682, 1988.

9. Miller, P.J. Assessment of joint motion. In Rothstein, J.M., ed., *Measurement in physical therapy.* New York: Churchill Livingstone, 1985, p. 103.

10. *Webster's new collegiate dictionary,* 150th ed. Springfield, MA: Merriam-Webster, 1973, p. 1282.

11. Lamb, R.L. Manual muscle testing. In Rothstein, J.M., ed., *Measurement in physical therapy.* New York: Churchill Livingstone, 1985, p. 47.

12. Kendall, F.P. and McCreary, E.K. *Muscle testing and function,* 3rd ed. Baltimore: Williams and Wilkins, 1983, p. 189.

13. Walker, M.L., Rothstein, J.M., Finucane, S.D., and Lamb, R.L. Relationship between lordosis, pelvic tilt, and abdominal muscle performance. *Physical Therapy* 67:512, 1987.

14. Moffroid, M., Whipple, R., Hofkosh, J., Lowman, E., and Thistle, H. A study of isokinetic exercise. *Physical Therapy* 49:735, 1969.

15. Mayhew, T.P. and Rothstein, J.M. Measurement of muscle performance with instruments. In Rothstein, J.M., ed., *Measurement in physical therapy.* New York: Churchill Livingstone, 1985, p. 57.

16. Rothstein, J.M., Lamb, R.L., and Mayhew, T.P. Clinical uses of isokinetic measurements. *Physical therapy* 67:1840–1844, 1987.

17. Murray, D.A. and Harrison, E. Constant velocity dynamometer: An appraisal using mechanical loading. *Medical Science Sports and Exercise* 18:612–624, 1986.

18. Winter, D.A., Wells, R.P., and Orr, G.W. Errors in the use of isokinetic dynamometers. *European Journal of Applied Physiology* 46:397–408, 1981.

19. *Standards for educational and psychological tests.* Washington, DC: American Psychological Association, 1974.

20. Payton, O.P. *Research: The validation of clinical practice.* Philadelphia: F.A. Davis, 1979.

21. Lovett, R.W. and Masten, E.G. Certain aspects of infantile paralysis and a description of a method of muscle testing. *Journal of the American Medical Association* 66:729, 1916.

22. Malone, T., Blackburn, T.A., and Wallace, L.A. Knee rehabilitation. *Physical Therapy* 60:1602–1610, 1980.

23. Davies, G.J. *A compendium of isokinetics in clinical usage and rehabilitation techniques,* 2nd ed. La Crosse, WI: S & S Publishers, 1984.

24. Donaldson, W.F., Warren, R.F., and Wickiewicz, T. A comparison of acute interior cruciate ligament examinations: Initial versus examination under anesthesia. *American Journal of Sports Medicine* 13:5–10, 1985.

25. James, S.L., Bates, B.T., and Osternig, L.R. Injuries to runners. *American Journal of Sports Medicine.* 6:40–49, 1978.

26. Elveru, R., Rothstein, J.M., and Lamb, R.L. Goniometric reliability in a clinical setting: Measurements of subtalar neutral and plantar and dorsiflexion. *Physical Therapy* 68:672–677, 1988.

27. McKenzie, R.A. *The lumbar spine—Mechanical diagnosis and therapy.* Worikanae, New Zealand: Spinal Publishers, 1981.

28. Vassos, B.H. and Ewing, G.W. *Analog and digital electronics for scientists.* New York: Wiley, 1972.

29. Kerlinger, F.N. *Foundations of behavioral research,* 2nd ed. New York: Holt, Rinehart and Winston, 1973.

30. Linton, M. and Gallo, P.S. *The practical statistician: Simplified handbook of statistics.* Monterey, CA: Brooks Cole, 1975, chap. 11.

31. Gage, N.L., ed. *Handbook of research on teaching.* Chicago: Rand McNally, 1963.

32. Campbell, D.T. and Stanley, J.C. *Experimental and quasi-experimental designs for research.* Chicago: Rand McNally, 1963.

33. Schumacher, H.R. *Primer of the rheumatic disease,* 9th ed. Atlanta, GA: Arthritis Foundation, 1988.

3

THE USE AND PROTECTION OF HUMAN AND ANIMAL SUBJECTS

Ernest D. Prentice and Ruth B. Purtilo

During the last fifty years we have experienced such a tremendous knowledge explosion in the fields of medicine and allied health that our medical armamentarium includes techniques and instruments only dreamed about a few years ago. Liver, heart, and bone marrow transplants are relatively common therapies, and "high tech" equipment such as surgical lasers, computerized axial tomograph (CAT) scanners, and nuclear magnetic resonance (NMR) machines are found in most major hospitals in the United States. In the field of physical therapy one need take only a cursory look around a physical therapy clinic to observe how technically sophisticated the profession has become. Indeed, it is anticipated that medical knowledge will continue to grow at an ever-escalating rate as we approach the twenty-first century.

Knowledge, in general, is advanced through the dedicated efforts of scientists and others engaged in a variety of scholarly pursuits. And, while observation and thinking are invaluable in the search for new knowledge, experimentation is crucial. A growing body of literature, including this book, expresses the commitment of physical therapists to sound clinical and basic science research approaches in order to further knowledge relevant to the practice of physical therapy.

In the biomedical fields, experimentation usually involves human and/or animal subjects. This chapter provides a survey of key ethical and legal responsibilities of investigators who use either humans or vertebrate animals in their research endeavors. The information presented is based upon various ethical codes and federal regulations that govern human or animal research. The codes and regulations that pertain to research, however, often include necessarily vague abstractions in order to permit flexibility in both interpretation and application. The authors, therefore, assume responsibility for liberties taken with respect to interpretation.

Because the ethics and regulation of research are intertwined and difficult to separate, we have chosen to concentrate on the roles of university and hospital review committees charged with ensuring that human and animal research is ethically conducted in full compliance with federal requirements. Because the ethical considerations germane to a review committee are equally relevant to the investigator, this chapter should prove helpful to physical therapists involved in human or animal research in the field of physical therapy as well as other disciplines.

One final comment on the scope of this chapter. It is obviously not meant to provide a comprehensive treatment of the subject. There are literally thousands of articles dealing with informed consent alone, and the federal regulations that apply to human and animal research are substantially longer than this entire book. Therefore, we have attempted to present only the most salient points concerning the use and protection of human and animal subjects.

THE USE AND PROTECTION OF HUMAN SUBJECTS

Evolution of the Institutional Review Board

The first significant worldwide focus on human subjects abuse is usually dated to 1946, when the Nuremberg Trials[1] brought to the world's attention the abuses that Nazi "scientists" carried out under the guise of medical research. The Nuremberg Code,[2] which addresses the ethics of human experimentation, was formulated as a reaction to the Nazi "medical" experiments conducted on prisoners in concentration camps such as Dachau and Buchenwald. In 1964, after nearly two decades of greatly expanded biomedical research and little attention to human subject protection, the Eighteenth World Medical Assembly adopted the Declaration of Helsinki[3] as a code of ethics for experiments involving human beings.

Less than one year after the Declaration of Helsinki, human research once again became a public issue when the press reported the Jewish Chronic Diseases Hospital study concerning transplant rejection.[4] This study, which involved the subcutaneous injection of live cancer cells in debilitated patients without their knowledge, provoked widespread public concern. In 1972, public opinion was inflamed further by the infamous Tuskegee Syphilis Study,[5,6] in which 399 black males with diagnosed syphilis were recruited without informed consent, misinformed about the nature of the research, and purposely left untreated even after penicillin therapy became available in the 1940s. Incredibly, this study, begun in 1932 and sponsored by the United States Public Health Service (USPHS), was in full progress during the 1960s at the time the USPHS and Department of Health, Education and Welfare (DHEW) began formulating the federal regulations governing human subjects research. The Tuskegee Syphilis Study was finally halted in 1972 after accounts of it appeared in the national press.

At approximately the same time the Tuskegee Syphilis Study achieved public notoriety, other reports of human subject abuse precipitated increased public and judicial attention to individual rights. Thus, it was in a highly charged emotional climate fueled by public concern and indignation that the United States Congress established in 1974, by Public Law 93-348, The National Commission for the Protection of Human Subjects in Biomedical and Behavioral Research.[7] During five years of dedicated and thoughtful study concerning various ethical issues and a detailed review of the first edition of the DHEW regulations (45 CFR 46) issued in

1974, this commission published a series of reports[8-14] that contain ethical principles and guidelines for the protection of human research subjects. The commission's reports serve as the basis for the final Department of Health and Human Services (DHHS) Regulations 45 CFR 46[15] and the Food and Drug Administration (FDA) Regulations 21 CFR 50, 56.[16] These regulations now govern federally funded and FDA-regulated human subjects research and the operation of the thousands of university and hospital institutional review boards (IRBs) that must review and approve the studies.

Role of the IRB

The National Commission in its report on IRBs[12] articulated the primary purpose of the IRB: "Investigators should not have sole responsibility for determining whether research involving human subjects fulfills ethical standards. Others who are independent of the research must share this responsibility, because investigators are always in positions of potential conflict by virtue of their concern with the pursuit of knowledge as well as the welfare of the human subjects of their research." The IRB, therefore, exists to aid the investigator in the protection of the rights and welfare of human subjects. The investigator, however, still bears the principal responsibility for the protection of his or her research subjects.

Ethical Review of Human Subject Research

The logistics of IRB review varies from institution to institution, but the major principles underlying IRB review do not. Before a human subject research protocol is implemented the IRB should thoughtfully and thoroughly consider the following factors which, taken together, reflect the ethical sensitivity of the investigator in designing the project.

The Prospective Subject Population

The prospective subject population must be appropriate with respect to the nature and goals of the research. In addition, the investigator should be guided by the principles that lead to an equitable selection of subjects with regard to the potential risks and benefits of the research. The IRB, therefore, should examine carefully the characteristics of the subject population. Factors such as the required number of subjects, age range, sex, ethnic background, and health status should be considered. The utilization of any vulnerable class of subjects, such as sick persons, pregnant women, fetuses, prisoners, children, elderly persons, mentally incompetent persons, and persons of low socioeconomic status, should be clearly justified.

Naturally, there are exceptions to the principle of "equitable selection of subjects." For instance, research involving the study of a disease to which only one ethnic or racial group is susceptible would not require the application of this principle. Two examples are sickle cell anemia in the black population and Tay-Sachs disease, which affects Jewish people.

Identification of Potential Risks

A risk is a potential harm (injury) associated with the research that a reasonable person, in what the investigator knows or should know to be the subject's position, would be likely to consider significant in deciding whether or not to participate in the research. The concept of risk includes discomfort, burden, or inconvenience a subject may experience as a result of the research procedures. Underlying the consideration of risk is the implicit moral guideline that an investigator has a duty not to harm the subjects.

The five major types of risks are: (1) physical risk (e.g., infection associated with venipuncture, adverse reactions to drugs, muscle soreness as a consequence of Cybex testing, heart attack induced by a maximal exercise test); (2) psychological risk (e.g., depression and confusion as a result of administration of hallucinogenic drugs, feelings of guilt precipitated by a sensitive survey); (3) social risk (e.g., invasion of privacy, loss of community standing); (4) legal risk (e.g., criminal prosecution, revocation of parole); and (5) economic risk (e.g., loss of employment, loss of potential monetary gain).

Risks also can be classified as minimal and greater than minimal. Federal regulations define minimal risk, saying, "The probability and magnitude of harm or discomfort anticipated in the research are not greater in and of themselves than those ordinarily encountered in daily life or during the performance of routine physical or psychological examinations or tests." Application of this classification does not, however, require consideration of the risks inherent in each subject's life. Indeed, such specific considerations would require a multitude of standards, effectively resulting in no standard.

Both the immediate and latent (delayed) risks of any procedure involving human subjects should be identified. In addition, risks should be minimized to the greatest extent possible and the estimated probability, severity, average duration, and reversibility of any potential harm should be determined according to available empirical data. Furthermore, since certain populations of vulnerable subjects may be at greater risk than others, the analysis of the risks should take into consideration the potential risk characterization of the subject. Pregnant women and their fetuses, for example, may be at greater risk in drug studies.

Identification of Potential Benefits

A benefit is a valued or desired outcome. Benefits associated with participation in research can be classified generally as those that accrue to the subject directly (e.g., improvement of health status) and those that accrue to society (e.g., acquisition of knowledge). The investigator should identify anticipated/expected benefits to the subject or to others. In addition, benefits should be maximized through proper protocol design to the greatest extent possible. Therefore, an underlying moral notion of "beneficence" should guide the investigator. Financial or other forms of remuneration should not be considered a benefit to be derived from research participation. Although the subject may consider financial compensation a desirable outcome this fact should not be used in the risk/benefit analysis.

Risk/Benefit Analysis

Once the potential risks and benefits are identified, an ethical review of research requires an examination of the relationship of the risks to the benefits. Risks and benefits cannot be considered parallel constructs, so no one formula can be applied. The various ethical codes and regulations, however, require a favorable balance between harm and benefit. To assist the investigator and the IRB in assessing the risk/benefit relationship, the following is a series of principles which take into consideration the vulnerability of the subject and whether or not the research is therapeutic in nature.

1. In research that has no likelihood or intent of producing a diagnostic, preventive, or therapeutic benefit to the subject (nontherapeutic research), the potential risk to the subject must be outweighed or balanced by the potential benefit to the subject and/or by the knowledge to be gained.

2. In research involving the study of the efficacy of a therapeutic or diagnostic method and the intervention is, therefore, not designed solely to enhance the well-being of the subject (therapeutic research), the potential risk should be outweighed or balanced by the potential benefit to the subject. In addition, the relation of the anticipated benefit to the risk must be at least as favorable to the subject as that presented by alternate standard therapies available to the subject in the nonresearch context. No subject should be allowed to continue participating in a research protocol if therapy of proven superior nature becomes available to the subject.

3. In research where a standard therapy not part of the research protocol is employed solely for the benefit of the subject along with additional procedures performed solely for research purposes, the anticipated benefits of the therapy should not be used to justify exposing subjects to the risks associated with the research procedures. Such risks can only be justified in light of the potential benefits of the research procedures. Conversely, only the risks associated with the research procedures should be used in determining the risk/benefit ratio.

4. In child research involving greater than minimal risk with no prospect of direct benefit to the subject, the following conditions should be met: *(a)* the risk represents only a minor increase over minimal risk; *(b)* the research will likely result in an increase in generalizable knowledge which is of vital importance for understanding the subject's disorder, condition, or state of health; and *(c)* the intervention or procedure presents experiences to the subject that are reasonably commensurate with those inherent in their actual or expected medical, dental, psychological, social, or educational situation.

5. In research involving pregnant women as subjects, the following condition should be met: *(a)* the purpose of the research is to meet the health needs of the mother, and the fetus will be placed at risk only to the minimum extent necessary to meet such needs; OR *(b)* the risk to the fetus is minimal. Only those research procedures that would be acceptable for a fetus going to term should be performed. In addition, whenever there is a potential conflict of interest (e.g., likelihood of abortion or planned abortion), the investigator

must not be involved in any decision as to the timing, method, and procedures used to terminate the pregnancy or in the determination of viability of the fetus at termination of pregnancy.

Investigator Qualifications

The IRB should review investigator qualifications and must be assured that *(a)* the investigator has the appropriate qualifications and/or licensure to carry out the procedures involving human subjects with an acceptable degree of potential risk; and *(b)* the investigator has adequate facilities and equipment to conduct the research with an acceptable degree of potential risk.

Informed Consent of the Subject

Finally, one of the most important functions of the IRB is to assist the investigator in the design and conduct of the consent process. Since "informed consent" is such a rich and complex doctrine, a separate section of this chapter deals with the considerations surrounding it. In addition, a sample consent form for a physical therapy research protocol is provided.

The Consent Process

Although there are federal regulations requiring the subject or the subject's legally authorized representative to give consent prior to the subject's participation in an experiment, the principal reason for informing subjects about an experiment is that they have a moral right to know what is to be done to them and what risk this entails before they give their consent. Human beings are considered autonomous, and the requirement of informed consent is designed to uphold the ethical principle of "respect for persons."[17,18] The use of human subjects is a privilege—a favor—granted to the experimenter, not a right. An experiment is something that is done to the subject, and therefore differs from the usual medical practice in which something is done solely for the patient.

In order for consent to be legally and ethically valid it must meet the requirements stated in Principle I of the Nuremberg Code: "The voluntary consent of the human subject is absolutely essential. This means that the person involved should have legal capacity to give consent; should be so situated as to be able to exercise free power of choice, without the intervention of any element of force, fraud, deceit, duress, over-reaching or other ulterior form of constraint or coercion; and should have sufficient knowledge and comprehension of the elements of the subject matter involved as to enable him to make an understanding and enlightened decision."

The Consent Form

The legal documentation of informed consent is the consent form signed by both the subject and the investigator (see the box, "Sample Informed Consent Form"). The ethical and, indeed, legal validity of the consent form is, however,

SAMPLE INFORMED CONSENT FORM

COMPARISON OF STRENGTH AND RANGE OF MOTION IN RELATION TO DIFFERENT SURGICAL PROCEDURES USED TO REPAIR ANTERIOR SHOULDER DISLOCATIONS

Invitation to Participate

You are invited to participate in a research study of the effects of different surgical repairs of shoulder dislocations on strength and range of motion.

Basis of Subject Selection

The reason you are invited to participate in this study is because you are 18 years of age or older and you have had a surgical repair of your shoulder following dislocation. In addition, it has been at least one year since your surgery.

Purpose of the Study

The purpose of this study is to determine which surgical procedure used to repair a shoulder dislocation allows patients to regain the greatest range of motion and develop the maximum possible shoulder strength.

Explanation of Procedures

You will be asked to complete a brief survey which asks questions concerning your shoulder injury. Following that you will be asked to move your arms through the entire range of motion which involves six different normal movements of your arm. You will then be tested for strength of the shoulder muscles by using the Cybex II Isokinetic Dynamometer. This machine allows you to perform five maximal contractions of your shoulder muscles during each of the six movements tested. You will be tested at both a slow and a fast speed. All testing will be done in the Physical Therapy and Sports Rehabilitation Center, University of Nebraska Hospital. The total time that will be required of you is approximately one hour.

Potential Risks and Discomforts

During the study you might experience some slight muscle fatigue and/or muscle discomfort. The time allowed for rest between each set of testing will minimize the risk of soreness and fatigue. All soreness and fatigue should be resolved within 24 to 48 hours.

Potential Benefits

You will receive no direct benefit from participating in this study. The results of this study may tell us which type of surgical repair for shoulder dislocation is best. This information, in turn, may help future patients.

Financial Obligations

All testing done will be provided to you at no cost. The only expense you will have is transportation to and from the university hospital and parking fees during the study.

Assurance of Confidentiality

Any information obtained in connection with this study will be held in strict confidence. Any information obtained in this study may be published in appropriate journals or presented at professional meetings. In such publications or presentations, your identification will be kept strictly confidential.

Continued

SAMPLE INFORMED CONSENT FORM *(Continued)*

In Case of Injury

In the event of a research related injury, please immediately contact Eric Bottjen, R.P.T., at 402/559-4000.

If you suffer an injury as a direct consequence of the research procedures described above, the emergency medical care required to treat the injury will be provided at the University of Nebraska at no expense to you, providing that the cost of such medical care is not reimbursable through your health insurance. However, no additional compensation for physical care, hospitalization, loss of income, pain, suffering, or any other form of compensation will be provided. None of the above shall be construed as a waiver of any legal rights or redress you may have.

Withdrawal from the Study

Participation is voluntary. Your decision whether or not to participate will not affect your present or future relationship with the University of Nebraska Medical Center. If you decide to participate, you are free to withdraw your consent and to discontinue participation at any time.

Offer to Answer Questions

If you have any questions, please do not hesitate to ask. If you think of questions later, please feel free to contact one of the investigators listed below.

If you have any questions concerning the rights of research subjects, you may contact the University of Nebraska Institutional Review Board (IRB), telephone 402/559-6463.

YOU ARE VOLUNTARILY MAKING A DECISION WHETHER OR NOT TO PARTICI-PATE IN THIS RESEARCH STUDY. YOUR SIGNATURE CERTIFIES THAT YOU HAVE DECIDED TO PARTICIPATE HAVING READ AND UNDERSTOOD THE INFORMATION PRESENTED. YOUR SIGNATURE ALSO CERTIFIES THAT YOU HAVE HAD AN ADE-QUATE OPPORTUNITY TO DISCUSS THIS STUDY WITH THE INVESTIGATOR AND YOU HAVE HAD ALL YOUR QUESTIONS ANSWERED TO YOUR SATISFACTION. YOU WILL BE GIVEN A COPY OF THIS CONSENT FORM TO KEEP.

_____   _____
Signature of Subject   Date

MY SIGNATURE AS WITNESS CERTIFIES THAT THE SUBJECT SIGNED THIS CON-SENT FORM IN MY PRESENCE AS HIS/HER VOLUNTARY ACT AND DEED.

_____   _____
Signature of Witness   Date

IN MY JUDGMENT THE SUBJECT IS VOLUNTARILY AND KNOWINGLY GIVING INFORMED CONSENT AND POSSESSES THE LEGAL CAPACITY TO GIVE INFORMED CONSENT TO PARTICIPATE IN THIS RESEARCH STUDY.

_____   _____
Signature of Investigator   Date

INVESTIGATOR
Erick J. Bottjen, R.P.T.   402/559-4000

(Courtesy of E. Bottjen, R.P.T., University of Nebraska Medical Center, Omaha, Nebraska.)

dependent upon the process of informed consent which requires the investigator to engage in dialogue or negotiation with the prospective subject in accordance with Principle I of the Nuremberg Code. The consent form, therefore, should be used by the investigator as an instrument to guide the negotiations with the prospective subject.

The informed consent form must embody the elements of informed consent contained in the DHHS and/or FDA regulations, which have essentially the same requirements regarding consent. The following guidelines reflect those requirements, and can be used by the investigator and the IRB in the construction and review of the consent document.

Language, Style, and Level

The federal regulations do not require any particular style of writing. In our opinion, however, the informed consent form should usually be written in the second person throughout. When combined with conditional language and the invitation to participate, using the second person communicates that the investigator believes there is a choice to be made by the prospective subject. Use of the first person may be interpreted as presumption of subject consent before consent has been legally obtained.

The informed consent form should be written in simple enough language that it is readily understood by the least educated, least sophisticated of the prospective subjects. The language should consist of short, concise sentences. Remember that although terms commonly used by members of a profession are a part of the professional's language, many people outside that profession do not understand the language. Common words in medicine, such as *catheter, intravenous, IV, prognosis,* and *symptomatology,* are not understood by many laypeople. Terms in the field of physical therapy, such as *Cybex, isokinetic, isotonic,* and *goniometry,* are equally misunderstood. If there is any doubt that a term may not be understood, add a definition. If some of the anticipated subject population does not understand English, provide appropriate translation.

If the consent form will be used for parents or other legally authorized representatives consenting on behalf of minors or other legally incompetent subjects, the consent form should be written in a style that reflects the fact that the minor or other subject is the participant and the consentor is agreeing to allow said subject to participate in the study.

The informed consent form must not contain any exculpatory language through which the subject or the subject's representative (1) is made to waive or appear to waive any of the subject's legal rights; or (2) releases or appears to release the research investigator, the sponsor, the institution, or its agents from liability for negligence.

Elements of Informed Consent

The elements of informed consent represent the information that should be communicated to the prospective subject. The arrangement or sequence of the elements in the consent form provides structure to the consent form and serves to guide the negotiations between the investigator and the prospective subject. We recommend that each element be identified by a subheading that helps to increase the readability of the consent form. In addition, the information content of each element should be restricted to information relevant to that element.

Invitation to Participate

The consent form should logically begin with an invitation to the prospective subject to participate in the research study. The invitation should not contain any language that is coercive or would be interpreted as a demand or request.

Basis for Subject Selection

The consent form should state why the prospective subject has been selected (e.g., subjects with specific diseases, conditions, characteristics, backgrounds). This statement should help the subject to assess the nature and importance of participation. When appropriate, the approximate number of subjects involved in the study should be stated. When appropriate, criteria for subject exclusion should be stated (e.g., pregnancy, age limitations, health restrictions).

Overall Purpose

The consent form should contain a clear statement of the overall purpose of the research which should help the subject assess the importance of the study relative to individual values.

Explanation of Procedures

The explanation of the procedures section of the consent form should include, where appropriate, the following.

1. A description of the study design (e.g., longitudinal, single-blind, double-blind, placebo), method of subject assignment to groups (e.g., randomization), and probability of assignment (e.g., 50-50 chance). Despite the fact that subjects may be kept unaware of treatment assignments in blinded studies and research involving placebos, subjects must be made aware of all the possible interventions and the method of assignment. Thus, prospective subjects are invited to remain ignorant of treatment assignment without the element of deception.
2. A description of each procedure to be applied to human subjects and how often it will be performed. All procedures, both experimental and nonexperimental, should be described or disclosed. Procedures that are experimental and/or performed for research purposes should be identified as such (e.g., a subject will undergo routine knee surgery for therapeutic reasons, and a series of CAT scans will be performed for research purposes. The surgical procedure should be described as normal prescribed therapy, and the CAT scans should be identified as a procedure performed for research purposes).
3. Identification of the individual(s) who will perform the procedures and/or interact with the subject.

4. A statement of where the research will be conducted, when the research will be conducted, and how much time (per session/in total) will be required of the subject.
5. A statement concerning any medications, therapeutic regimens, foods, or other substances that are contraindicated or disallowed.

Potential Risks and Discomforts

Both immediate and latent risks of each procedure should be clearly described in the consent form. Disclosure of risks should be based upon what a reasonably prudent prospective subject might wish to know. Risks should not be understated or overstated, and if there are no potential risks this should be so stated. Prospective subjects should also be told whether participation in the study precludes participation in other programs or therapeutic regimens that may be beneficial to them and the extent to which this may constitute a risk.

Potential Benefits

Both immediate and delayed benefits of the research should be clearly stated in the consent form. The potential benefits must not be overstated, coercive, or guaranteed. If there are no benefits to the subject or to society, it should be so stated.

Alternatives to Participation

When a component of the protocol is designed to enhance the well-being of the subject, the consent form should state any appropriate alternative procedures or course of therapy that might be advantageous to the subject.

Financial Obligations

This section of the consent form should state clearly all financial obligations of the subject with respect to both the study and any related medical therapy (e.g., financial responsibility for physician and physical therapist fees, hospital charges, medication, laboratory tests, posttreatment follow-up). If there is the potential of additional cost to the subject as a result of participation in the study, it must be disclosed. If there is no cost to the subject and that fact is not obvious, it should be so stated.

Financial Compensation

Any economic incentives or rewards for participation should be clearly stated in the consent form. Economic incentives are usually cash payments but may also include, when appropriate, free physical examinations, free treatment, free medications, treatment at lower cost, and so forth. Cash payments should be stated in dollar amounts and any conditions, such as partial or no payment for early termination and bonuses for completion, should be stated. The nature and amount of financial or other compensation should not constitute undue inducement of the subject (e.g., the compensation alone should not serve as sufficient inducement for the subject to volunteer). When establishing the amount or type of compensation, the investigator should consider the background and socioeconomic status of the subject population.

Assurance of Confidentiality

This section of the consent form should state that any information obtained in connection with the study that could identify the subject will remain confidential and will be disclosed only with the subject's permission. If the investigator intends to release any information, the consent form should state the person(s) or agency to whom information will be furnished, the nature of the information to be furnished, the purpose of the disclosure, and whether the subject's name will be used as an identifier. It is strongly recommended that a code be used to identify subjects. When appropriate, the ultimate disposition of data should be described.

In Case of Injury

For research involving more than minimal risk, the consent form should contain an explanation of whether or not compensation and medical treatment are available if injury occurs, and, if so, what this consists of.

Withdrawal from the Study

The consent form should contain a noncoercive disclaimer that permits the subject to withdraw from the study at any time without penalty or loss of benefits to which the subject is otherwise entitled.

Offer to Answer Questions

The consent form should contain an offer by investigators to answer all immediate and subsequent questions that the subject may have regarding the research and a research subject's rights.

Concluding Consent Statements

The consent form should contain concluding consent statements that clearly indicate that both the subject's signature and the investigator's signature certify voluntary and informed agreement on the part of the subject to participate in the study. In addition, there should be a witness certification statement.

Signature Blanks

The consent form should contain dated subject, investigator, and witness signature blanks.

Identification of Investigators

The consent form should list the names and telephone numbers of the investigator(s) to assist the subject in contacting the investigator(s) should any questions arise.

Consent/Assent Procedures for Minors

Research involving children is governed by 45 CFR 46:401-409 which provides additional protection for children involved as subjects in research. The DHHS regulations reflect, with some discrepancies, the National Commission's report and recommendations regarding child research.[10] Children are considered a vulnerable research population because their intellectual and emotional capacities are limited. Subjects who are children, therefore, should be afforded special protection from the risks and burdens of research. Accordingly, the National Commission recommends that, where appropriate, prior to involving younger children, studies be conducted first on animals and adult humans, and then on older children. Adults are perceived as less vulnerable than older children who are, in turn, considered less vulnerable than younger children.

Legally, children cannot give consent on their own behalf. The consent of their parent(s) or a legal guardian is, therefore, required before they can participate in research projects. Under special circumstances, however (e.g., research involving neglected/abused children), the IRB may approve a waiver of parental consent. If the research involves only minimal risk activities (e.g., venipuncture, skin biopsy, EEG, ECG, urine collection, moderate exercise, standard psychological testing), the consent of only one parent is necessary. If, however, the research involves greater than minimal risk activities, the consent of both parents should be obtained (1) unless one parent is deceased, unknown, incompetent, or not reasonably available, or (2) when only one parent has the legal responsibility for the care and custody of the child.

In addition to obtaining parental/legal guardian consent, the investigator should also solicit the assent of child subjects. This requirement is based upon the ethical premise that society should respect the developing autonomy of children. Although the federal regulations do not specify an age of assent, the IRB is charged with determining this by taking into account the age, maturity, and psychological state of the children involved. The National Commission, however, suggests seven as the age at which a child with normal cognitive development becomes capable of meaningful assent.

The federal regulations also do not specify the elements of assent that must be transmitted to prospective child subjects. Many of the elements of informed consent that are required on adult consent forms are not relevant to assent of children. For instance, the Compensation in Case of Injury clause and the Financial Obligations of the subject statement are probably not important factors in the child's decision whether or not to assent. Certainly, a child assent form should contain, at a minimum, simplistic descriptions of the purpose of the study, procedures, risks, benefits, and confidentiality safeguards. Additional elements can be included according to the child's level of understanding and the relative importance of the element to the child.

Although the federal regulations address assent, they do not provide for the possibility that a child may object to participating in research. The National Commission, however, suggests that a child's deliberate objection should usually be regarded as a veto of his or her involvement in the research. Of course, parents or guardians may override a young child's objections to interventions that hold the prospect of direct benefit to the child.

Alterations and Waiver of
Informed Consent

Under special circumstances, DHHS regulations permit investigators to use a consent procedure that does not include, or which alters, some or all of the elements of informed consent. Before a waiver can be issued, the IRB must determine that all of the following conditions exist: (1) the project involves no more than minimal risk; (2) the rights of the subject will not be significantly infringed upon; (3) the research could not practically be carried out without the waiver or alteration; and (4) if possible, the subject will be fully informed after the project has been completed.

The IRB may waive the requirement of the investigator to obtain a signed consent form for some or all subjects (or parents/guardians) if it finds that either (1) the only reason linking the subject and the research would be the consent document, and the principal risk would be potential harm resulting from a breach of confidentiality; or (2) the research presents no more than minimal risk of harm to subjects and involves no procedures for which written consent is normally required outside the research context.

THE USE AND PROTECTION OF
ANIMAL SUBJECTS

Evolution of the Institutional Animal Care
and Use Committee

Most of the countries in the Western world have addressed at various times and in various ways the ethics of animal experimentation. Indeed, the question of what constitutes appropriate animal welfare in the research context has been debated with considerable fervor for more than a century. In the United States, animal welfare currently is a major societal issue which has precipitated numerous protests, violent confrontations, and laboratory raids. During the last decade the protest activities of various animal welfare groups, such as the radical Animal Liberation Front (ALF) and the more moderate People for the Ethical Treatment of Animals (PETA), have escalated. These protests and the concomitant media attention have, in turn, raised the level of public sensitivity and governmental consciousness regarding animal welfare. Legislative authorities at the local, state, and federal level have responded in various ways, passing policies, bills, and amendments to existing legislation that address laboratory animal welfare.

At the national level, in 1985 the DHHS issued its new Public Health Service (PHS) Policy on Humane Care and Use of Laboratory Animals.[19] This policy specifically requires the establishment of Institutional Animal Care and Use Committees (IACUCs) responsible for approving the animal experimentation sections of grant applications to the PHS. In conjunction with publication of the new PHS policy, the National Institutes of Health (NIH) issued its fifth revision of the "NIH Guide for the Care and Use of Laboratory Animals."[20] The new guide, which serves as an adjunct to the PHS policy, also requires the establishment of IACUCs and addresses the quality of animal care to a much greater extent than did previous editions. In 1986 the DHHS again revised its PHS Policy on Humane Care and Use of Laboratory Animals[21] to incorporate changes required by the Health Research Extension Act of 1985.[22] The mandated changes increase the responsibilities of the IACUC, particularly in terms of the training of scientists, animal technicians, and other personnel involved in animal care, treatment, or use. Also in 1985 an amended Animal Welfare Act[23] both strengthened and extended laboratory animal welfare standards and United States Department of Agriculture (USDA) enforcement of those standards through its animal welfare rules, which were issued in final form in 1989 and 1991.[24]

Role of the IACUC

Without doubt, the most significant provision of both the PHS policy and the amended Animal Welfare Act is the requirement of prior institutional review of animal research by the IACUC. As a society we have an ethical imperative to make thoughtful decisions regarding the use of animals in the pursuit of knowledge. It is, therefore, the IACUC that now shares with the investigator the responsibility for ethical decision making with regard to the use of laboratory animals. There is, however, a lack of consensus regarding what constitutes the appropriate social balance between the needs of science and animal welfare. Since neither the PHS Policy nor the Animal Welfare Act contains explicit criteria concerning acceptable use of animals, each institution must formulate its own ethical criteria to be applied to animal experimentation. Federal guidelines allow considerable flexibility in the IACUC protocol review process, and each committee functions with relative autonomy.

Ethical Review of Animal Research

The following are the ethical principles concerned with animal welfare that have been adopted by the University of Nebraska Medical Center (UNMC). These principles provide guidance to investigators and serve as the protocol review criteria employed by the UNMC IACUC.[25]

1. When live animals are used in research or biological testing, there must be a reasonable expectation that such utilization will contribute to the enhancement of human or animal health, the advancement of knowledge, or the good of society. The relative value of the study is a particularly important consideration in potentially painful experiments where there is an ethical imperative that the benefits of the research clearly outweigh any pain, discomfort, and distress experienced by the animals.

2. It is recognized that in many research protocols there is simply no alternative to the use of live animals. Despite this social imperative for animal experi-

mentation, all investigators have an ethical obligation to explore ways in which animals can be partially or totally replaced by other biological systems or mathematical/computer models. When a research question can be pursued using reasonably available nonanimal or in vitro models and still result in sound scientific conclusions, the investigator should choose these alternatives.

3. Selection of an appropriate animal model is an important consideration, particularly at a time when alternative models of animal research are being emphasized. It is the investigator's responsibility, therefore, to select the optimal species for a particular project. In addition, the number of animals utilized in a protocol should be minimized, consistent with sound scientific and statistical standards. It is also the investigator's responsibility to consider the source of the animal and to ensure that all animals used for experimental purposes are lawfully acquired.

4. When animals are used in a research project, the investigator has an ethical obligation to seek the least painful techniques feasible that will allow the protocol objective(s) to be pursued adequately. If a procedure has associated pain, discomfort, or distress, it is imperative that the investigator estimate the probable occurrence, magnitude, and duration of the pain, discomfort, or distress. The investigator should distinguish between acute and chronic pain as well as pain that will be alleviated versus pain that cannot or will not be reduced or alleviated.

5. In potentially painful procedures, the investigator must take all necessary steps to assess and monitor pain as well as discomfort and distress. In assessing pain, the investigator should use behavioral signs based on the normal behavior pattern of the species under study. In some circumstances physiological parameters may be used (e.g., plasma cortisol, catecholamines, white blood cell counts, and cardiovascular parameters).

6. If a procedure will cause more than momentary slight pain or distress to the animal, the pain must be minimized in both intensity and duration through the administration of appropriate anesthetics, analgesics, and tranquilizers consistent with acceptable standards of veterinary medicine. It should be emphasized that the requirement for the alleviation/reduction of pain applies not only when the procedure is being conducted but also following the procedure until such time when the pain is either alleviated or reduced to an acceptable tolerance level.

7. In no case should potentially painful experiments be conducted on an awake animal who is under the influence of a paralytic or curarizing drug without the concomitant use of an appropriate anesthetic.

8. Research in which painful stimuli are used should be so designed as to provide a means of escape from that pain by the animal.

9. It is recognized that in certain research protocols the administration of appropriate anesthetics and/or analgesics will compromise the scientific validity of the experiment. Such experiments must be justifiable in terms of scientific design and value, and the deletion of these drugs should be based not on intuition but on referenceable scientific fact or experimental data. In

addition, pain, discomfort, and distress levels should be carefully monitored. There is a limit to the pain to which an experimental animal may be exposed. An animal observed to be in a state of severe pain that cannot be alleviated or reduced to an acceptable tolerance level should be immediately euthanized.

10. No animal should be subjected to multiple survival surgeries, except when they are interrelated and essential to the primary research objective.

11. Whenever possible, alternatives to the LD_{50} test should be utilized.

12. Physical restraint procedures should be used on awake animals only after alternative procedures have been considered and found to be inadequate. If a restraint will be utilized, the animal should, via positive reinforcement, be trained or conditioned to the restraining device prior to the beginning of the experiment. The restraining device should provide the minimum restraint consistent with the maximum security and comfort of the animal. In addition, the restraining device should provide the animal with the greatest possible opportunity to assume its normal postural adjustments. Awake animals should not be subjected to prolonged physical restraint.

13. It is the responsibility of the investigator to ensure that adequate postsurgical/procedural care is provided to all animals. This care must meet acceptable standards in veterinary medicine and must be provided as long as necessary, including during nonduty hours.

14. Euthanasia is the act of inducing painless death. The proposed method of euthanasia must be consistent with recommendations of the American Veterinary Medical Association (AVMA) Panel on Euthanasia. Accordingly, the following criteria should be employed in choosing a method of euthanasia: the method's ability to produce death without causing pain; the length of time required to produce loss of consciousness; the time required to produce death; reliability; the hazard to personnel; the potential for minimizing psychological stress; the compatibility with the requirements and purpose of the research; the emotional effect on observers or operators; economic feasibility; compatibility with histopathological evaluation; and drug availability and abuse potential. If an animal will not be subjected to euthanasia at the completion of a research protocol, it is the responsibility of the investigator to ensure that the final disposition of the animal is both humane and acceptable.

15. Procedures involving the use of animals should be performed by or under the immediate supervision of an individual with the appropriate qualifications and experience relative to the procedures to be carried out on live animals.

SUMMARY

The development of ethical and legal guidelines for human and animal subjects research has led to increased awareness of acceptable practices. The sometimes laborious process to which the individual practitioner must submit him- or herself in the development of a research protocol and the shadow that sometimes falls between idealism and reality are a necessary but small price to pay for the increased security that human subjects today will not be subjected to unreasonable and unjustifiable potential harm and that animals will be utilized in experiments that are scientifically justified and humane.

Many questions and problems relative to the ethics of research still exist. The search for greater understanding of the issues continues, however, in the health professions, the basic sciences, and the field of medical ethics. A recently completed President's Commission established for the study of ethical problems in medicine and research devoted four of its nine volumes of reports explicitly to the refinement of many of the key issues discussed in this chapter. Undoubtedly, the physical therapist will increasingly be asked to justify the scientific basis for the various treatments and diagnostic procedures he or she uses. Therefore, these issues will be even more pressing with time.

REFERENCES

1. *United States v. Karl Brandt et al.* Trials of War Criminals Before the Nuremberg Military Tribunals under Control Council Law No. 10 (October 1946–April 1949).

2. *Trials of war criminals before the Nuremberg military tribunals under control council law no. 10,* Vol. 2. Washington, DC: U.S. Government Printing Office, 1949, pp. 181–182.

3. World Medical Assembly, 1964, Human experimentation: Code of ethics of the World Medical Association, declaration of Helsinki. *British Medical Journal* 2:177, 1964.

4. *Hyman v. Jewish Chronic Diseases Hospital,* 206 N.E. 2nd 338 (1965).

5. Brandt, A.M. Racism and research: The case of the Tuskegee syphilis study. *Hastings Center Report* 8 (No. 6), 1978, pp. 21–29.

6. Public Health Services Report, 1973. Tuskegee Syphilis Study Ad Hoc Advisory Board. Washington, DC: U.S. Government Printing Office.

7. Public Law 93-348. The National Research Act.

8. The National Commission for the Protection of Human Subjects of Biomedical and Behavioral Research: *Research on the fetus: Report and recommendations* (DHEW Publication No. (OS) 76-127, Appendix, DHEW Publication No. (OS) 76-128). Washington, DC: U.S. Government Printing Office, 1975.

9. The National Commission for the Protection of Human Subjects of Biomedical and Behavioral Research: *Research involving prisoners: Report and recommendations* (DHEW Publication No. (OS) 76-131; Appendix, DHEW Publication No. (OS) 76-132). Washington, DC: U.S. Government Printing Office, 1976.

10. The National Commission for the Protection of Human Subjects of Biomedical and Behavioral Research: *Research involving children: Report and recommendations* (DHEW Publication No. (OS) 77-0005). Washington, DC: U.S. Government Printing Office, 1977.

11. The National Commission for the Protection of Human Subjects of Biomedical and Behavioral Research: *The Belmont report: Ethical principles and guidelines for the protection of human subjects of research* (DHEW Publication No. (OS) 78-0012; Appendix I, DHEW Publication No. (OS) 78-0013; Appendix II, DHEW Publication (OS) 78-0014). Washington, DC: U.S. Government Printing Office, 1978.

12. The National Commission for the Protection of Human Subjects of Biomedical and Behavioral Research: *Institutional review boards: Report and recommendations* (DHEW Publication No. (OS) 78-0008; Appendix, DHEW Publication No. (OS) 78-0009). Washington, DC: U.S. Government Printing Office, 1978.

13. The National Commission for the Protection of Human Subjects of Biomedical and Behavioral Research: *Report and recommendations: Ethical guidelines for the delivery of health services by DHEW* (Publication No. (OS) 78-0010; Appendix, DHEW Publication No. (OS) 78-0011). Washington, DC: U.S. Government Printing Office, 1978.

14. The National Commission for the Protection of Human Subjects of Biomedical and Behavioral Research: *Research involving those institutionalized as mentally infirm: Report and recommendations* (DHEW Publication No. (OS) 78-0006; Appendix, DHEW Publication No. (OS) 78-0007). Washington, DC: U.S. Government Printing Office, 1978.

15. DHHS Regulations 45 CFR 46, March 8, 1983.

16. FDA Regulations 21 CFR 50, 56. Fed Reg 46 (17), January 27, 1981.

17. Lebacqz, K. and Levine, R.J. Respect for persons and informed consent to participate in research. *Clin Res* 25:101–107, 1977.

18. Lebacqz, K. and Levine, R.J. Informed consent in human research: Ethical and legal aspects. In Reich, W.T., ed., *Encyclopedia of bioethics.* New York: Free Press, 1978, pp. 754–762.

19. PHS policy on humane care and use of laboratory animals. *NIH guide for grants and contracts* 14(8), June 25, 1985.

20. NIH guide for the care and use of laboratory animals. *NIH guide for grants and contracts* 14(8) June 25, 1985.

21. PHS policy on humane care and use of laboratory animals. Revised September 1986.

22. Health Research Extension Act of 1985. Public Law 99-158, November 20, 1985.

23. U.S. Congress. The Animal Welfare Act 1966 (Public Law 89-544). Amended 1970 (Public Law 91-579), 1976 (Public Law 94-279), 1986 (Public Law 99-198).

24. USDA. Animal Welfare, Final Rules. 9 CFR Parts 1, 2, and 3. Fed Reg 54(168). Thursday, August 31, 1989, Fed Reg 56(32), February 15, 1991.

25. Prentice, E.D., Zucker, I.H., and Jameton, A. Ethics of animal welfare in research: The institution's attempt to achieve appropriate social balance. *The Physiologist* 29:17–20, 1986. Reproduced with permission of *The Physiologist.*

4

CRITICAL REVIEW
OF PUBLISHED RESEARCH

Katherine F. Shepard

The ability to critique research literature is a skill that is fundamental to all research endeavors. Skill in critiquing research leads to skill in doing research. In this chapter I discuss the nature of the critique process and describe how to critique a research article. I hope to share with you the intellectual challenge, intrigue, and fun of critiquing research.

THE CRITIQUE PROCESS

We must approach reading and critiquing research with the recognition that we have two ways of thinking and feeling (mindsets), each of which may hamper our ability to critique effectively. The thinking, or cognitive, mindset concerns our belief in the written word. The emotional mindset has to do with our "gut feelings" as well as with learned reactions to criticism.

The written word is a powerful medium in our culture. We more frequently confuse the written word with truth than the spoken word, because we believe that if something has been published, then greater minds than ours put their stamp of approval on it. Undoubtedly our education system has played a strong role in this belief. Teachers use classroom textbooks with which they ideologically and prag-matically agree. It was the unusual teacher in our formative years who taught us to question an author's presentation of reality in our biology, English, and history books. In college we became adept at taking essay exams by knowing which authors our professors agreed with and not criticizing these authors' views too harshly. And how many of us as novices in our chosen profession ever criticized the experts (though the experts may often be overheard criticizing other experts)? From reading newspapers and magazines, we learned to disagree with *opinions* because we had fine role models in columnists and political cartoonists, but we are still hesitant to disagree with information presented as fact. Even when it is a misquote, there is nothing like a "fact," especially if numerical, to give credence to one side of an argument.

So, a new mindset to acquire before you begin to critique research is to recognize that written words, including all facts, are naturally fallible. Fallibility comes from an author's sources of information (which are themselves fallible), from an author's naturally incomplete experiences, and from an author's current perceptions of and beliefs about a particular phenomenon. It is entirely possible that the day after a manuscript was published, the author had another experience or accepted a new thesis that was contrary to what she or he had just published. Thus we should respond to written words, especially the written words in research articles, as if they are a somewhat temporary and always dynamic form of communi-cation. Much to the frustration of researchers in today's world of rapidly changing technology, their theories and findings may well have become out-of-date in the time it took to submit, process, and finally publish their work. To be effective researchers, they must remain skeptical and flexible. And so must the reader.

The second mindset has to do with criticism. The word *criticism* has a trouble-some connotation for us. Criticism conjures up images of finger-wagging parents, pursed-lipped teachers, and clergy glaring down from pulpits, often implying

God's criticism as well as their own. The problem, which begins in childhood, is that criticism is seldom given as information. Words that convey disagreement with our actions are most often accompanied by nonverbal parental admonitions; a person's eyes, tone of voice, facial expressions, and body posture convey more accurately than words that an offense has been committed.

We grew up learning to avoid criticism. It hurt. Criticism was especially painful when our basic character was called into question ("You are the most inconsiderate child I have ever seen!") and when we could produce no argument to prove our innocence or redeem ourselves. If we could not avoid criticism, we learned to defend ourselves against it, saying, "No it wasn't me"; "You don't understand"; "I didn't mean. . . ." We learned to fight back by trying to discredit those who criticized us ("He doesn't know anything." "She wasn't there.").

As we become adults and take on the responsibilities of health care professionals, we still perceive criticism primarily as a threat. We are upset by patients who are critical of their health care; we avoid conversations with colleagues who we feel are "negative"; and we spend uneasy nights worrying about the implications of negative words from authority figures. Unfortunately, we carry our memories about criticism and the concomitant feelings of rejection and shame with us as we engage in research.

To critique research effectively one must also learn to give and receive criticism in a way that is emotionally healthy. This can be achieved by entering into the critique process with two cognitive behaviors. The first is that all research should be critiqued on the basis of its facts: Who did what? What did they do? Why did they do it? When? Where did they do it? and, most important, How did they go about doing it? and How did they interpret what they found out? The critique of research must be *specific* to these points and not irritatingly global. It must not merely say, for example, "This is poorly done research." These critique points will be elaborated later in this chapter.

The second cognitive behavior to assume is *constructive criticism*. Constructive criticism means that for every idea, fact, or interpretation of fact one criticizes, he or she suggests a well-founded alternative. If you do not have a well-founded alternative, you must say so, thus admitting you can do no better than the author. Unsubstantiated criticism is worthless, and unfounded alternatives discredit the critic, not the author. For example, nearly every clinical research paper published could be blindly criticized for not having a larger sample size. The question is not the number itself but the *hows*, *what*, and *whys* of the sample relative to the author's interpretation of his or her findings. In sum, criticism should be thoughtful and constructive, focused on facts, and delivered in a professional manner.

These behaviors for becoming engaged in the process of research critique are implied in the American Physical Therapy Association's document, *Integrity in Physical Therapy Research*:

Criticism

1. Physical therapists should comment critically, objectively, constructively, and openly on any reports of research which they consider to be professionally or scientifically unacceptable.

a. Constructive criticism of research should be well-founded and should include suggestions for enhancing the acceptability of the research.
2. Physical therapists whose reports of research are criticized as representing research which is professionally or scientifically unacceptable should respond objectively to the criticism, and without recrimination or reprisal, as part of the process of the search for truth.[1]

Why Critique?

The most important reason for learning to critique research is to discover which research findings have merit and which do not. For those in clinical practice, research findings have powerful patient care consequences, because findings that are well founded can be used to increase our effectiveness in evaluating and treating patients. On the other hand, findings that are unfounded may be used benignly (and be no more effective than current clinical practices) or they may have tragic consequences to patients in terms of their physical or psychological health.

Another reason to become proficient in critiquing research is that you simultaneously become better at designing, conducting, and interpreting your own research. You will ask richer questions, frame clearer hypotheses, become more meticulous in setting up your methods, work with a deeper understanding of alternative research designs, and learn to state and discuss conclusions with confidence relative to other research in the area. In addition, the critique process opens one's eyes to new avenues of research.

A third reason for learning to critique is to develop professional reading and writing skills. After initially reading *every* word of a research article, one begins to read more swiftly, scanning for major points in key sentences, noting clever ways of writing and illustrating difficult concepts, learning new words, and improving grammatical skills. Eventually, you find yourself silently reorganizing and rewriting research articles as you read. Thus, learning to critique well results in an improved ability to discern useful and well-founded knowledge, to create and carry out valid research, and to employ a scientific writing style.

CRITIQUING A RESEARCH ARTICLE

The type of research designs with which we are most familiar is related to quantitative data collection and analysis. This research may be descriptive, experimental, or quasi-experimental. The use of qualitative data in research is relatively new, and we have fewer well-developed techniques on how to critique studies that use qualitative data, such as ethnographies or qualitative case studies.

In this section I will focus on the type of research critique that is common in the biological and physical sciences and is most pertinent to the majority of articles published in the health professional literature. Then, in the next section I will introduce some thoughts and techniques on how to critique qualitative research. Qualitative research has its origins in the social and behavioral sciences. This type of research will open up a new arena of research methodologies that can immeasurably enhance our skill in collecting, analyzing, and interpreting patient outcome data.

Many checklists outline the relevant questions to ask in evaluating each section of a research paper. The list in Appendix 4-A was compiled from many others. I use this simplified form to teach students the critique process. Another list of guideline questions, located in Appendix 4-B, was published by the American Physical Therapy Association (APTA) Committee on Research. These guidelines are used for analyzing research reports presented at annual conferences of the APTA. A third source of information for evaluating research papers is the manual for authors and editors published by the American Medical Association.[2]

I present here an approach to critiquing research articles that has worked well for me and the graduate students and clinicians I have worked with over many years. It is, however, only one approach. From these guidelines, you will evolve your own unique approach to critiquing research that is comfortable and effective for you.

Getting Started

Sitting down to critique a research article should not feel like a forced reading of *War and Peace*. Approach reading research with the anticipation of reading an intriguing mystery. Every piece of research has flaws. Flaws are inherent in research. How skillful will you be in uncovering the flaws? Will the flaw be a misquote of prior research on the topic, a subtle design problem, or suggested unrealistic clinical implications? Critiquing research is serious, but it is also fun.

The first thing to do is reproduce the entire research article you are about to critique, including all figures, the bibliography, and the appendixes. This will become your worksheet. As you critique, make notes in the margins, put question marks and exclamation points near questionable statements or outrageous claims, diagram procedures, and jot down memos to yourself. If you are critiquing a number of articles prior to beginning a research project, discard the college practice of capturing the essence of an article on index cards. You no longer want to capture the essence of a research article. Rather, you want to dissect it to uncover its strengths and weaknesses and decide whether or not you agree with the research techniques used as well as the findings. So, reproduce and set out to grapple with the article.

To effectively critique a research article, you must understand and critique each part of the article as well as the article as a whole. The critique process does not need to be undertaken in a linear fashion, that is, starting with the abstract and reading through to the summary. Some parts of the manuscript (e.g., method) are more important than others; you will move back and forth between other sections (information reported in the introduction as compared with findings interpreted in the discussion); and reading some sections (e.g., results section based on an implausible method) will not be worth your time. Thus, when you have finished your critique, you should have knowledge of the worth of specific components as well as a sense of the merit of the entire piece of research.

Title

Computers have affected our lives in many ways, including our ability to locate and glean information from the research archives. In order to retrieve research articles from a computer database, the key words that note major topics contained in an article must be clearly identified. Thus, the titles of research articles have become increasingly more specific and descriptive. No longer do we have catchy but meaningless titles such as "The Paramecium as a Master Robot." Instead, the research question is often turned into the title. For example, the research question, What is the energy cost of walking with hip joint impairment? becomes the title "Energy Cost of Walking with Hip Joint Impairment." The computer key words for this article are: Energy expenditure: Hip joint; Joint instability; Kinesiology/biomechanics, general; Locomotion.[3] The question, What distinguishes an experienced clinician from a novice clinician? becomes "The Novice versus the Experienced Clinician: Insights into the Work of the Physical Therapist." The computer key words for this article are: Model, theoretical; Physical therapy profession, professional issues: Professional practice; Professional-patient relations.[4] Thus the title of an article should contain key words and phrases that reflect the essence of the article and allow computer coding of the article in such a manner that the interested reader can locate it.

Abstract

The abstract is a short summary of the article (about 150 words) that usually includes the purpose of the research, an overview of the method, and the major findings. Abstracts are helpful only for further identifying whether the article is one you might be interested in reproducing and critiquing. An abstract should *never* be used to make decisions about the potential clinical usefulness of the results presented because it does not contain sufficient information about the method. Without a careful review of the research method, the reader is unable to determine whether or not the findings are of any value. This is a serious issue in clinical settings where research abstracts may be circulated to staff with the good intention of presenting new ideas and keeping the staff up-to-date. The abstract, at best, gives only an inkling of what was done. You should no more think of applying results obtained from a research abstract than you would think of using a piece of equipment in clinical practice for which only anecdotal reports exist.

Introduction

Purpose

The first thing to do in the introduction section is locate the purpose of the study and any specific hypotheses that have been developed for testing. The purpose is usually located either in the first paragraph of the introduction (usually the last sentence) or in the last paragraph of the introduction (often the first sentence). Sometimes, especially if the introduction is lengthy, two similarly stated purposes will be found: (1) a general purpose in the first or second paragraph of the introduction to focus the reader; and (2) a more specific purpose in the last paragraph to set the stage for reading the method section. The null or research hypotheses are usually located in the last paragraph of the introduction after the purpose statement.

A well-written, definitive purpose and testable hypotheses convey positively an author's ability to clearly define and carry out research. Conversely, ill-defined purposes and untestable hypotheses make the reader uneasy about whether the author is clear about what he is doing and how carefully he will proceed.

Literature Review

The literature review should give a good sense of how well the author knows the research literature in the chosen topic. Here the author should build a case for why the research should be done. I stopped trying some years ago to ask the traditional question, To whom is this research important? People become involved in research because the quest is fascinating to them. Almost always, it is also fascinating to someone else. Not every reader may be particularly interested in the subject, but the author who is fascinated with and committed to a research topic will usually do good research. The author who does research because someone else is interested in it betrays that motivation by a sketchy literature review, ill-defined methods, and a half-hearted discussion of findings.

In reading the introduction, keep the author's reference list in front of you. In fact, it is impossible to read an introduction without constantly referring to the reference list. The reference list is a map of where and how extensively the author traveled to find background information. The author has the responsibility to do a thoughtful and careful job of literature selection and review for the reader.

Ask yourself, Who are the authors? (Are they well known in the field or first-time researchers?) In what journals is the information published—scientific journals that meet the standards for citation in indexes such as the *Index Medicus* or less rigorous nonindexed journals? When was the article published? Has the author used only articles published ten years ago? Remember, however, that a recent publication date may be a good criterion—but not always. Some classic theories still pertinent today were first published 40 or 50 years ago. How long is the article? Several pages in length usually suggests anecdotal, commentary, or brief case study evidence. How much of the reference list is filler—articles with almost identical titles, by the same group of authors, published in different journals; broad, peripherally related references; or, worse, textbooks? In summary, given a rich literature on the subject, has the author selected the most pertinent and the most powerful references?

The more you know about your field of interest, the more fun it is to read reference lists in the article you are critiquing. You recognize authors and articles as old friends. Often you have critiqued a work cited and thus know how valid the background information is. You discover new articles and new colleagues in your area of interest. And, perhaps most importantly, you can tell how thorough the author has been. Thoroughness in background preparation bodes well for thoroughness in research design.

If you are just beginning your research endeavors and are unfamiliar with the literature in your chosen topic area, it is imperative that you not simply accept the author's interpretation of literature review findings. An astonishing amount of the research literature is misquoted. Although authors usually do not deliberately misconstrue facts or attempt to mislead the reader, neither do they perform literature reviews from a totally objective, disinterested standpoint. Remember that researchers do not poke around in the literature trying to find a research topic. They come with a question in mind (and often a strong hunch of what the answer might be). Thus, when reading the literature, they are attempting to confirm whether what they have chosen to do has been done before, how well it has been done, and what the results were. They will then use this information to make a case for why they are doing this particular research and why it is important. You may even find the same reference citations used to support two totally different points of view!

Thus, you should locate and critique references which are unfamiliar to you. This is especially true if you have concerns about the validity of the methods used or any suspicions that too strong a case has been made based on too little evidence. One technique used by some authors, which is very helpful to the reader, is to provide in the introduction section a brief critique (one or two sentences) of the references most central to their study. If authors were routinely asked to offer a critique of their background materials, perhaps there would be less error reported in the introduction.

Method

The method section (not the results) is the heart of the research article. A poorly done method will yield worthless results. Thus, the quality of the method section will determine whether or not you even want to finish reading the article. If there are serious errors in instrumentation or procedure, think about skimming the discussion section to see if the author is aware of the methodological errors. If the author appears to be unaware and the research topic is one you are both interested in, you may want to contact the author to discuss your concerns.

In some scientific journals, the method section is curiously designed. Information is put into small type, indented on both sides, and sketchily presented—as if it were of less consequence than other parts of the article! Do not be misled by this. If the method section is difficult to read, have an enlargement made and proceed with your critique.

For illustrative purposes, Displays 4-1 and 4-2 contain parts of method sections taken from actual research articles; identifying names and numbers from these articles have been altered. These will be referred to for examples of common problems found in method sections.

Subjects

Subjects must be described by the researcher in enough detail so that you are clear about not only who the subjects are but also as to what population the results can be generalized. Obviously, if the study was done on healthy, college-age females, the results cannot be generalized to patient care populations. Describing subjects in sufficient detail includes:

1. Subject criteria. Who are they? The criteria the authors used to select the subjects to be included in the study (inclusive criteria) might include age, sex, and disability. Criteria upon which subjects were excluded from the study (exclusive criteria) might include congenital deformities or surgeries in a sample from a patient population or dedicated athletes in a sample from a normal population. In Display 4-1, note that the inclusive and exclusive criteria for subject selection are not clearly stated. For example, was employment an inclusive criterion? What is meant by the criterion "an injury of sufficient severity to have disrupted the worker's daily life"?
2. The number of subjects included in the entire study and in each group. Are there enough subjects in each group so that analytical statistics can be used?
3. Selection of subjects. How were the subjects selected? Was selection by random sample, cluster sample, or sample of convenience? In Displays 4-1 and 4-2 there is no indication how the samples were selected from the larger population. Thus there is no way of knowing how biased or unbiased the sample selection was.
4. Group assignment. How are subjects assigned to groups? Does it appear that subjects were selected and assigned to groups in such a way that the results would be favorable, not only because of the intervention but because of who the subjects were? For example, normal subjects selected from a college population might be healthier and more aware of their bodies, or better educated about or more interested in the research being undertaken than normal subjects from the general population.

Variables Under Study

What data were collected from the subjects? What were the descriptive data variables? These variables might include age, sex, height, educational level, or disability. What were the independent and dependent variables? These variables might be pain, strength, flexibility, or amount of learning. Or what was the phenomenon under study, for instance, cultural responses to illness, professional socialization, or patient adherance to home programs?

Do the variables being studied relate specifically to the purpose of the study? Can they be used to directly test the hypotheses established in the introduction? Are these variables appropriate for measuring what is being studied? In Display 4-2 the independent variable was the type of treatment (facilitation or traditional exercise techniques) received by patients who had a diagnosis of stroke. The dependent variable used to measure change between the two groups was a combined manual muscle test and range-of-motion test. What do you think about the use of this tool for measuring changes in patients with a stroke? Is such a patient able to isolate specific muscle groups? Should muscle strength and joint flexibility be measured as a single variable?

DISPLAY 4-1
EXAMPLE OF A METHOD SECTION FROM A DESCRIPTIVE STUDY

Purpose of the Study: The purpose of the study was to explore the relationship among occupational development, occupational performance, and social support as they relate to the return to work in the hand-injured patient.

Subjects: Forty-four subjects with hand injuries were selected from three facilities: a large urban hospital, a small, rural private hospital, and a private practice clinic. All subjects were regularly employed before their trauma. To be involved in the study, the subject's hand injury had to qualify as an injury of sufficient severity to have disrupted the worker's daily life. The majority of the subjects had at least one surgical intervention and had been admitted to the hospital.

Procedure: A chart audit and an interview schedule designed by the author were used to determine activities of daily living status, work status, social support systems, and referral to physical therapy, occupational therapy, and vocational counseling. The subjects were interviewed one time individually, not less than 2 months after the injury. All of the subjects were in advanced stages of rehabilitation but had not yet completed their treatment programs.

Instrumentation

Is the equipment used described in sufficient detail or displayed in a figure so that you clearly understand what it is and how it was used? In descriptive research, the instruments may be standardized scales, questionnaires, or interview schedules. These should be described in sufficient detail, or a reference should be given, or they should be included in an appendix so readers know what questions were used to elicit which data.

In the method example in Display 4-1, the author states that a chart audit and an interview schedule designed by the author were used to collect data. In reviewing this narrative information, however, we are left with many questions. What information was derived from the chart audit and what from the interview? What was the specific phrasing of the interview questions? Were they designed to elicit specific information (e.g., by answers like yes/no) or broad information (e.g., patient perceptions)? Were follow-up probe questions asked in order to clarify and verify patient-reported information? In what context did the author mean "social support systems"?

Are reliability and validity of the instrument reported? It is not sufficient to report that an instrument has been subjected to validity and reliability studies without citing specific information. For example, if an instrument is reported to be valid, the type of validation that was done should be reported. If reliability of the instrument or interrater reliability has been established, test–retest coefficients or Kappa coefficients should be reported. Note the author's lack of such validity and reliability citations for the manual muscle test that was used in the Display 4-2 method example.

DISPLAY 4-2
EXAMPLE OF A METHOD SECTION FROM QUASI-EXPERIMENTAL RESEARCH

Purpose of the Study: The purpose of the investigation was to evaluate the effectiveness of both the traditional approach and the facilitation technique approach to therapeutic exercise in a sample of stroke patients.

Sample: A total of 64 adults (38 men and 26 women) were admitted to Allegheny Hospital between January 1980 and January 1981 with a diagnosis of stroke. Each of these patients (subjects) was selected from a larger population of approximately 400 stroke patients admitted with a diagnosis of stroke within the time period noted.

Criteria for inclusion were (1) stroke documented by CT scan within seven weeks of onset and prior to therapy being initiated; (2) medically fit to participate in a nonrestricted program as determined by the attending physician and documented by electrocardiogram and lab analyses; and (3) informed consent.

Procedure: Neurological examinations, CT scans, and other lab tests were conducted on all subjects. The 64 patients who met the study criteria were randomly assigned one of two treatment groups for remediation of motor loss in the affected lower extremity, with either facilitation (Bobath and Rood) or traditional exercise techniques. In order to standardize treatment techniques, the physical therapy staff of 14 was divided into two groups of seven, each assigned the task of defining therapeutic exercise techniques. Examples of agreed upon facilitation techniques included bilateral weight-bearing and weight-shifting exercises, use of reflex-inhibiting patterns, and tactile, vibratory, and vestibular stimulation activities. Examples of agreed-upon traditional treatment-techniques included assistive, active, and progressive-resistive exercises as well as the use of skateboards, reciprocal pulleys, and springs. Once consensus was reached between the two groups, all physical therapists and all occupational therapy staff were instructed in facilitation and traditional exercise therapies. The occupational therapy staff were allowed to use facilitation techniques on the upper extremities during self-care training for both groups.

Among the study groups, the lower extremity exercise program was generally no less than one hour a day and usually not more than one-and-a-half hours a day in addition to other components of the stroke rehabilitation program.

To quantify lower extremity muscle strength, an abbreviated manual muscle test was administered on admission and discharge. This manual muscle test has been judged to be both valid and reliable. The test scores ranged from a high of 7 (part moves through complete range of motion (ROM) against gravity with normal resistance) to a low of 0 (no movement of the part; no contraction can be palpated).

Operational Definitions

The absence of clear definitions for terms, procedures, and techniques is very common in research articles. What is perfectly clear to an author actively engaged in patient care and research is often perfectly unclear to the reader. In Display 4-2, treatment activities are identified that distinguish between facilitation techniques and traditional techniques. However, we do not have sufficient information about "other components of the stroke rehabilitation program." What components is the author referring to? In Display 4-1, the statement "All of the subjects were in advanced stages of rehabilitation but had not yet completed their treatment programs" also lacks sufficient definition. Without operational definitions, it is very difficult to understand clearly or to replicate the research method.

Procedure

The step-by-step procedures the subjects go through should be listed in chronological sequence. The approximate length of time required for subjects to undergo procedures should be noted. Instructions given to each subject should be stated. Exactly how each group was treated alike or differently should be very clear. You should be able to close your eyes and visualize what is happening to the subject at each step: what he is being asked to do, how she is responding, what data are being collected. In the Display 4-1 example, were the subjects interviewed by someone who was also directly involved in their treatment program? How much longer than 2 months after injury were the subjects interviewed? Do you think the length of time between injury and data collection might interfere with validity or reliability of the data gathered? In the Display 4-2 example, when and how many times were the subjects tested? And what type of instruction did the physical and occupational therapists receive on facilitation and traditional exercise therapies?

The person(s) doing the data collection and coding should also be stated. If one person is gathering data, *intrarater reliability* should be established. If two or more people are involved in data gathering, *interrater reliability* should also be established. An intrarater or interrater reliability check halfway through the data gathering assures you that those gathering the data are aware of how important consistency is to the credibility of the study design. Note that in the method sections presented in Displays 4-1 and 4-2 no mention was made of intrarater or interrater reliability.

Finally, evidence that subjects are participating in research under informed consent of their rights and under guarantee of full disclosure of the benefits and risks of the study should be stated.

Data Analysis

At the end of many results sections, the author informs the reader of the statistics used to analyze the data. It is up to you to judge whether or not these statistics are appropriate for responding to the purpose of the study and for testing the hypotheses stated. If you are unfamiliar with a variety of analytical statistics, an invaluable resource is Huck, Cormier, and Bounds.[5] This book provides examples of the many types of statistics used in research papers, under what conditions the statistic should be used, and how to read tabled data. One example is their discussion of the use of two different *t*-tests:

Two Forms of the t-*Test*

There are two forms of the *t* test for comparing group means, one for independent samples and one for correlated samples. The *independent samples t test* is used in situations in which the scores in one group have absolutely no logical relationship with the scores in the other group. In the IQ example none of the Master's level IQ's could be logically related (paired) with any of the Ph.D. level IQ's. More generally, the two samples will be independent whenever (1) a large group of subjects are randomly assigned to two subgroups (possibly an experimental group and a control group) or (2) the subjects in the groups are selected at random from larger populations (as was the case with the hypothetical IQ study).

The second form of the *t* test is the *correlated samples* t *test*, which is also referred to as the matched *t* test, the correlated *t* test, and the paired *t* test. This *t* test is appropriate for three situations in which each of the data observations in the first group is logically tied to one of the scores in the second group. The first of these is the research situation in which a single group of subjects is measured twice, for example, measured under two different treatment conditions or before and after a common experience. Each score in the first group is logically tied to a specific score in the second group because it is obtained from the same person. (pp. 52–53)

If a statistic that is not well known is used by an author, a reference source should be provided. Probability levels that will be accepted by the author are also stated here. The most common probability level accepted is $p \le .05$. However, it is the author's prerogative (even if you disagree) to set a higher probability level (and thus incur a greater chance of a Type II error). For further information on probability levels and Type I and Type II errors, refer to Huck, Cormier, and Bounds, pages 44–45.[5]

Results

Tables and Figures

It is a good idea to review the tables and figures presented in the results section *before* reading the narrative. Both descriptive and analytical data are displayed in these tables and figures. Thus, the quickest and most accurate way to find the results is to look at the actual data. Those critiquing the research literature often shy away from tabled data. Initially, many tables look foreboding and many figures unintelligible, especially to someone who had prior difficulties understanding math or who has math anxiety.

Remember, it is the author's responsibility to present data clearly. If you cannot understand figures because the labeling is incomplete or too much data is presented, or if the data is presented in type too small to read, your cognitive abilities are not at fault. See Figure 4-1 for an example of ineffective data presentation and Figure 4-2 for an example of effective data display.[6,7] If you need help deciphering data in the table, turn again to examples in Huck, Cormier, and Bounds.[5] Remember, as with acquiring any skill, you will become less overwhelmed and more adept at reading tables with each article.

Another reason to peruse tables and figures before reading the results narrative is that besides having a first-hand look at the data, you have the opportunity to

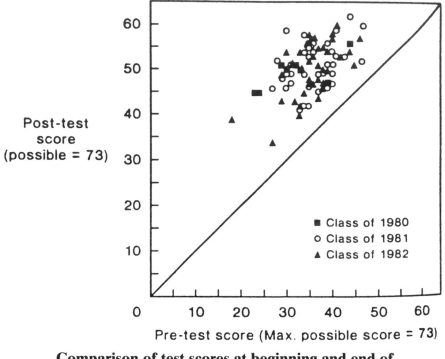

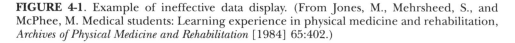

Comparison of test scores at beginning and end of three-week clerkship in PM&R.

FIGURE 4-1. Example of ineffective data display. (From Jones, M., Mehrsheed, S., and McPhee, M. Medical students: Learning experience in physical medicine and rehabilitation, *Archives of Physical Medicine and Rehabilitation* [1984] 65:402.)

interpret the data yourself, before the author tells you what he or she found. You will be surprised how often you find information in tables that the author overlooked in the narrative report and subsequent interpretation of the data. For example, the author may have cited the "three highest values." In your review of the table, you notice that the top four values are within three points of each other, while the fifth highest value is 12 points away. In this case, it would make sense for the author to have grouped and reported the top four values. As another example, you may find standard deviation values so broad that comparing mean values, as the author may have done in the narrative, is inconsequential. As a third example, you may find that your interpretation of a chi-square analysis table is startlingly different from the author's.

Results Narrative

Once you have conquered the tables and figures, reading the results is easy because you do not have to stop and try to figure out each table while simulta-

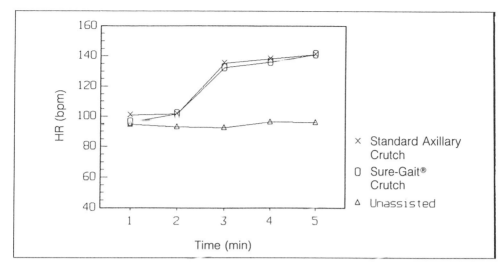

Effect of crutch type on heart rate (HR) during level ambulation. Crutch walking was initiated at end of minute 2.

FIGURE 4-2. Example of effective data display. (From Annesley, A., Almada-Norfleet, M., Arnall, D., and Cornwall, M., Energy expenditure of ambulation using the Sure-Gait (R) crutch and the standard axillary crutch, *Physical Therapy* [1990] 70:18–23. Reprinted from *Physical Therapy* with the permission of the American Physical Therapy Association.)

neously struggling through the narrative. Remember, the author should *highlight* tabled data in the narrative, not repeat it. The highlighted data should be the most powerful data that the author will discuss, relate to prior research, and draw implications from.

If the author stated hypotheses in the introduction, he or she should also state early in the results whether or not the hypotheses were supported or not supported by the data. Analytical values should always be presented along with probability levels, for example, $r = .36$; $p \leq .05$.

The use of simple, powerful statistics should be the rule of thumb for all researchers analyzing their quantitative data. Be wary of the author who uses a multitude of analytical statistics, all of which seem to be making the same point. Remember how easy it is for computers to run statistical packages. Unfortunately, if the author is uneasy with the use of statistics or has been baffled by an over-exuberant statistical consultant, you may witness repetitive statistical findings that serve to confuse rather than enlighten.

Discussion

Critique of the research article is all downhill after the review of the results section. You are aware of the author's goals (purpose, hypotheses) and background information relevant to those goals, understand the method, and have seen and processed the results. In the discussion section, the author can take the liberty of exploring his or her findings and concomitant observations, sharing hunches, decrying pitfalls, and making judgments about the worth and usefulness of the findings. The discussion section is also where you can take the liberty of reflecting on your own judgment regarding the merits of the study, and agreeing or disagreeing with the author's explanation of findings, the clinical or educational usefulness of those findings, and how those findings relate to prior research in the field.

Reading the discussion is much like reading the introduction. In both instances, you look for what information the author included and muse about alternatives for interpreting this information. Thus the introduction and discussion sections are read differently than the method and results sections. In method and results, the critique process involves a more linear form of questioning focused on what the author did, how the author did it, and the legitimacy of what the author did.

There are some specifics to look for in discussion sections: Does the author integrate descriptive and analytical data? Does the author compare this inter-related data with the findings of other researchers reported in the introduction section? If this integration and comparison is done, the discussion section is richly informative. If it is not done, the discussion is a shallow, uninteresting repetition of the results section.

Neither author nor the reader should succumb to the temptation to generalize the results beyond the population from which the sample was drawn. Relative to the significance of the findings, does the author distinguish between statistical significance and clinical significance? For example, a 6-degree range-of-motion difference may be statistically significant but how significant is that to the evaluation and treatment of patients?

Does the author state what he or she might do differently next time, thus recognizing design problems as well as identifying pitfalls for others doing research on this topic? Unfortunately, many researchers feel that if their results did not come out as they intended or if major design difficulties were encountered, it is wise not to mention the difficulties or, perhaps, not even publish. How unfortunate this perception is! How many untold hours of subsequent research could be put to better use if pitfalls were identified in the literature! How many innovative ideas about cause-and-effect relations or the whys of a phenomenon could be generated if more unanticipated results were presented and discussed! How much more rapidly could we grow as effective researchers if we had the courage to disclose our research "failures" and seek input from colleagues in our own and other disciplines.

Does the author offer interesting and plausible ideas for future research? No one has thought more about follow-up research than the person who has just completed a research study. It is to be hoped that some of these ideas are elaborated upon at the end of the discussion section.

Conclusion

The conclusion appears to be an antiquated carryover from the traditional research writing format used before the advent of the abstract. There is nothing in the conclusion that has not been stated elsewhere in the body of the paper. Additionally, the main summary points have already been highlighted for you in the abstract. It is not necessary that you read the conclusion.

REVIEW OF QUALITATIVE RESEARCH PAPERS

Qualitative research papers such as ethnographies or cross-comparison case studies are quite different in format and content from the type of research papers discussed so far. In a qualitative research paper, the introduction section may be quite brief. This is because there are so few qualitative studies in health care professions research upon which to build. The research design or method section is expanded to include a theoretical framework. The results and discussion sections usually become a single, combined research findings section of 20 or more pages, which includes examples drawn from extensive field notes that comprise the qualitative research data. The presentation and discussion of theory is also a strong component of the research findings section.

A brief discussion of how to critique the research design (method) and research findings sections of qualitative studies follows. Reading chapter 5 on qualitative research, by Beverly Schmoll, and other qualitative research papers will help you to understand the following critique process. See also, for example, Jensen, Shepard, and Hack.[4]

Research Design

The qualitative researcher gains information both from field sites (e.g., an out-patient clinic or an academic institution) and from subjects. The subjects may be participating directly in the process (e.g., by being interviewed) or indirectly (e.g., by being observed). The author should describe these sites and subjects, noting number, pertinent characteristics, and the reasons these particular sites and subjects were selected for study.

The conceptual or theoretical framework for the study should be clearly identified. This includes explicating specific categories or themes under study and explaining how they fit into a broader theoretical framework (e.g., a theoretical framework that explains patient compliance or professional socialization). The categories and themes identified in the theoretical framework are drawn from theory, prior research findings, and the researcher's own perceptions and experiences.

As in the procedure section of quantitative research designs, the data collection strategy and sequence should be carefully outlined. The *data collection strategy* includes the situational context—who participated and under what circumstances. The *data collection sequence* includes what happened and when.

Specific methods for obtaining field data should be described. These methods may include participant observation of situations, events, or people; interviews with key people (informants); use of standardized tests or rating scales; collections of case studies; or information obtained from written records. Through a process known as *triangulation*, skilled qualitative researchers use multiple sources to verify information and to ensure validity of their data. Look for these multiple verifying data sources during your critique.

The author should clearly identify how people are trained to collect and code the qualitative data and should outline explicit procedures that were used to reduce and categorize data. Look for checks and balances. Did the author establish and reaffirm interrater reliability among the data coders? Did more than one person verify the placement of data in predefined categories? Was there any check on data accuracy through review of the data by a key informant who gave the original data to the researcher?

Other points pertinent to the critique of *any* research study should not be overlooked. Are operational definitions clear? Is there evidence of subject protection? Is instrumentation pictured or included in an appendix to the study?

Research Findings

Extensive anecdotal information about the environment, events, and people under study will comprise the major research findings. This information will usually be in the form of direct quotes and detailed observations. Although the researcher has collected thousands of pieces of field data, the field notes presented in the research paper will be for the purpose of illustrating the major themes that emerged as the data was coded, reduced, and categorized. All field notes cited should be labeled by subject, time, and event for verification. The author not only presents the field data but explains and interprets the data in light of the theoretical framework he or she is working with. Some categories that emerge from the data may be displayed in qualitative or quantitative descriptive data tables. Tabled data should be critiqued similarly to tables and figures found in other types of research designs.

Data collection and codification problems that may have interfered with the reliability or validity of the data should be honestly stated. In any qualitative research paper, the author might also present examples of data that did not fit neatly with other data into summary categories. Once these examples are presented, of course, the author is obligated to attempt an explanation or to suggest additional research that may give a more comprehensive picture of the phenomenon under study.

Finally, the author should present to the reader a summary of major findings relative to modified or newly developed concepts or theories. This is an exciting section of the qualitative research paper and is rich in ideas for ways to think imaginatively about profound social and behavioral health care-related phenomena.

As in all research papers, the qualitative researcher discusses how the findings may be applied to clinical or educational settings and presents ideas for future research. In addition, the qualitative researcher, who does not ordinarily set out to confirm specific hypotheses, may establish a series of post hoc hypotheses to be studied in the future, usually by more quantitative research methods. These, like all hypotheses, should be stated in an unambiguous, clearly testable format.

THE LAST STEP

Finally, you want to pause after your section-by-section critique of any research article and reflect upon the entire article. Was it a superb piece of research? Relatively good? Relatively poor? Disgraceful? Remember how easy it is to tear apart *any* piece of research. Think of what was done well, as well as what was poorly done. Were the errors major or minor? Were the errors identified by the author or overlooked? What knowledge did the author have to offer that you did not already hold? Were you challenged to consider alternative theories or to broaden your perceptions and beliefs?

It takes courage to do research—and even more courage to publish it. Remember your own research can and will be critiqued the same way. Use a scholarly mind and a gentle voice.

REFERENCES

1. American Physical Therapy Association. *Integrity in physical therapy research.* Alexandria, VA: APTA, adopted 1985; revised 1987.

2. American Medical Association. *Manual for authors and editors: Editorial style and manuscript preparation.* Los Altos: Lange Medical Publications, 1981.

3. Gussoni, M., Margonato, V., and Ventura, R. Energy cost of walking with hip joint impairment. *Physical Therapy* 70:295–301, 1990.

4. Jensen, G., Shepard, K., and Hack, L. The novice versus the experienced clinician: Insights into the work of the physical therapist. *Physical Therapy* 70:314–323, 1990.

5. Huck, S., Cormier, W., and Bounds, W. *Reading statistics and research.* New York: Harper and Row, 1974.

6. Jones, M., Sinaki, M., and McPhee, M. Medical students: Learning experience in physical medicine and rehabilitation. *Archives of Physical Medicine and Rehabilitation* 65:401–403, 1984.

7. Annesley, A., Almada-Norfleet, M., Arnall, D., and Cornwall, M. Energy expenditure of ambulation using the Sure-Gait (R) crutch and the standard axillary crutch. *Physical Therapy* 70:33–37, 1990.

APPENDIX 4-A
Critical Reading of Published Research

Introduction

Purpose/research question clearly defined?

Well-documented supportive rationale for importance of carrying out the study?

Null or research hypotheses (statement of expected results) testable?

Method

Subjects

Subjects adequately described: number, characteristics, inclusive/exclusive criteria?

Method of subject selection and assignment clear?

Sample bias avoided?

Design

Sufficient detail or references for replication of the study?

Intervention appropriate to answering the research question?

Instrumentation

Equipment described or pictured; reliability and validity reported?

Data collection instruments described?

Operational definitions clear?

Procedures

Describes steps (procedures) subjects go through and time required of subjects?

Instructions given to subjects?

Describes who will collect the data; intrarater and interrater reliability established?

Evidence of patient protection (informed consent)?

Data Analysis

Appropriate and adequate for type of study and data collected?

Information given or references provided to understand less common analytical statistics?

Acceptable probability levels set?

Results

Presented in such a way as to confirm or disprove hypotheses?

Relevant critical values and probability levels for descriptive and analytical statistics included?

Includes only findings pertinent to problem; does not include method or discussion?

Data in figures and tables are correctly displayed and agree with text?

Text highlights and summarizes but does not extensively repeat tabled data?

Discussion

Speaks to (discusses) acceptance or rejection of a priori hypotheses?

Integrates descriptive and analytical data, and draws conclusions and reports implications?

Generalizes results correctly to the suggested population (external validity)?

Discusses findings relevant to related research cited in introduction?

Highlights clinical relevance of findings and makes practical suggestions for clinical application of results?

Suggests follow-up research?

Conclusion

Brief paragraph on key findings and implications?

Abstract

Includes purpose, method (subjects and design), and results?

Suggests clinical relevance?

Briefly presented in 150 words or less?

Communication

Precise and concise expression?

Logical sequence of and understandable relationships among ideas?

Correct grammar and professional terminology (no jargon)?

Figures, tables, and references follow correct journal style?

An understandable "fit" among various sections of the paper?

APPENDIX 4-B
Guidelines on Critically Considering Research Papers

Critically considering a research report means analyzing the report for the purpose of deciding whether to agree with the author's conclusion. These guidelines, posed in the form of questions, provide a systematic approach for analyzing most research reports presented orally, by poster or published in literature. Critically considering a research report also means providing constructive criticism of the report when warranted. These guidelines are intended to stimulate and guide objective and constructive criticism of research reports.

The guidelines are necessarily brief. No attempt is made in these guidelines to provide information on the principles and logic of research design and statistical analyses of data. Sources for further study are suggested at the end of the guidelines.

Advice on Giving Criticism: *The person who gives constructive criticism orally, in response to a research report presentation, is advised to avoid speaking in a vengeful, demeaning, or sarcastic manner. The purpose of constructive criticism, as an important part of the process of searching for truth, is to help others and one's self learn, not to belittle the presenter or to practice one-up-manship in public.*

THE QUESTION: What question is the study designed to answer?
1. Is it important, and to whom? Does the presenter make a good case for the importance of the question?
2. Does the presenter state hypothesis(-es) and reasons for hypothesis(-es)?

THE METHOD: What was done to answer the question?
1. The subjects: who; how many? Were they appropriate for the phenomenon studied? Was the number adequate for the phenomenon studied and for the design of the study?
2. How many groups of subjects were in the study? If there were two or more groups of subjects, how did the subjects get into the different groups? Was the method of assigning the subjects to the different groups free from bias?
3. Over and above any measurements that were taken, was anything done to the subjects in the study?
4. If there were two or more different groups of subjects in the study, in what ways were the groups treated alike and in what ways were the groups treated differently?
5. Is the description of what was done in the study clear enough so you could duplicate (replicate) the study?
6. What was the sequence of events in the study? If the presenter does not do so, would you be able to draw a block diagram of the sequence of events in the study?

7. If any experimental manipulation of treatment was done in the study, was the manipulation of treatment (were the different treatments) appropriate for answering the question? If NO, what would you have done?

8. What was the variable measured in the study? Was the variable appropriate for answering the question? If NO, what would you have measured? If any experimental manipulation of treatment was done in the study, was the variable measured appropriate for detecting the effects of the different treatments? If NO, what would you have measured?

9. What method of measurement was used, and what kind of data were obtained, in the study? Was the method of measurement appropriate for the variable(s) measured? If NO, what method of measurement would you have used? Were the data appropriate for answering the question? If NO, what kind of data would you have collected?

10. What method of statistical analysis was applied to the data obtained in the study? Was the method of statistical analysis appropriate for the kind of data obtained in the study, and was the application of the method appropriate for answering the question? If NO, what method of statistical analysis would you have used, and how would you have applied it?

THE RESULTS: What did the investigator find?

1. What summary data were presented, and in what form?
2. Do summary data answer original question? What do summary data suggest/indicate relative to original question?
3. What do statistical analyses show? What is the probability that the results of the study could have occurred by chance?

THE DISCUSSION AND CONCLUSION: What does the presenter say about the results?

1. Are results explained? Are results attributable to what was done? If NO, to what might the results be attributable?
2. Are results tied back to hypothesis(-es) and reasons for hypothesis(-es)? Does the presenter discuss relationship of results to findings of other pertinent studies?
3. Is a conclusion presented? What is it? Do you agree? If NO, why not?
4. Are any conclusions offered that are not supported by what was done and found in the study? If YES, which conclusions?
5. Given the original question, the method, and the obtained data, were any important analyses overlooked? If YES, what? Were any important or alternative conclusions overlooked? If YES, what?

OVERALL EVALUATION: What is your judgment of the study?

1. Was the original question answered? If YES, was the question answered convincingly?

2. Does the study make an important contribution to knowledge or practice?
3. Is the study worth replicating (repeating) or extending? If extended, what would you do next?

(Adapted from *Guidelines on Critically Considering Research Papers*, APTA Committee on Research, 1985, 1989.)

SOURCES FOR FURTHER STUDY

Design of Research and Analysis of Data in the Clinic: An Introductory Manual for Clinical Research. APTA, 1985.
Design of Research and Analysis of Data in the Clinic: Introduction to Factorial Designs and Analysis of Variance. APTA, 1985.
Research: An Anthology. APTA, 1983.
Reading Tips for Reports on Research—An Anthology. APTA, 1986.
Using and Understanding Surveys: An Introductory Manual. APTA, 1985.

APTA Committee on Research
January 1989

PART II

TYPICAL CLINICAL RESEARCH DESIGNS

5

QUALITATIVE RESEARCH

Beverly J. Schmoll

OVERVIEW OF QUALITATIVE RESEARCH
Characteristics of Qualitative Research

TYPES OF QUALITATIVE RESEARCH
Case Studies
Historical: Life History
Ethnography
Grounded Theory Methodology
Selecting a Qualitative Research Approach
Combining Qualitative and Quantitative Research

DESIGN ELEMENTS OF QUALITATIVE RESEARCH

GETTING STARTED
Identifying a Topic
Posing Research Questions
Reviewing the Literature

COLLECTING DATA
Observations
Training
Direct Observation
Participant Observer
Observation Settings
Informed Consent
What to Observe

Amount of Observations
Recording Observations
Interviews
Types of Interviews
Types of Questions
Conducting the Interview
Unobtrusive Data

ANALYZING THE DATA
Constant-Comparative Process: An Overview
The Constant-Comparative Process Illustrated
Raw Data from Interviews
Memos Based on Raw Data
Themes from Data
Memos Based on Memos
Development of Concepts
Development of Theory

ADDRESSING RELIABILITY

ADDRESSING VALIDITY

REPORTING THE DATA
Structure of the Report

LIMITATIONS OF QUALITATIVE RESEARCH

QUALITATIVE RESEARCH IN PHYSICAL THERAPY
Existing Qualitative Research in Physical Therapy
Applications of Qualitative Research Processes to the Development of
Therapeutic Interventions
Future Applications of Qualitative Research in Physical Therapy

ENDING NOTES

Qualitative research has historically been identified with the fields of anthropology and sociology. Today, this form of research is gaining greater recognition among health care professionals who are interested in addressing questions about the "human" or qualitative aspects of their profession and practice.[1-4]

Qualitative research enables physical therapists to gain a better understanding of human factors that are not quantifiable but undoubtedly influence many facets of physical therapy practice. This form of research is suitable for addressing questions involving a multitude of factors (variables) that are impossible to anticipate, control, or eliminate. Generally, questions involving human variables are difficult to study because of either ethical concerns or the inability to control for the variables in a manner that assures valid and reliable findings. Qualitative research is an approach that can be used to address relevant questions without compromising ethical standards. Issues of validity and reliability are addressed in qualitative research via a constant-comparative process that accommodates the multitude of confounding variables inherent in clinical practice. The ability to conduct clinical studies and to discover and explain clinical phenomena without the need to control variables is a compelling reason for physical therapists to use qualitative research methodology.

This chapter introduces the reader to the suitability of qualitative research in physical therapy and is designed to provide a starting point for the reader who wishes to pursue qualitative studies in physical therapy. It should be noted that research that uses descriptive statistical analysis is not addressed in this chapter. For the purposes of this chapter, qualitative research is distinguished from quantitative forms of research. The research approach described here does not rely upon quantitative data or quantitative forms of analysis. The chapter is organized into four major sections: (1) overview of qualitative research; (2) types of qualitative research; (3) design and implementation of qualitative research; and (4) qualitative research in physical therapy. Greatest attention is given to design and implementation of qualitative research.

OVERVIEW OF QUALITATIVE RESEARCH

Qualitative research commonly is referred to as *phenomenology*. The derivatives of this word are "phenomen(a)," meaning observable experiences or how things appear, and "ology," meaning study of. Phenomenology means the study of experiences or how things appear. Anthropologists and sociologists describe phenomenology as the study of situations, events, persons, interactions, and observed behaviors.[5] Qualitative research seeks "to describe, decode, translate and otherwise come to terms with the meaning, not the frequency, of certain more or less naturally occurring phenomena in the social world."[6]

The purpose of qualitative research is to address the same questions posed in quantitative research: Who? What? Where? How? and Why? in relation to qualitative, nonquantifiable aspects of human behavior and experiences. The answers to the questions are derived by collecting multiple types of data via observations, interviews, and unobtrusive data sources. Analysis of the data is done through multiple comparisons of multiple data sources until main themes and prevalent concepts emerge from the multiple sources of data. Analysis of relationships among concepts results in the generation of theory.

The inverted pyramid depicting the phases of qualitative research in Figure 5-1 highlights the inductive process used for analysis of data. Themes, concepts, and theory are grounded in *all* data collected. Unlike quantitative approaches to research, data are not compared to hypotheses nor are possible answers to ques-

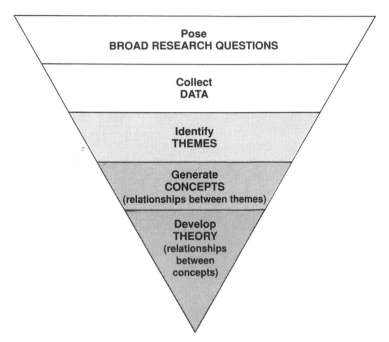

FIGURE 5-1. Phases of qualitative research.

tions posed at the outset of the study. Rather, concepts and theory emerge that are consistent with data collected during the study. All data are regarded as legitimate, and thus none are discarded. This aspect of qualitative research makes it viable and useful in a clinical setting teeming with variables that are considered confounding and unacceptable for analysis in other research approaches. The findings from qualitative research are reported through rich written descriptions. The descriptions include actual examples of data collected to support and explain the findings of the study.

Characteristics of Qualitative Research

Several characteristics of qualitative research distinguish it from quantitative research. The differences in the characteristics of qualitative and quantitative research are summarized in Display 5-1. The differences in design elements are addressed in detail later in the chapter.

Each dimension common to qualitative and quantitative research varies between the two approaches to research. In qualitative research, the questions are broad and general. The questions may be refined or altered during the course of the study. Questions are not translated to hypotheses against which data are compared. Rather, data influence the revision or addition of questions. Data are compared to data throughout the study, resulting in themes, concepts, or theory which are continually compared to all of the data as it is collected. The phases of

DISPLAY 5-1
COMPARISON OF CHARACTERISTICS
OF QUALITATIVE AND QUANTITATIVE RESEARCH

Dimensions	Qualitative	Quantitative
Research questions	Focus on qualitative aspects of human experiences	Focus on physical events and quantifiable aspects of human behavior
Researcher expectations	To discover information To describe human experiences To develop concepts, theories To explain and interpret human behavior or events	To test hypotheses and theories To verify hypotheses and theories To predict physical or human events
Role of person being studied	Active participant Participant behavior spontaneous Participant behavior is both means and end	Subject Behavior prescribed by researcher Subject behavior is a means to an end
Study approach	Inductive process Data guide study All variables part of study Dynamic, systematic process using constant comparisons	Deductive process Hypotheses guide study Specific variables studied Fixed, systematic process
Data	Reflect perceptions of persons being studied Collected throughout study In form of "words" for analysis	Independent of perceptions of persons studied Collected in designated time frame In form of "numbers" for analysis
Research environment	Data collected in settings natural to persons being studied No manipulation of environment by researcher	Data collected in controlled environment Researcher manipulates environment to control for variables
Outcomes	Written descriptions of findings that are highly valid	Numerical accounts of data that are highly reliable

qualitative research depicted in Figure 5-1 are not pursued in a linear fashion but occur simultaneously throughout the study.

The roles of persons being studied and the role of the researcher are different from those in quantitative approaches to research. The persons being studied are in the role of a participant rather than that of a subject. The behavior of participants and the perceptions of participants are among the sources of data in qualitative research that are analyzed to identify concepts and generate theory. Thus, participant behavior represents both a means and an end in qualitative research. In quantitative research, subject behavior serves as a source of data which is a means for verifying or rejecting a hypothesis.

The researcher does not manipulate the environment in qualitative research. The interactions between researcher and participant are not clearly prescribed at the outset of the study. Qualitative researchers expect to interact with study participants and scrupulously document all interactions with participants. The interactions between the researcher and study participants are a source of data. These data are compared with all other sources of data.

Although both qualitative and quantitative research approaches share the common goal of adding to a body of knowledge and ultimately contributing to the development of theory, the processes used and the final study outcomes are decidedly different. Qualitative research utilizes an inductive process to reach its outcome, while quantitative research utilizes a deductive process to reach its outcome. The inductive process (inverted pyramid) rests on all data being regarded as legitimate and allowing the data to guide the study. The deductive process used in quantitative research controls data to address issues of validity and reliability and analyzes data in relation to hypotheses. The qualitative research approach is dynamic and systematic. The quantitative research approach is fixed and systematic. Qualitative research accommodates the fluid, unpredictable human behaviors, interactions, and situations inherent to clinical practice. Quantitative research, while most worthy and useful in testing quantifiable phenomena in clinical practice, is not capable of managing multiple, confounding variables inherent to clinical practice in a systematic, rigorous manner.

Quantitative research generates numerical data, analyzes the data through a variety of statistical and descriptive measures, and reports numerical findings that can be highly reliable because of the fixed, systematic process used for analysis. Validity is addressed in quantitative research by establishing criteria for the types of data to be collected and the types of data acceptable for inclusion in analysis. Qualitative research, on the other hand, generates verbal data (oral and written), analyzes verbal data through a constant comparison process, and results in written descriptions of findings that are highly valid because they are soundly grounded in all data collected. The inclusion of all data and comparisons of all data at several levels of analysis result in findings that explain and interpret qualitative aspects of human behavior, situations, or events.

The differences in characteristics of the two approaches, in large measure, influence the researcher's selection of one approach over the other. One form of research is not preferable to another. Both research approaches add to bodies of knowledge, and both can be used to develop concepts and theories that explain commonly observed phenomena. The key issue is to select the research approach most suitable for addressing the research questions to be studied. Quantitative research addresses questions that are quantifiable and are appropriately analyzed through statistical analysis. Qualitative research addresses questions that focus on the qualitative aspects of human behavior and experiences and are appropriately analyzed through a comparative process. Qualitative, inductive research aims to discover while quantitative, deductive research aims to check out what we think we may already know.[7]

TYPES OF QUALITATIVE RESEARCH

There are four major types of qualitative research: (1) case studies; (2) life histories, a form of historical research; (3) ethnography; and (4) grounded theory methodology. All four types share the characteristics that have been described. Each type of qualitative research, however, possesses a unique orientation to studying human behavior and human experiences.

Case Studies

The case study describes in detail and from a holistic perspective a single entity, phenomenon, social unit, or behaviors of a single individual.[8] In physical therapy, case studies are used to describe patients who present unusual diagnostic findings, who respond to therapeutic intervention in an unusual manner, or who are recipients of a unique therapeutic intervention. The case study as a form of qualitative research differs from the case study presented as single-subject research in the quantitative approach. In quantitative research, the case study focuses on quantifiable measures and analysis. In qualitative research, the case study focuses on the qualitative aspects of human behavior, situations, and events that are not quantifiable and cannot be analyzed in terms of numerical data.

Typically, qualitative case studies are reported with rich, detailed descriptions. Case studies attempt to describe the patient and the intervention so that the reader can vicariously share the described experiences. The case study report, ideally, results in the reader identifying with the experience as one that is relevant and valid given what the author and readers "know" about current physical therapy practice.

A case study can be a significant beginning to in-depth qualitative research. Case studies can be used to share unique experiences and, more importantly, to generate sources of data that can be subjected to constant-comparative analysis. A compilation of case studies that represent experiences with patients within a clinical setting and across clinical settings can serve as rich data sources to identify concepts common to given patient populations, multiple patient populations, given forms of interventions, and multiple forms of intervention. Further comparison of concepts generated from case studies describing multiple patient groups, clinical settings, physical therapists, and modes of intervention across time frames can be the basis for developing theory in physical therapy.

A mistake made in regard to case studies is to treat them as single, isolated incidents. In addition, only unusual case studies tend to be reported. If we begin to report case studies that represent the "ordinary" physical therapy intervention and the "typical" patient, then physical therapists can begin to develop concepts and theory that are highly relevant to physical therapy practice. Imagine the possibilities!

Historical: Life History

Although the design of historical research is typically consistent with quantitative research designs, it can be adapted to a qualitative research design. The life history is a form of qualitative historical research that is particularly relevant to physical therapy. Leininger describes the life history research approach as it relates to nursing practice.[2] Leininger describes the purpose of a life history as obtaining a "personalized and longitudinal account of an individual's health, care, and illness patterns from a lifetime perspective" (p. 119). This type of research uncovers the chronological sequence of persons' perceptions and experiences related to (1) their health; (2) care given to themselves, by others, or to others; and (3) their illnesses.

Life histories can be self-disclosures, that is, self-produced in an autobiographical format, or they can be biographical, as accounts taken and reported by a researcher. Autobiographical life histories are common. Biographical life histories, undertaken with the purpose of adding to the body of knowledge in a discipline, are uncommon.

The life history is initiated with a set of questions. The questions are pursued via extensive interviewing of the person(s) being studied. Other documents and artifacts can also be examined and compared to data collected during interviews. Highly skilled interview techniques are needed to engage in this type of research. As with other types of qualitative research, the outcome is a rich, detailed, written description of the information collected from the person being studied. Major themes or concepts are derived from the historical account provided by the individual being interviewed. Leininger describes a life history protocol which may be of interest to the reader planning to pursue this type of research.[2]

Although the life history is similar to a case study, it covers a life span and multiple events rather than a specific point in time or a specific event. Like case studies, life histories when accumulated represent rich sources of data that can be subjected to comparative analysis to establish concepts and theory related to health, care, and illness.

In physical therapy, life histories can be used to address questions concerning psycho-social reactions to disability, patterns of behavior common to chronic conditions, therapeutic management of chronic conditions, appropriate timing for physical therapy interventions, availability of health care services, access to health care services, significance of support systems (family and professional services), impact of family constellation on coping skills, stresses associated with injury and disability, and prevention of injury and disability.

The life history as a type of qualitative research represents a useful approach to discovering the efficacy of physical therapy intervention and the nature of other aspects of physical therapy practice. This type of research is, to date, rarely reported in health care. Given physical therapists' familiarity with and skill in taking histories as part of the evaluation of patients, this type of research utilizes existing "research" skills possessed by physical therapists.

Ethnography

Ethnography is identified strongly with the social sciences. It has been a mainstay of research conducted in the fields of anthropology and sociology. An example of ethnographic research likely to be familiar to many is the research conducted among primitive cultures by Margaret Mead. She lived among the persons of the primitive cultures, participated in the customs of the people, and kept detailed notes on the behaviors she observed and on her own experiences while living with the persons she studied.[9]

Ethnography, as described by Agar, is both a process and a product.[10] He describes the process as (1) learning something by collecting data; (2) trying to make sense out of the data through analysis; (3) checking one's interpretations of the data made during analysis by collecting more data; (4) determining if initial interpretations continue to make sense in light of the additional data; (5) refining one's interpretations through more analysis; and (6) continuing the process of collecting data, analyzing data, and checking one's interpretations of the data until the analyses of the data repeatedly result in the same interpretations. The product of this process is an account of events, situations, and interactions that is congruent with the perceptions of the people being studied.

The process and outcome of ethnography are essentially the same as that for other forms of qualitative research. A factor that distinguishes ethnography from other forms of qualitative research is the long-term association of the researcher with the persons or groups being studied. Ethnographers (persons who conduct ethnographic research) collect data through observations and participation in the everyday affairs and experiences of the persons being studied. Denzin[11] describes three aspects of an ethnographer's role. First, the ethnographer shares in the life and activities of the persons being studied. Second, the ethnographer participates in the symbolic world of the participants by becoming familiar with their linguistic and behavioral rules and patterns. Third, the ethnographer assumes a role distinct enough from the participants to maintain integrity of intent to document a cultural milieu, yet sufficiently integrated with the life of the participants to allow meaningful participation in their symbolic world. Given these aspects of the ethnographer's role, the ethnographer must guard against being identified with a particular group or segment of a group being studied.

The ethnographer transfers direct observations and experiences into descriptions of behavior that the persons being studied agree are possible explanations for what is occurring. Some researchers claim ethnographic techniques may gather information about human behavior that is impossible to obtain by quantitative research methods.[12]

In physical therapy, an ethnographic research approach is appropriate, for example, in addressing questions concerning the differences in physical therapy services in hospital settings versus ambulatory care or home settings; interpersonal interactions among/between patients, physical therapists, family members, or other health care professionals; patient compliance with therapeutic regimens; environmental factors influencing the therapeutic process; physical therapists' roles in various practice settings; the nature of clinical education experiences; professional socialization; decision-making processes within departments or health care teams; and group dynamics. Any question that demands that considerable time be spent with persons being studied in order to provide a holistic description of their experiences and perspectives is appropriate for ethnographic investigation.

Grounded Theory Methodology

Grounded theory methodology is associated primarily with the field of sociology. Many persons may be familiar with the use of this methodology as described by Glaser and Strauss in their books *Awareness of Dying*[13] and *Time for Dying.*[14] Glaser and Strauss describe grounded theory methodology as focusing on the generation of theory rather than on the verification of theory.[15] Theory generated via this qualitative research approach is related to social and psychological phenomena.[1] The theory is derived from data rather than deduced from an existing body of theory. The end product of a study using this approach is a theory or set of hypotheses that account for much of the relevant human behavior that comprises the data collected during the study.

Glaser and Strauss contend that theory based on data can rarely be refuted completely by more data or replaced by another theory.[15] Grounded theory stands the test of additional data because it meets four essential criteria for a practical theory: (1) fit of concepts/theory to data; (2) relevance to practitioners; (3) workability; and (4) modifiability. A theory's fit refers to the fit between the data collected and the conceptual elements of a theory. All of the conceptual elements must be consistent with all of the data collected. This is in contrast to deductive forms of research in which data are considered in relation to existing theory or preestablished hypotheses.

The criterion of work, according to Glaser, refers to a theory's ability to "explain what happened, predict what will happen and interpret what is happening" in the area of study.[16] This is met through the use of a systematic process that involves validation of data by the persons who are actually being studied. Closely related to the criterion of work is the criterion of relevance. The study findings are relevant if the readers of the findings can (1) identify with the conceptual elements described and (2) regard the findings as worthwhile to them in their social or practice world. Last, the criterion of modifiability is met if the findings or theory can expand or change in response to additional data. The researcher who uses this approach views theory as an "ever-developing entity not a perfected product."[15]

The research process used in grounded theory methodology is similar to that used in ethnographic research. A distinction between the two is that the grounded theorist (a researcher employing grounded theory methodology) does not necessarily engage in prolonged contact with the persons being studied within their natural environments. In addition, the findings in grounded theory methodology describe relationships between concepts that emerge from the data rather than the people or events observed. Both approaches include descriptions of actual observations or information derived from interviews, documents, or other artifacts; but grounded theory reporting focuses on descriptions of relationships between concepts and how the concepts interrelate to form a theory rather than providing written descriptions of human experiences with the emphasis on capturing the totality of the experiences per se.

In physical therapy, a grounded theory methodology is appropriate, for example, in addressing questions concerning the influence of cultural differences in persons seeking or responding to physical therapy interventions; the development and nature of various forms of interpersonal relationships; determining the efficacy of quality assurance mechanisms; the nature of patient education; the identification and handling of ethical issues; the influence of technological advances on physical therapy practice; the development of therapeutic interventions; the passage of patients into health care settings; and the role of patient.

Grounded theory methodology is suited for studying questions that have not been studied previously. Most importantly, it is an ideal research approach for developing theory in physical therapy. Its comprehensive, systematic process of analysis handles confounding variables across a breadth of settings, persons, and situations. Grounded theory methodology is ideal for translating physical therapy practice into theories of practice.

Selecting a Qualitative Research Approach

While each of the four types of qualitative research described is somewhat unique, they share common characteristics, as outlined in Display 5-1. The characteristics of each research approach influence, in large measure, the selection of a qualitative versus quantitative research design. If the research questions require collecting numerical data and subjecting the data to statistical analysis, a qualitative research approach is not appropriate. Nor is qualitative research appropriate for testing or verifying hypotheses or theories.

Qualitative research is appropriate for addressing questions related to qualitative aspects of human behavior and human experiences. Many research questions related to clinical practice cannot adequately be addressed if confounding variables must be eliminated because of logistical and ethical considerations. Such questions can be addressed in a systematic, rigorous manner via a qualitative research approach. Constant-comparative analysis and triangulation, which serve as the basis for data analysis in qualitative research, allow the inclusion of confounding variables without skewing the concepts and theory that emerge from this type of research. These forms of analyses enable the researcher to discover, describe, and explain human behavior and human experiences that cannot adequately be studied via quantitative research designs.

The suggestions for research questions accompanying each type of qualitative research described in this chapter can be addressed by any of the approaches. The determination of which type of qualitative research approach to use is based on (1) how a question is posed; (2) the number of persons to be studied; (3) the timespan of experiences to be studied; (4) the importance of experiencing first-hand a person's or group's experiences; (5) the availability of sources of data and access to

data sources; (6) past, present, or future time orientation; and (7) logistical considerations such as travel, cost, and time away from one's work setting. Collectively,
these considerations guide the researcher in selecting the primary type of qualitative research to be used in a study.

The researcher also can choose to combine the various types of qualitative
research methodology. For example, multiple case studies or life histories can be
analyzed through a grounded theory methodology. Grounded theory methodology
can be combined with ethnographic research. Ethnographic research can be combined with case studies or life histories. The combination of approaches often is
most appropriate for addressing qualitative research questions and ensuring that
findings describe and explain what is happening.

Combining Qualitative and Quantitative Research

A researcher may choose to combine qualitative and quantitative research
designs. There are pitfalls, however, to combining the approaches.[17-19] First, the
focus of qualitative research is different from the focus of quantitative research.
Second, there is a temptation to subject qualitative data to statistical or numerical
analysis. Third, the researcher is faced with managing two different sets of expectations. On the one hand, the qualitative researcher's expectations are to describe
and interpret human behavior and human experiences as they unfold without
purposeful manipulation of the research environment so we can better understand
human phenomena. On the other hand, the quantitative researcher expects to test
and verify hypotheses or theories about various phenomena that require manipulation of the environment to control for variables. These different expectations
create conflict and are not likely to be compatible within a single research study.
Fourth, data guide qualitative research. Hypotheses guide quantitative research.
Finally, qualitative data reflect the perceptions of the persons being studied, while
quantitative data are collected independent of the perceptions of the persons
being studied. The quantification of qualitative data places a researcher at risk of
presenting data out of "real-life" context and thus undermining the very strengths
and significance of qualitative research. If the researcher can conduct two studies
simultaneously and be rigorous in carrying out each research approach or can
collect two separate sets of data subjected to appropriate analyses, subsequent
discussion of the commonalities or differences in research findings can be most
worthwhile and significantly contribute to the body of knowledge in an area
of study.[20]

DESIGN ELEMENTS OF QUALITATIVE RESEARCH

The design of qualitative research reflects its focus on the qualitative aspects
of human experiences. Its design elements share the systematic, rigorous qualities

of quantitative research. The processes employed to ensure the reliability and validity of research findings, however, are achieved through a set of processes different from those used in quantitative research.

The design elements of qualitative research are presented in six major sections: (1) starting the research; (2) collecting data; (3) analyzing the data; (4) addressing the issue of reliability; (5) addressing the issue of validity; and (6) reporting the data. A discussion of the limitations of qualitative research follows the descriptions of the major design elements.

GETTING STARTED

General criteria for selecting a qualitative versus quantitative research approach and criteria for selecting a specific qualitative research approach were described above. This section discusses (1) identifying a topic; (2) posing research questions; and (3) reviewing the literature.

Identifying a Topic

At one time or another, every physical therapist has made a statement such as, "It seems to me that . . ." or "My experiences suggest that . . ." These statements reflect clinical experiences. Commonly, discussions with colleagues help determine if one's clinical experiences seem to coincide with others'. If a topic in question is important and of high interest, one might review articles on the topic or attend an educational program related to the topic. Usually, these activities are pursued by clinicians to seek affirmation of their impressions or hunches or to glean further information on a topic. When a topic of interest is related to human behavior and if one's hunches are reaffirmed by multiple clinical experiences, the experiences of others, and educational pursuits, one has the basis for embarking upon a qualitative research study.

Posing Research Questions

The next step is to pose questions related to the topic. The statements made initially about a topic must be translated into questions. The questions are refined to address a manageable area of inquiry for the researcher to study. Questions used to guide qualitative research are more global than those used to establish hypotheses. A degree of specificity is needed in the questions, however, to provide an initial focus for the study. The questions are specific in regard to the setting, persons, events, or behaviors to be studied.

Example: How do the behaviors of a physical therapist influence a patient's compliance in carrying out a home program?

In this example of a research question, the persons and their behaviors are described from a global perspective. The specific persons and behaviors are not addressed in the question. Specificity emerges in an evolutionary manner during the course of the study. As data are collected, the researcher may refine and modify the initial research questions and add other research questions to be explored.

Reviewing the Literature

In qualitative research, a review of literature serves as a source of inspiration, represents a source of data, or helps the researcher make initial decisions regarding data collection. A review of the literature can spark interest in a topic area and help determine the types of questions used to guide a study. The literature confirms the importance of studying a topic and provides insights and support for assumptions made in the study. A lack of literature on a topic is one criterion for choosing a qualitative research approach.

A review of the literature can take place throughout a qualitative study. As such, it can serve as a source of data to be analyzed in relation to the data collected in a study. The use of the literature as a data source is valuable, particularly when a grounded theory methodology is used for developing theory.

A review of the literature is useful also in determining how initial data are to be collected. It can guide the researcher in decisions about the setting and the techniques to be used for data collection. Collectively, these decisions help determine which type of qualitative research will be used for the study.

In summary, qualitative research begins with an interest in a topic related to qualitative aspects of human behavior. Most often, the topic emerges from personal experiences, discussions, educational activities, or a review of the literature. The topic to be studied is phrased into research questions that are global but also provide enough specificity to focus the study initially. The nature of the questions and literature review determine which type of qualitative research is to be used. Next the qualitative researcher plans for data collection.

COLLECTING DATA

The selection of techniques for collecting data depends on the research questions. All qualitative research uses observations or interviews to collect data. Observations are used if the focus of the study is to describe a setting, situations, people, or human experiences that require of the researcher long-term observations and interactions with the persons being studied. Interviews alone are appropriate if the focus of the study explores a topic that spans an extended period of time or focuses on events people have experienced in varying time periods. Frequently, observations and interviews are combined. In addition, unobtrusive data, for example, documents and artifacts, are used in combination with observations and interviews, if they are accessible and available. The collection of multiple forms of data is common in qualitative research.

In summary, there are three major techniques for collecting data in qualitative research: observations, interviews, and use of unobtrusive data sources.

Observations

Two types of observation can be used to collect data: indirect observation and direct observation. The discussion that follows relates to direct observation. Indirect observation is described later as a type of unobtrusive data.

Training

Using observations as a means of collecting data requires considerable training and preparation. Observations are more than ordinary looking. Physical therapists possess the observation skills needed for this type of data collection, for they become highly skilled observers in their clinical roles. These same skills are applicable to qualitative research.

Direct Observation

Direct observation involves observation by the researcher, with his or her presence known to the persons being observed. The researcher's presence is confined to observation, and there is no interaction with the persons being observed. This form of observation is common in quantitative research but is seldom the form of observation used by qualitative researchers.

Participant Observer

In qualitative research, the researcher often uses a technique referred to as *participant observation*. The researcher interacts with the persons being studied and participates in their experiences while collecting observational data. The researcher's participation allows the researcher to share in the life and activities of the persons in the study, thereby gleaning a sense of their symbolic world. The researcher, however, must guard against being identified with a particular group or segment of a group being studied. In addition, the researcher must strive to be nonjudgmental and nonthreatening during interactions with the persons or groups being studied.

Observation Settings

Observations take place in settings in which the persons being studied ordinarily live and function. Observations in natural settings are often referred to as *naturalistic observations* or *field work*. The researcher does not manipulate the environment to alter events or attempt to control events. Persons are allowed to live and function as though the researcher was not present.

Informed Consent

Informed consent and review by a human subjects review process is essential for pursuing qualitative research methodology. Informed consent and human subjects review should be obtained when using any type of qualitative research methodology. These activities are easily managed when using case studies, historical research, or grounded theory methodological approaches. Ethnographic methodology is more complex when observations involve multiple persons within a cultural group or general practice setting. Reynolds suggests,

> If there is no deliberate attempt to change or manipulate the participants or their environment, or to disguise the nature of the research or its existence, concerns over the moral appropriateness will be minimized and will focus primarily upon indirect effects.[21]

Given the nature of qualitative research, informed consent is desirable and necessary if the participants can be identified prior to data collection. If prior identification of study participants is not possible, as may be the case in some ethnographic studies, the researcher should inform the leaders or the key persons who make others available for the research of the research intent and ensure that all persons who participate become aware of their role in the project before or after the fact. In either case, participants should have the prerogative of agreeing or not agreeing to be part of the research project. In the rare instances when an informed consent is not possible, there must be a documented absence of any type of manipulation by the researcher. An example of such a circumstance is when an investigator is observing behavior in a natural setting such as in a waiting area or treatment area and noting behavior as it occurs in the general course of events. Even under this circumstance, all involved persons should be informed and should give consent to have the data they provide through action or word used for research.

In general, the researcher should seek permission to be present and discuss the research with the persons involved in the study. It is important to describe the nature of the study and the role of the researcher in observation, and to discuss and assure confidentiality of the data collected through observations. It is advisable to describe how the data will be used, analyzed, and reported. It is important to inform persons in order not only to meet ethical requirements but also to minimize fear or concerns about participation in the study.

What to Observe

Observations in qualitative research are comprehensive. The purpose of the observations is to describe in detail a setting, activities/events, people, human behavior, and the meanings people attach to the setting, the events, and their experiences. To accomplish this purpose, observations are made in several spheres as described by Denzin:[11]

1. Physical environment. Observations are made of the physical environment. Aspects of the environment to be noted are:
   a. dimensions of the setting
   b. color of walls, equipment, accessories
   c. type and intensity of lighting
   d. type of furniture and equipment

e. floor plan of area
f. location of the setting in relation to the larger environment of which it is a part.
2. Social environment. Observations are made of the persons in the setting. The aspects of the social environment to be noted are:
   a. the number of persons present, and the variations in numbers of persons during various time frames
   b. how people organize themselves into groups and subgroups
   c. patterns (where, when) of action and nonaction within and among groups
   d. form (e.g., formal, informal, planned, unplanned) and content of verbal interactions among participants
   e. form and content of verbal interactions between participants and researcher
   f. frequency of interactions
   g. nonverbal behavior
   h. backgrounds of people (e.g., age, sex, positions held, physical characteristics).
3. Events and activities. Observations are made of events and activities that are part of the persons' experiences within the setting. Aspects of events and activities to be noted are:
   a. type of event/activity
   b. time of day, week, year the event/activity occurs
   c. frequency and duration of like events/activities
   d. persons involved in events/activities
   e. context of event/activity (i.e., what happened prior to event/activity, what follows)
   f. reaction of persons to event/activity.

Amount of Observations

The amount of time spent in observation varies with the research questions. The researcher plans to spend as much time in observation as is needed to collect relevant data. Extensive observation over several months usually is required to capture the totality of any situation and the human experiences common to the setting being studied. It is important to plan observations for various times of the day, week, or year so that data representing as many variables as possible may influence the findings. Typically, the exact amount of time to be spent in observation is not predetermined. In part, the decision to end observation depends on the outcome of analysis of the data that is occurring simultaneously with the observations. Thus, observations are concluded when the data no longer influence or alter the concepts that have emerged from analysis of the data.

Recording Observations

The recording of observations is commonly referred to as *field notes*. Field notes can be likened to progress notes, but they are far more comprehensive. Field notes contain detailed descriptions of what is observed. The descriptions are objective accounts of behavior. Direct quotations are cited to minimize the researcher's interpretation of verbal interactions. Although each researcher develops a personal method for recording observations, all use a systematic process and exercise discipline in objectivity.

The researcher's feelings and impressions of observations are also recorded in field notes. These interpretations, however, should be recorded separately from the objective recordings of the observations. Single interpretations of behavior by the researcher do not stand alone. The interpretations must repeatedly be grounded in actual data collected through observations or other data-collection techniques. Ultimately, the written accounts of the observations must represent what persons being studied confirm are possible interpretations of what actually is occurring.

In summary, observation, with varying degrees of participation by the researcher, is an effective technique for collecting data related to human behavior. It allows the researcher to note several aspects of behavior within the total context in which the behavior unfolds. Only through extensive observation can a researcher provide detailed accounts of behavior, persons, events, and settings that are relevant and useful in better understanding the dynamic qualities of human behavior. The researcher requires skills in observing and in taking meticulous field notes. High levels of objectivity and discipline are essential for rigorous observation by the researcher. The researcher should expect to spend as much time writing accounts of observations and writing memos, as part of the analysis of the relationships between data, as is spent in actual observations.

Interviews

Observations are rarely used as the only technique to collect data in qualitative research. In order to describe the "meanings" people attach to interactions, settings, and events, monitoring and testing of observations are accomplished by interviewing the persons being studied.

Types of Interviews

A researcher uses three types of interview formats to collect data. First, unstructured interviews can be used to collect data via informal conversations. This type of interview is unplanned and spontaneous. Researchers in the role of participant-observer frequently use this type of interview to validate their observations and initial interpretations of what is being observed.

The second type of interview is semistructured. Semistructured interviews are planned. Broad areas of inquiry are identified and all persons interviewed are asked questions related to the same areas of inquiry. The researcher may ask the same initial questions of all persons and follow with questions to address areas of inquiry not spontaneously addressed during the respondents' responses to the initial question. Open-ended questions are used for this type of interview. The questions do not have a planned sequence, but all areas of inquiry are addressed through the course of the interview.

The third type of interview is standardized and structured. Specific questions are designed and asked of all persons in an identical sequence. In qualitative research, the questions used in a structured interview are open-ended and designed to avoid yes and no responses.

The researcher may select one or more interview formats to collect data. The unstructured interview is commonly used in combination with observations. The semistructured and structured interviews used may also be in combination with observations or as a primary technique for collecting data. Most importantly, the framework chosen for the interviews needs to permit respondents to express their own understandings of behavior and events and to convey the "meanings" they attach to the behaviors, events, and settings under study.

Types of Questions

Six types of questions can be used to collect data. Following is a list of the types of questions outlined by Patton[5] and examples of each type.

1. Experience/behavior. These questions seek information that would be observed if the researcher observed the respondent.
   To a physical therapist: If I followed you through a typical day in the clinic, what would I see you doing?
   To a patient: If I accompanied you to physical therapy, what experience would I observe you having?
2. Opinion/value. These questions seek information about what people are thinking. They focus on cognitive views.
   To a staff member: What would you like to see happen in this department?
   To a patient: What is your opinion of physical therapy?
3. Feeling. These questions seek information about people's emotions. They focus on affective experiences.
   To a student: Describe your feelings when you find yourself in that situation. Do you feel frustrated? Angry? Challenged?
   To a patient: Describe how you feel when you leave your physical therapy treatment. Do you feel calm? Agitated?
   [Note: It is useful to follow the question with adjectives to obtain a description of feelings. Frequently, affective experiences (feelings) are confused with opinions, which are based on cognitive processes.]
4. Knowledge. These questions focus on factual information rather than on beliefs or feelings.
   To a patient: How long have you been receiving physical therapy?
   To a physical therapist: What is the protocol for admitting persons who are on a waiting list to physical therapy?
5. Sensory. These questions focus on the senses: vision, sound, smell, taste, and touch.
   To the patient: Describe what you saw, heard, or smelled as you entered the physical therapy clinic the first time.
   To the patient: How does your physical therapist sound to you when he or she greets you upon arrival for treatment?

[Note: The questions should contain specific types of sensory stimuli to avoid responses that reflect opinions or feelings.]
6. Background/demography. These questions focus on characteristics of the persons being interviewed. They may be asked in person or submitted in a questionnaire format. Questions of this type are asked of patients routinely when they are admitted to physical therapy. Information which might be included:
   a. age
   b. sex
   c. education
   d. occupation
   e. previous injuries or illness
   f. previous physical therapy.

Any or all types of these questions can be used during interviewing. It is important that the interviewer be clear about what type of information is being sought. The phrasing of questions influences the type of response. Generally, a broad, open-ended question is used to initiate an interview. Follow-up questions and probing questions guide the respondent toward providing the information the interviewer is seeking. Leading or loaded questions must be avoided, however. An example of a leading question is, How satisfied are you with your physical therapy treatment? Including the word "satisfied" directs or leads the respondent to describe a degree of satisfaction. If asked, What is your opinion about physical therapy treatment? respondents can choose to respond in a manner that reflects their opinions.

An example of a loaded question is, How would you describe the conflicts between physical therapists and physicians in this facility? This presumes that there are conflicts. Another way to phrase the question is, How would you describe the working relationship between physical therapists and physicians in this facility? This question permits respondents to share their perspectives. Interview questions in qualitative research should be designed to be truly open-ended and neutral in tone to ensure capturing the perceptions of the respondents.

Conducting the Interview

Establishing rapport with the person being interviewed is essential for effective interviewing. Part of establishing rapport is seeking permission to talk with the person and to explain why the interview is being requested. As with observations, it is wise to describe the nature of the study, how the interview is to be conducted, and how the information from the interview will be analyzed and reported. Confidentiality must be assured, unless written consent is provided to identify interview responses with the respondent.

Creating rapport also involves a bit of casual conversation while interviewer and respondent prepare for the interview. This should be limited, however. Nonverbal behavior of the interviewer also influences rapport. A warm smile, sincere handshake, or friendly posture from the interviewer helps to create a relaxed, comfortable atmosphere. The setting for the interview is important, too. A private, uninterrupted setting is ideal.

Active listening skills are required in order to obtain rich data via interviewing. Eye contact, nodding, and verbal interjections, such as "uh huh" and "I see," encourage the respondent to continue sharing information. Pauses at the end of responses allow respondents to catch up with their thoughts. Respondents frequently share additional information if given an opportunity to reflect for a moment. Restating or paraphrasing the person's responses is essential for validating the data collected during interviewing. Restatements are repetitions of responses in the interviewer's own words. This technique ensures that the interviewer's perceptions of the responses match the intent and perceptions of the respondents. If the restatements do not reflect the perceptions of the respondents, the respondents are provided an opportunity to clarify their intent so the interviewer captures the meaning of what is related by the respondents from the respondents' point of view.

Audio recordings of interviews provide a permanent record of the interview and ensure that accurate quotations are used by the researcher during analysis of the interview data. As with the interview, permission must be granted by the respondents for the use of an audio recorder during the interview. Note taking can be kept to a minimum when audio recordings accompany the interview, which allows the interviewer to engage in more effective active listening and enhances the interviewer's ability to concentrate totally on the respondent. Notations can be limited to respondents' nonverbal behaviors, such as gestures and facial expressions which further convey their perceptions.

In a semistructured interview format, an interview note-taking worksheet eases the recording of key phrases or nonverbal behavior. Note-taking worksheets can be organized into columns which represent the major areas of inquiry. The worksheets can then serve as an outline for the interviewer and help to ensure that the interviewer probes all areas of inquiry. The worksheets are also useful in data analysis.

Interviewing is a technique for collecting data and is essential for monitoring and testing the researcher's interpretations of what is observed. Interviews can also be used as a primary technique for collecting data. Six types of questions can be used within three formats of interviewing. The questions and interview format are designed to discover information related to the research questions. The strength of interviewing as a means of collecting data rests with the researcher's interview skills, particularly active listening skills. Information collected during interviews is validated with the use of restatements. Audio recordings of interviews provide permanent evidence of both the responses and the researcher capturing the perceptions of the persons being studied via restatements throughout the interview.

Unobtrusive Data

Unobtrusive data are often overlooked because of their obvious presence. The advantages of using many forms of unobtrusive data are their ready accessibility and their accessibility without prior consent. Webb et al.[22] describe three major forms of unobtrusive data: (1) physical traces, (2) written materials, and (3) observations. A fourth form of unobtrusive data which can be added to the list is audiovisual sources.

1. Physical traces. Physical evidence not generated specifically for purposes of being studied can become a valuable data source for the researcher. Two types of physical evidence are described by Webb et al.: (*a*) evidence of erosion, and (*b*) evidence of deposit.[22]

    a. Evidence of erosion. Physical therapists commonly use evidence of erosion as a data source when they examine the bottom of shoes to determine if patterns of wear coincide with a patient's physical status. In fact, if a patient demonstrates an appropriate gait pattern in the clinic, but the wear pattern on the bottom of his shoes does not match the wear pattern of an appropriate gait pattern, the physical therapist can be certain the desired gait pattern is not transferred to everyday activity outside of the clinic. This type of physical evidence is not scientific, but it serves as a valid data source. Other examples of evidence of erosion in the physical therapy clinic might include traffic patterns as determined by wear of floor coverings, repair rate of equipment, and use of disposable products.

    b. Evidence of deposit. Evidence of physical deposit is used by physical therapists when assessing the effectiveness of cleaning procedures of hydrotherapy tanks. Cultures are taken of the tanks. If the bacteria count deposits are higher than acceptable, a need to modify or increase frequency of the cleaning procedures is indicated. Other examples of evidence of deposit in the physical therapy clinic are the contents of wastebaskets and items appearing on work counters or in office spaces. Artifacts also represent evidence of physical deposit. Storage rooms frequently are filled with artifacts representing aspects of physical therapy practice from years long past.

2. Written materials. Several types of written materials can provide valuable data for the qualitative researcher. Written materials that are relevant and useful data sources for physical therapy research include:

    a. medical records
    b. department statistics and reports
    c. policies and procedures
    d. home programs
    e. treatment protocols
    f. admissions protocols
    g. quality assurance reports and summaries
    h. curriculum plans
    i. newspapers, magazines, journals, and books
    j. telephone directories, especially the Yellow Pages
    k. mail
    l. faculty, staff, and student performance appraisals
    m. surveys.

    This list is not inclusive, but it does suggest that multiple sources of written materials are available as data sources for physical therapy research in practice, administration, and education.

3. Observation. Direct observation and participant observation by researchers, with their presence known to persons being studied, has been described as a technique for collecting data. Indirect observation, without the knowledge of persons being studied, can also serve as a technique for collecting data. Observations in public settings are an example of using this technique. This author has noted the differences in behavior of groups of persons as they arrive at conference sites: physical therapists, for example, engage in more touching upon greeting one another than do other groups observed. This observation is based on observing physical therapists arriving and greeting one another over a twenty-five year period, encompassing 85 or more conferences. The observations of this behavior have been casual and indirect.

   Other types of indirect observations are made through hidden cameras or two-way mirrors. Hidden cameras are commonly used as security devices, but the recordings from such cameras represent a data source for the researcher. The use of two-way mirrors is more familiar to physical therapists. They are present in many educational and medical settings. Both hidden cameras and two-way mirrors allow observations without influencing the behavior of persons being observed. The use of hidden cameras and two-way mirrors poses ethical considerations to be addressed by the researcher, however.

4. Audiovisual materials. Audiovisual materials that represent unobtrusive data sources include:
   a. Audio recordings. The use of audio recordings in combination with interviewing has been described. Audio recordings of conversations and instructional materials are also data sources.
   b. Video recordings. Videotapes can be used in combination with observations and interviews, in which case permission must be granted by the persons being studied. Instructional and commercial videotapes can also be used as sources of data.
   c. Photographs, films, slides, posters, displays, and models. These types of audiovisuals represent possible unobtrusive data sources. Like written materials, they can provide the researcher with information about current and past practices in physical therapy.

Unobtrusive data frequently are overlooked by the researcher. They reveal much about human behavior and human experiences. Generally, unobtrusive data serve as a primary source for retrospective research. They also enhance studies that use observation and interviewing as primary techniques for collecting data.

In summary, the three major techniques for collecting data are (1) observation, (2) interviewing, and (3) use of unobtrusive data sources. Qualitative research demands that data be collected from multiple sources using one or more of these techniques. The qualitative researcher requires skill in observation, interviewing,

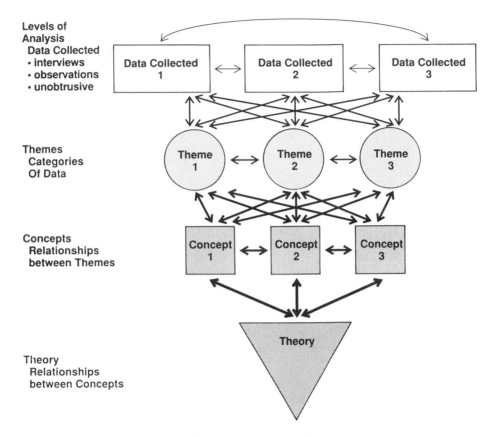

Levels of Analysis
Data Collected
• interviews
• observations
• unobtrusive

Themes
Categories
Of Data

Concepts
Relationships
between Themes

Theory
Relationships
between Concepts

FIGURE ─ ⁹ Constant-comparative process.

note taking, and identifying unobtrusive data sources that relate to the topic of study. Data derived from multiple techniques, persons, and settings over an extended period of time or across various points in time permit extensive analysis through multiple comparisons. The process of constant-comparative analysis will be described next.

ANALYZING THE DATA

Constant-Comparative Process: An Overview

Analysis of data is accomplished in qualitative research through a constant-comparative process. This analysis occurs simultaneously with data collection throughout the span of the study. Concurrent collection and analysis of data is a design element that distinguishes qualitative research from quantitative research. The constant-comparative process involves three levels of analysis leading to the generation of theory (Figure 5-2).

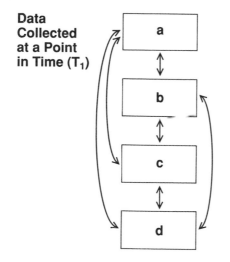

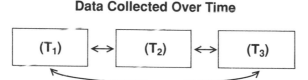

FIGURE 5-3. Temporal analysis. Each datum (a, b, c, d) is compared to every other datum within a point in time (T_1) and over time (T_1, T_2, T_3). The arrows represent comparisons between data at a point in time and comparisons of data collected at multiple points in time. This process continues throughout the study with data and memos generated from the data.

The first level of analysis requires comparisons of data. Data collected at a point in time and over time are compared (Figure 5-3). Comparisons of data collected from a number of persons or a variety of data-collection techniques are also made as illustrated in Figure 5-4. The comparison of data from two or more sources often is referred to as *triangulation.* The term *triangulation* is borrowed from a navigational technique in which several reference points are used to locate the exact position of an object. Triangulation, as part of the constant-comparative process for analysis, uses several types of data, persons, and events at a point in time and across points in time to interpret and understand the meanings of human phenomena. Triangulation is accomplished by using (1) a variety of data sources (e.g., interview or observation of several persons); (2) a variety of techniques for collecting data (e.g., interviews, observations, unobtrusive data); (3) a variety of researchers; and (4) multiple perspectives to interpret a single set of data (e.g., interviewing several persons who have experienced the same event).[11]

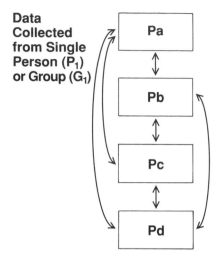

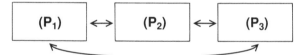

Data Collected across Persons or Groups

FIGURE 5-4. Person group analysis. Each datum (a, b, c, d) collected from a single person (P_1) or a single group (G_1) is compared to every other datum collected from a single person or group. Data collected from single persons (P_1, P_2, P_3) or single groups (G_1, G_2, G_3) are compared to each other. This process continues throughout the study.

The outcome of data analysis is the identification of main themes or categories of data. Themes represent several individual data that comprise a data cluster or data category as depicted in Figure 5-5. It is possible for an individual datum to be part of more than one data cluster, resulting in the identification of a theme.

The second level of analysis requires comparisons of themes that represent all of the data collected (Figure 5-2). Themes continue to be compared to additional data collected. If an initial theme does not "fit" additional data, the researcher eliminates or modifies the theme until it does represent the data. Comparisons of themes throughout the study result in the generation of concepts. Concepts represent the relationships between themes. Several themes result in generating concepts (Figure 5-5), and a given theme may result in the generation of one or more concepts.

THEME GENERATION

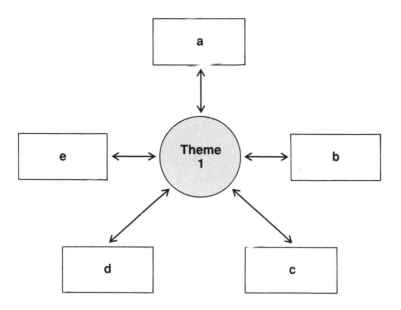

CONCEPT GENERATION

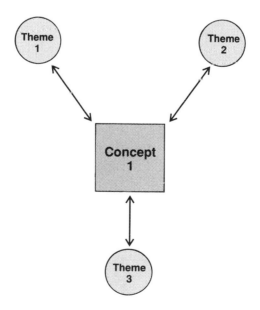

FIGURE 5-5. *(Continued on next page.)*

THEORY GENERATION

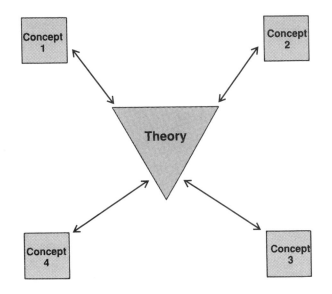

FIGURE 5-5. Theme, concept, and theory generation. Comparisons of individual data (a, b, c, d, e) derived from multiple persons/groups and multiple data collection techniques result in the identification of themes representing data. Similar comparisons of themes result in the generation of concepts, and comparisons of concepts result in theory development. The theory is grounded in data derived from multiple sources or data-collection techniques over the time of the entire study. Theory represents the relationships of all concepts.

The third level of analysis requires comparisons of concepts (Figure 5-2). Concepts continue to be compared to themes as themes are modified, and compared to data as they continue to be collected. Concepts are eliminated or modified if they do not "fit" the additional data and revision of themes. Comparisons of concepts to data and themes continue until concepts represent all of the data collected. These comparisons result in the generation of theory. Theory represents the relationships of all concepts that describe and explain the phenomena being studied (Figure 5-5, pp. 109–110).

The constant-comparative process is evolutionary and inductive in nature. The data guide the study throughout the study. Comparisons are made continually within and between the three levels of analysis. All data and thus all variables are included in the analysis. This aspect of qualitative research makes it particularly viable for clinical studies. The inclusion of all data (all variables) in the analysis results in findings that represent the dynamic, changing nature of clinical practice. Thus, qualitative research findings can be highly valid and readily applicable to physical therapy practice.

The Constant-Comparative Process
Illustrated

The constant-comparative process is illustrated further by using data and sharing examples of comparisons I made while studying mentor/mentee relationships.[23] A grounded theory methodology approach was used for the study. Data were collected by interviewing persons employed in helping professions (including physical therapy) who comprised mentor/mentee pairs.

Raw Data from Interviews

Examples of quotations noted during the interviews follow. Each quotation represents an individual datum.

A mentee says of a mentor:

"Never felt like only an employee or a low employee."

"Treated me well."

"(Mentor) identified me as someone he could work with, . . . tutored me. . . ."

The mentor of this relationship says of a mentee:

"We do an awful lot of talking together."

"The travel time for public appearances allowed a lot of time for informal discussions."

A second mentor describes the development of a relationship with a mentee:

"It began strictly professional and evolved into a more personal relationship."

Later, the mentor states:

"I became aware of him one year after joining staff. I liked what he represented professionally."

And later in the interview, the mentor states:

"We worked closely together. Always spent a lot of time together."

The mentee of this relationship made the following statements:

"Spent a lot of time together . . ."

"(Mentor) shared privy information with me."

"(I) shared the banner with (mentor)."

Memos Based on Raw Data

Following each interview, I wrote memos describing my general impressions about the data and these impressions were compared (grounded) to actual interview quotations. Memos were also written about each interview following the transcriptions of the interviews. Examples of memos are presented below.

About the first mentor/mentee pair, these excerpts are from a memo written on interview with mentee:

1a. Mentor seemed to single mentee out as one to groom.

Relationship evolved.

Initially, mentor teaching mentee, preparing mentee.

More and more sought advice from each other.

Evolved from one-way to two-way.

Excerpts of memo written on mentor:

1b. Early on mentee stood out from others.

Mentor impressed with work ethic, creativity, personality, and consistently good performance.

More and more, mentor brought mentee with him to public speaking engagements.

Had a chance to talk informally a great deal.

Could share confidential matters and know they would remain confidential until appropriate time.

On the second mentor/mentee pair, the following memos were written.

Excerpts of memo written on interview with mentee.

2a. Have always spent a lot of time together, as a student—later shared an office.

Made a good team.

Increasingly became colleagues and have shifted away from teacher-student mode.

Difficult to separate the personal from professional.

Excerpts of memo written on interview with mentor.

2b. The mentor called the mentee, inviting him to consider an opening for a position. He was gradually promoted, following in mentor's career track.

Mentor put a lot of time and effort into mentee.

Mentor shared things about (his/her) role with mentee which would be regarded as privy.

They shared an office—spend lots of time together.

Lots of time to talk.

Relationship also has personal-social component. They have dinner together. Mentor knows mentee's family.

Themes from Data

As raw data and the memos on each interview were compared, possible themes or categories of data began to emerge. Comparative analyses of data and memos were made at specific points in time of the study and across times throughout the study. Comparisons of data were also made within mentor/mentee pairs and between mentor/mentee pairs. Multiple quotations (data) made by mentors and mentees resulted in the generation of main themes. For example, from the raw data and memo excerpts shared thus far, the following themes began to emerge:

a. Mentor and mentee spend considerable time together.
b. Formal and informal time spent together.
c. Confidential information is exchanged.
d. Mentor "sees" something in mentee which makes mentee "stand out."
e. Relationships evolve from strictly professional to include a personal component.

The data and memos written on data within a mentor/mentee pair and across mentor/mentee pairs supported these themes.

Memos Based on Memos

After several additional interviews, memos based on the individual memos were written that reflected major themes or categories of findings present in multiple mentor/mentee pairs.

Here are examples of memos which related to the development of mentor/mentee relationships.

3. A key to development seems to be opportunity to talk with each other frequently. First two pairs have mentioned frequent encounters.

Also—time to talk is not just under formal conditions, but informal as well.

Time to talk about personal items, brainstorm, etc.

Informal, frequent communications seem to be a key as to whether this type of relationship develops or not. Organizational climate plays a role as to whether frequent encounters and dialogue are even possible or not.

A later memo:

4. Commonalities and opportunities are essential for mentor/mentee relationship to occur. Takes both for it to happen.

Building on the development of mentor/mentee relationships, after several more interviews a memo states:

5. Informal communications are significant to the development of the relationship and to the quality of the relationship.

   This is closely linked to qualities found in mentor/mentee relationships. Both persons have to be willing, receptive, open, and trustworthy.

   Trust and honesty—key qualities—these develop and feed into communications which feeds into an evergrowing sense of trust and honesty.

And a later memo states:

6. Mentor/mentee relationships develop like other close relationships. Persons have to be together. Informality. Amount of togetherness/proximity impacts development of relationship.

   Once relationship is established, relationship may be ongoing, even though mentor and mentee spend little time together. They will continue to communicate or see each other. They still feel a closeness, even though apart.

Development of Concepts

Memos 4, 5, and 6 illustrate how the researcher progresses in the constant-comparative analysis by analyzing the relationships between themes that have been generated from raw data. Themes that continue to be supported by additional data are then used to generate concepts. Concepts represent multiple themes that emerge from the study. Findings from qualitative research are presented as concepts when the study is preliminary in nature. Here is an example of a final finding representing a conceptual description, reported in this study:

The establishment and continuation of mentor/mentee relationships depends on the presence of a combination of characteristics common to mentors, characteristics common to mentees, characteristics common to mentor/mentee pairs, and environmental factors.

Development of Theory

This study resulted in the generation of concepts rather than theory, because it represented a preliminary investigation of a topic not previously subjected to systematic, rigorous study. Comprehensive studies or analysis of findings from multiple studies may result in the development of theory. Theory is generated from ongoing, multiple comparisons within and between all levels of analysis.

Constant-comparative analysis is time-consuming and demands rigor, patience, and discipline on the part of the researcher. The amount of data to be analyzed is usually quite great and can seem overwhelming to a novice of qualitative research. At each level of analysis, coding and sorting of the data is facilitated by using different colors of paper for writing memos and for distinguishing between themes and concepts.

Computer software is available to aid in each step of this analysis. Data can be entered, coded by content area, and sorted for multiple comparisons, thereby identifying major themes. Memos can be entered and retrieved to make further comparisons for the development of concepts. Memos written on concepts can be entered, retrieved, and sorted for the development of theory. The use of computer software eliminates the need for sorting through reams of paper. It also enables the researcher to compare themes, concepts, and theoretical schemes to the original data. A person skilled in the use of microcomputers can have a draft of the final report produced at the completion of the analysis. The improvements in micro-computer software hold promise for easing the analysis required in qualitative research.

In summary, the analysis proceeds from (1) accounts of observations, interviews, and unobtrusive data, to (2) the identification of themes, to (3) the development of concepts, and to (4) the development of theory. Triangulation is an integral component of the comparative process. Comparisons are made concurrently with data collection. Comparisons are made of raw data, memos written on raw data, and memos written on memos. The final concepts or theory are analyzed in relation to the raw data and reported with reference to quotations or vignettes of the original observations, interview findings, or unobtrusive data findings.

ADDRESSING RELIABILITY

The issue of reliability is addressed prior to the issue of validity because it represents the aspect of qualitative research that receives the greatest criticism from persons unfamiliar with the design and processes inherent in qualitative research. Reliability addresses the issues of replicability and consistency. If, according to Chenitz and Swanson,[1] a qualitative researcher is asked, "If I were to repeat your study, would I generate the same results?" the researcher would have to respond, "No." Exact replications of qualitative studies are not possible. In fact, any study relying upon human behavior, whether it be qualitative or quantitative, can not be *exactly* replicated.

If the researcher is asked, however, "If I apply your findings to a similar situation, will they help me to interpret, understand, and predict behavior or events?" the researcher can respond, "Yes." The test for reliability in qualitative research is the application of the findings or theory to similar groups, events, and settings over time.

Specific aspects of the qualitative research design address the issue of reliability. Collecting data from multiple persons or groups, across situations, and across timeframes tests for consistency of data and perceptions. Qualitative researchers continually test their impressions and interpretations of data against the perceptions of the persons being studied. During interviewing, questions are asked in several ways, and the researcher restates the responses throughout the interview to ensure reliability. Concurrent collection of data from observations, interviews, and unobtrusive sources with analysis over an extended time period ensures internal consistency of the data from which concepts and theory emerge.

Reliability in reporting is addressed by relating to the reader exactly how the findings/theory are derived from the study. The researcher provides a chain of evidence, like an audit trail, to demonstrate the reliability of the study. Generalization of the findings rests with the reader. Concepts and theory generated through qualitative research are generalizable to the extent that multiple readers deem them relevant and useful in explaining what happens, how it happens, and why it happens.

ADDRESSING VALIDITY

The issue of validity is addressed differently in qualitative and quantitative research because of their different purposes. In quantitative research, validity addresses the question, Do the findings represent what was purported to be measured? In qualitative research, validity addresses the question, Do the findings represent reality? Several design elements of qualitative research ensure that the findings of the study represent reality from the perspective of the persons being studied.

First, multiple forms of data are collected that are subjected to constant-comparative analysis. Data are collected via more than one technique, as in observations and interviewing. All data derived from each technique are compared for consistency. The researcher uses triangulation to determine if the various types of data result in a single theme, concept, or theory.

Second, except in retrospective studies, data are collected from the persons being studied. Observations are made in natural settings in which the persons being studied normally live and function. The researcher checks observations, interview responses, and unobtrusive data sources with the persons in the study. They are asked if the researcher's perceptions of an event represent their perceptions. During interviewing, the researcher repeatedly restates responses to ensure accuracy in interpreting the responses.

Third, data are collected from multiple persons or groups. The data are subjected to constant-comparative analysis to determine consistency and accuracy across persons or groups. Fourth, data are collected over a long time period until additional data no longer add to the themes and concepts that emerge from the study. Fifth, all data are treated as legitimate. Data are not discarded if they do not fit a theme or concept. Rather, the themes and concepts are modified to fit the data.

One aspect of qualitative research may negatively influence the validity of findings: if the researcher chooses to use only observation as a technique for collecting data. As Webb et al. note, the presence of an observer can impact the behavior of the persons in the study.[22] Because of this possible influence, the researcher must test observations by collecting data via interviewing or unobtrusive sources to verify observational data.

Using multiple forms of data, multiple data sources (e.g., persons or groups), triangulation, constant-comparative analysis, and ongoing monitoring and testing of data throughout the study addresses the issue of validity. The concurrent collection and analysis of data and analysis of data via a multiple comparative process result in highly valid study findings, which are a particular strength of qualitative research. Rigorous qualitative research can add to the body of knowledge in physical therapy by explaining and predicting the human aspects of practice and who, how, or what influences practice.

REPORTING THE DATA

The qualitative research report provides a detailed, rich description of the human behaviors, events, persons, and settings studied.

Full reports of qualitative research generally appear in doctoral dissertations, monographs, and books. The extensiveness of the data and the need to report the study findings in relation to the data generally preclude the inclusion of a full report in a journal. Instead, the researcher selects one or two aspects of the study for reporting in a journal article. These "pieces" of the study can be reported within the space constraints of a journal using the following outline.

Structure of the Report

The qualitative research report should include the following major sections:

1. Introduction. The introduction includes the major research question(s) that guided the study, the significance of the questions, and the assumptions for the study.
2. Review of literature. The review of literature presents the need for the study and supports the significance of studying the research question(s). It may also be used to describe both the choices made for techniques used in collecting data and the persons and settings selected for collecting data in the study.
3. Methodology. The methodology section describes the setting and persons studied. It also describes the techniques used to collect data and the process used to analyze the data.
4. Findings and discussion. The findings and discussion section presents the major concepts or theoretical scheme by including quotations or vignettes which explain them. The relationships between the major concepts are described to explain the development of the theory.
5. Implications. The implications section includes a discussion of the implications of the findings in relation to the existing body of knowledge and suggests further areas for inquiry.

One should strive for a balance between descriptions and quotations and analysis and interpretation of the findings. Descriptions and quotations should be sufficient to allow the reader to enter the setting and events experienced by the persons being studied, without being trivial or mundane.

Analysis and interpretation of the findings should allow the reader to appreciate how the data were analyzed and to comprehend the relationship between raw data and the final concepts or theory presented. If a study is reported effectively, the reader will relate to the findings and concur that the findings represent what happened and represent what might happen again under similar circumstances.

LIMITATIONS OF
QUALITATIVE RESEARCH

The limitations of qualitative research relate (1) to what appropriately can be expected from this research approach because of its purpose and design elements and (2) to cautions and demands that center on the role of the researcher. Although many of the limitations have been described throughout this chapter, they are presented here collectively to aid the reader.

Qualitative research is limited to studying qualitative aspects of human behavior and human experiences. As such, it is not an appropriate approach for measuring human phenomena and testing human phenomena through statistical analysis. Measures of validity and reliability associated with quantitative research are not appropriate for assuring validity and reliability in qualitative research. As stated earlier, a researcher does not expect to be able to exactly replicate qualitative research. The qualitative researcher does strive, however, for internal consistency—as is done in quantitative research—but through a different design process. Validity is centered not around rigor of measurement but around discovering reality from the perspective of persons being studied. Qualitative research is limited to describing and explaining human behavior and human experiences rather than testing, verifying, or predicting quantifiable aspects of human behavior.

The qualitative researcher must be sensitive to the possible influence of his or her presence on the behavior of persons being studied. He or she must exercise caution to avoid being identified with particular persons or groups and to avoid interactions that might be viewed as threatening or judgmental by study participants. These concerns are addressed by establishing trust with the persons or groups being studied.

Qualitative research, unlike quantitative research, is not conducted within a highly prescribed set of parameters. Instead, because of its evolutionary nature of design, qualitative research is initially framed by a loose set of parameters. Thus, the qualitative researcher must have a high tolerance for ambiguity and have considerable capacity to adjust data collection techniques as the study progresses. The researcher must exercise high levels of objectivity and self-discipline in collecting data and in making all possible comparisons of data. An open, receptive mindset is needed to accept all data as legitimate and to analyze data until themes, concepts, or theory truly fit the data. Data collection, memo writing, and constant-comparisons and triangulation of data demand considerable time and patience if pursued in a rigorous and accountable manner.

Qualitative researchers require high levels of skill in observation and interviewing. Meticulous recording of observations, interviews, and unobtrusive evidence is required to achieve reliable and valid findings. In addition, qualitative research requires that considerable time be spent in collecting data, recording data, and writing memos on data as part of the constant-comparative analysis. Fortunately, microcomputer software eases the time-consuming tasks of analysis and writing.

As must all researchers, the qualitative researcher must guard against bias and employ rigorous research processes to make meaningful and useful contributions to a body of knowledge.

QUALITATIVE RESEARCH IN PHYSICAL THERAPY

Qualitative research in physical therapy is limited to date. Many descriptive studies using quantitative data and descriptive statistics appear in the literature, but qualitative research is less common in physical therapy. In this section, applications of ethnographic and grounded theory qualitative research approaches conducted in the field of physical therapy are described.

Existing Qualitative Research in Physical Therapy

Scully and Shepard conducted an ethnographic study, using grounded theory analysis, to examine the process of clinical education from the viewpoint of clinical teachers.[24] Observations were made over a three-month period in five clinical settings. Observations were accompanied by interviews with clinical teachers to verify observations and the interpretations of observational data by the investigators. Simultaneous data collection and analysis of data resulted in the identification of two components of the clinical education process: (1) the clinical teaching situation, and (2) teaching tools used by clinical teachers. The findings are presented as major categories with specific examples of raw data collected during observations and interviews. The relationships of the categories are then presented as major concepts, and implications for the concepts are presented in the study report. This particular study report illustrates the nature of qualitative research reporting in a scholarly journal.

Another example of ethnographic research is that conducted by Yarbrough in which she studied physical therapists' behavior within a hospital setting.[25] She made observations three days a week for an average of 18 hours each week over a four-month time span. The observations were combined with informal interviewing and multiple unobtrusive data sources, including photographs, policy and procedure manuals, bylaws of the medical staff, annual reports, and questionnaires used to collect biographical data on the participants in the study. Constant-comparative analysis and triangulation occurred simultaneously with data collection throughout the study. The results of Yarbrough's study provide a richly detailed description of the factors influencing the perspectives toward their profession held by physical therapists in a given hospital setting. Analysis of the major themes resulted in central concepts which she described and discussed in relation to implications for curriculum development in physical therapy education. This study is an example of a comprehensive report appearing in a doctoral dissertation.

Tammivaara, Yarbrough, and Shepard conducted an ethnographic study to discover the determinants of quality in physical therapy education programs.[26] Participant observation was conducted during two three-day, on-site evaluation visits made in conjunction with the American Physical Therapy Association (APTA) accreditation process. In addition, a fourth investigator, Jensen, interviewed nine on-site team leaders using a structured interview format and analyzed unobtrusive data including on-site, team-training institute materials, APTA accreditation documents, and APTA accreditation reports. Data from the on-site fieldwork and that derived by Jensen were analyzed using a constant-comparative process and triangulation. The outcome of these collaborative studies is reported as concepts and skills required by on-site teams in the accreditation process and as a framework for assessing educational programs. A conceptual scheme for assessing the quality of physical therapy educational programs is presented in the study report. This study is an example of a comprehensive report appearing in a monograph.

Later, Jensen built on the pilot study reported in the 1986 monograph and proceeded to investigate how the APTA accreditation on-site visit served as a means for expressing the values of the profession.[27] She engaged in over 200 hours of nonparticipant observations to collect data during actual accreditation site visits and analyzed all accreditation documents prepared by on-site teams and the programs under accreditation review. A constant-comparative method was used for data analysis within the framework of a conceptual model that depicted the accreditation on-site process. Five main themes reflecting professional values were identified by the researcher. This study is an example of building theory through successive investigation.

Grounded theory methodology was used by Schmoll to discover the nature of mentor/mentee relationships among persons engaged in or preparing for professional roles.[23] Eleven of the fourteen mentor/mentee pairs studied were comprised of at least one physical therapist. Extensive interviews of the mentor/mentee pairs were conducted using a semistructured interview format. Restatements were made throughout all interviews and all interviews were audio recorded. Constant-comparative analyses were made within and among mentor/mentee pairs, among mentors, and among mentees. Major themes were identified and presented as characteristics and factors found in mentor/mentee relationships as described by the study participants. The conclusions of the study are presented as concepts and relationships among concepts. Implications of the concepts are discussed by the investigator. This study is an example of a comprehensive report appearing in a doctoral dissertation.

A study conducted by Jensen et al. used nonparticipant observations of physical therapist-patient treatment sessions to describe the work of the physical therapist and similarities or differences between novice and master physical therapy clinicians.[28] An initial conceptual framework comprised of practice environment components, tools used by physical therapists for intervention, actual therapeutic interventions, and patient outcomes was developed to guide this study on the work of physical therapists. Five themes were generated through coded data and field note observations. These themes represent dimensions of practice that initially differentiate novice and master clinicians. The study design lends itself to subsequent investigations so that theory can be developed through the findings from multiple studies.

These examples of qualitative research in physical therapy illustrate the components of qualitative research described in this chapter. Other examples of qualitative research in physical therapy appear under Selected Readings.

Applications of Qualitative Research Processes to the Development of Therapeutic Interventions

The use of qualitative research processes in the development of therapeutic interventions is common in physical therapy. The therapeutic interventions developed by Bobath,[29] Brunnstrom,[30] and Knott and Voss[31] were devised, in part, by systematic observations. These individuals carefully documented their clinical observations and compared their clinical observations over time. Their observations were compared with documented studies, which were subsequently compared with additional clinical observations. Ongoing observations and constant-comparative analysis of observations and studies conducted by other investigators resulted in the development of their respective clinical intervention approaches. Each type of intervention has been modified as the individuals gained new knowledge from additional observations and analysis of documented studies. This process is characteristic of qualitative research and highlights its appropriateness and usefulness in addressing clinical practice questions.

Future Applications of Qualitative Research in Physical Therapy

The qualitative studies conducted in the field of physical therapy have addressed important issues which impact the physical therapy profession. Qualitative studies to date have to a limited degree addressed patient/therapist interactions;[28] however, many clinical practice issues, patient/therapist interactions, aspects of the therapeutic process, and specific therapeutic interventions remain uninvestigated. Much remains to be "discovered," described, and interpreted. Qualitative research is a powerful tool for addressing a multitude of clinical practice issues. Dean's application of a psychobiological adaptation model to physical therapy can serve as the basis for identifying relevant clinical questions appropriate for qualitative study.[32] The model describes the relationship of primary and secondary factors that influence patients, therapists, and, subsequently, treatment outcomes. The secondary psycho-social factors relating to patients—sociology, stress management, lifestyle, and occupation/environment, as described in Dean's model—are appropriately studied via qualitative research. Dean identifies the primary clinical professional factors as therapeutic techniques, modalities, patient education, and prevention. The utility of qualitative research techniques has been described earlier in their application to the development of therapeutic interventions. In addition, the study of patient education and prevention are appropriately studied through qualitative research. The combination of patient factors and clinical professional factors are described as influencing treatment outcome in her model of physical therapy practice. This model provides an excellent starting place for identifying possible clinical questions to be addressed through qualitative research.

Qualitative research can become central to investigating clinical practice questions and issues. The focus and design elements of qualitative research enable physical therapists to address highly important and relevant clinical questions that cannot be addressed through other research approaches because of the inability to control confounding variables inherent in clinical questions. The inclusion of these variables as data in qualitative research not only makes some types of clinical research feasible, but helps to ensure that clinical research findings are valid in relation to the dynamic reality of clinical practice.

With greater attention given to aspects of qualitative research (e.g., observations and interviews) that are inherent in daily practice, physical therapists can systematically investigate their "hunches," which may result in findings that explain the qualitative aspects of human behavior and human experiences impacting physical therapy practice. The use of case studies and life histories as described in this chapter represent highly feasible and practical types of qualitative research for the physical therapists to pursue. Concepts and theory generated through qualitative research will result in descriptions and explanations of aspects of physical therapy practice that physical therapists must have to better meet the needs of patients and that are sought by others who challenge the efficacy of physical therapy.

ENDING NOTES

General Systems Theory says that each variable in any system interacts with other variables so thoroughly that cause and effect cannot be separated. A single variable can be both cause and effect. Reality will not be still. And it cannot be taken apart! You cannot understand a cell, a rat, a brain structure, a family, or a culture if you isolate it from its context. *Relationship* is *everything.*[33]

In the context of human behavior and human experiences this quotation summarizes the worthiness of qualitative research for physical therapy. The clinical world is brimming with variables that potentially represent cause and effect in the therapeutic milieu. Attempts to control the variables and label variables in terms of cause and effect under controlled situations provide skewed visions of reality. Reality is fluid. The qualitative research approach assumes that reality is dynamic and seeks to understand human behavior and experiences from the contexts in which they unfold. The relationship between the art and science of physical therapy is awaiting discovery!

REFERENCES

1. Chenitz, W.C. and Swanson, J.M. *From practice to grounded theory: Qualitative research in nursing.* Menlo Park, CA: Addison-Wesley, 1986.

2. Leininger, M.M., ed. *Qualitative research methods in nursing.* Orlando, FL: Grune & Stratton, 1985.

3. Shepard, K.F. Qualitative and quantitative research in clinical practice. *Physical Therapy* 67:1891–1894, 1987.

4. Schmoll, B.J. Ethnographic inquiry in clinical settings. *Physical Therapy* 67:1895–1897, 1987.

5. Patton, M.O. *Qualitative evaluation methods.* Beverly Hills, CA: Sage Publications, 1980.

6. VanMaanen, J., ed. *Qualitative methodology*. Beverly Hills, CA: Sage Publications, 1983.

7. Mentzberg, H. An emerging strategy of "direct" research. In VanMaanen, J., ed. *Qualitative methodology*. Beverly Hills, CA: Sage Publications, 1983.

8. Merriam, S.B. *Case study research in education: A qualitative approach*. San Francisco, CA: Jossey-Bass Publishers, 1988, p. 16.

9. Mead, M. and MacGregor, F. *Growth and culture*. New York: Putnam, 1951.

10. Agar, M.H. *The professional stranger: An informal introduction to ethnography*. New York: Academic Press, 1980.

11. Denzin, N. *The research act*, 2nd ed. New York: McGraw-Hill, 1978.

12. Wilson, S. The use of ethnographic techniques in educational research. *Review of Educational Research* 47:245–265, 1977.

13. Glaser, B.G. and Strauss, A.L. *Awareness of dying*. Chicago: Aldine Publishing Co., 1965.

14. Glaser, B.G. and Strauss, A.L. *Time for dying*. Chicago: Aldine Publishing Co., 1966.

15. Glaser, B.G. and Strauss, A.L. *The discovery of grounded theory*. Chicago: Aldine Publishing Co., 1967.

16. Glaser, B.G. *Theoretical sensitivity*. Mill Valley, CA: Sociology Press, 1978.

17. Morse, J.M. *Qualitative nursing research: A contemporary dialogue*. Rockville, MD: Aspen Publishers, 1989, p. 137.

18. Bednarz, D. Quantity and quality in evaluation research: A divergent view. *Evaluation and Program Planning* 8:289–306, 1985.

19. Smith, J.K. and Heshusius, L. Closing down the conversation: The end of the quantitative-qualitative debate among educational inquirers. *Educational Researcher* 15:4–13, 1986.

20. Firestone, W.A. Meaning in method: The rhetoric of quantitative and qualitative research. *Educational Researcher* 16:16–21, 1987.

21. Reynolds, P.D. *Ethics and social science research*. Englewood Cliffs, NJ: Prentice-Hall, 1982, p. 65.

22. Webb, E.J., Campbell, D.T., Schwartz, R.D., and Sechrest, L. *Unobtrusive measures: Nonreactive research in the social sciences*. Chicago: Rand McNally & Co., 1966.

23. Schmoll, B.J. A description of mentor/mentee relationships among persons engaged in or preparing for professional roles (unpublished doctoral dissertation). East Lansing, MI: Michigan State University, 1981.

24. Scully, R. and Shepard, K. Clinical teaching in physical therapy education. *Physical Therapy* 63:349–358, 1983.

25. Yarbrough, P. An ethnography of physical therapy practice: A source for curriculum development (unpublished doctoral dissertation). Atlanta: Georgia State University, 1980.

26. Tammivaara, J., Yarbrough, P., and Shepard, K. *Assessing the quality of physical therapy education programs*. Alexandria, VA: Department of Education, American Physical Therapy Association, October 1986.

27. Jensen, G.M. The work of accreditation on-site evaluators: Enhancing the development of a profession. *Physical Therapy* 68:1517–1525, 1988.

28. Jensen, G.M., Shepard, K.F., and Hack, L.M. The novice versus the experienced clinician: Insights into the work of the physical therapist. *Physical Therapy* 70:314–323, 1990.

29. Bobath, B. *Abnormal postural reflex activity caused by brain lesions*, 3rd ed. Rockville, MD: Aspen Systems, 1985, pp. ix–3.

30. Brunnstrom, S. *Movement therapy in hemiplegia: A neurophysiological approach*. Hagerstown, MD: Harper and Row, 1970, pp. vii–5.

31. Knott, M. and Voss, D.E. Proprioceptive neuromuscular facilitation, 2nd ed. New York: Harper and Row, 1968, pp. xi–5.

32. Dean, E. Psychobiological adaptation model for physical therapy practice. *Physical Therapy* 65:1061–1068, 1985.

33. Ferguson, M. *The aquarian conspiracy: Personal and social transformation in the 1980s.* Los Angeles: J.P. Tarcher, 1980, pp. 156–157.

SELECTED READINGS

Barritt, B., Beekman, T., Bleeker, H., and Mulderij, K. *Researching educational practice.* Grand Forks, ND: Center for Teaching and Learning, University of North Dakota, May 1985.

Beveridge, W.I.B. *The art of scientific investigation.* New York: W. W. Norton and Co., 1957.

Bryman, A. The debate about quantitative and qualitative research: A question of method or epistemology? *British Journal of Sociology* 35:75–92, 1984.

Cox, R.C. and West, W.L. *Fundamentals of research for health professionals,* 2nd ed. Laurel, MD: RAMSCO Publishing Co., 1986.

Jensen, G. and Denton, B. Teaching physical therapy students to reflect: A suggestion for clinical education. *Journal of Physical Therapy Education* 5:33–38, 1991.

Louis, K.S. Multisite/multimethod studies—An introduction. *American Behavioral Scientist* 26:6–22, 1982.

Piaget, J. *The construction of reality in the child.* New York: Ballantine Press, 1954.

Raz, P., et al. Perspectives on gender and professional issues among female physical therapists. *Physical Therapy* 71:530–539, 1991.

Stainback, S. and Stainback, W. Broadening the research perspective in special education. *Exceptional Children* 50:5, 1984.

Williams, D.D., ed. *Naturalistic evaluation.* San Francisco: Jossey-Bass Publishers, 1986.

6

SINGLE-SUBJECT, BEHAVIORAL, AND SEQUENTIAL MEDICAL TRIALS RESEARCH

Otto D. Payton

SINGLE-SUBJECT DESIGNS
   Designs
   Method
   Interpretation
   Example from the Literature
   Statistical Analysis

SEQUENTIAL MEDICAL TRIALS

It is sometimes difficult or even impossible, on a practical level, to meet some of the requirements of extensive group designs. In clinical practice settings, for example, it is usually not possible to select a truly random sample from a population. It is also frequently impossible to identify experimental and control groups of 20, 30, or more subjects at one time and assign them randomly to treatments. Faced with these practical concerns, one may choose to weaken the generalizability of one's conclusions by offending against some of the assumptions of a group parametric statistical design; or one may look for designs that do not make such assumptions.

A more serious concern relates to the ethics of withholding treatment from a control group in order to study the effects of the treatment on the experimental group. Public concern over this issue has expressed itself in stricter regulations governing informed consent and human rights, and it is sometimes difficult to "sell" control group participation to patients and third-party payers. *Single-subject designs* and *sequential clinical trials designs,* while not completely free from ethical issues, may be less troublesome than group designs in many circumstances, as will be discussed below, and they may better serve the interests of the clinical scientist.

SINGLE-SUBJECT DESIGNS

The most pervasive concern behind the development of single-case, or single-subject, designs is the serious loss of information on individual differences that routinely occurs in group designs in which there is significant variability among subjects in their response to the treatment variable.[1] The behavioral sciences, such as psychology, were, in the mid-twentieth century, the first to become acutely aware of this problem. Although a number of published studies indicated no significant changes in groups as a result of therapy, careful analysis of the data revealed that some patients got better and others got worse. The group design canceled out this information. Clearly, there was a need to study individual responses to therapeutic interventions.

Single-subject designs emerged in response to this need.[2] A delightful story comparing single-case and group designs is found in Parsonson and Baer.[3] Agnew and Pyke have developed an analogy for group designs which suggests that describing a human population on the basis of a random sample is like describing the creatures in the ocean on the basis of a two-hour fishing sample taken at a depth of 200 feet off the west coast of Florida.[4] Unlike laboratory rats, people have diverse characteristics.

Single-case designs are useful for dealing with both intersubject and intrasubject variability.[5] Group designs tend to average out both of these sources of variability, thereby creating a great deal of difficulty for the clinician who needs to know that *this* patient got better whereas another got worse in response to the same treatment. Repeated measures provide information on variability before, during, and after the treatment (i.e., intrasubject variability); clinicians deal with this kind of variability every day as they evaluate patient response to treatment. Single-case designs allow these observations to enter into experimental studies. By repeating single-case experiments on other patients, intersubject variability can also be approached in an experimental mode.

Generalizability of results is an important issue in both group and single-case designs. There are at least three important types of generality:[5] Will these results generalize to other subjects? Will these results work in the hands of other therapists? Will these results transfer to other settings? Barlow and Hersen contend that single-case designs will, in the long run, produce greater generality than will group designs because they *account for* variability, rather than average it out: "The more we learn about the effects of a treatment on different individuals, in different settings, and so on, the easier it will be to determine if that treatment will be effective with the next individual walking into the office. But if we ignore differences among individuals and simply average them into a group mean, it will be more difficult to estimate the effects on the next individual, or 'generalize' the results" (p. 49). "It is our further contention that, in terms of external validity or generality of findings, a series of single-case designs in similar clients in which the original experiment is directly replicated three or four times can far surpass the experimental group/ no-treatment control group design" (p. 57).[5]

Single-case, or single-subject, designs are often called *intensive designs* because they look at one "unit" in great detail. Similarly, group designs are called *extensive* because they include a number of cases. Single-subject designs are often called *interrupted time-series designs* because measurements are taken at specific time intervals rather than continuously; and they are also called *intrasubject replication designs* because of the repeated measures involved. Hersen and Barlow describe single-case designs as the scientific study of behavioral change, and they compare and contrast the experimental study of a single case with uncontrolled case studies.[2] Time-series designs are the quasi-experimental pre-post design described by Campbell and Stanley,[6] applied to a single subject.

These designs emphasize the idiographic features of human response, and they permit the researcher to examine the process as well as the outcome of the therapeutic intervention. They may be used, for example, to validate the treatment plan for one individual, which can be of practical interest to third-party payers and in quality assurance studies. Intensive experimental designs such as those that follow may be used in clinical problems that are characterized by wide variability in behavioral responses, for example, cerebral palsy.[7] These designs are useful when groups are not available in sufficient numbers to permit group designs, when the within-subject variability is greater than the variability between experimental and control groups, when one is exploring an area and is not sure of the appropriate questions or designs for a group study, and when one may want to change treatment in response to patient reactions to beginning procedures, that is, to individualize treatment as therapy proceeds (see ABC design, Figure 6-4). For example, if the first independent variable only introduced stability into the measured dependent variable, as illustrated in Figure 6-7, the experimenter might decide to introduce a second independent variable to try to increase the response measured.

Designs

Figure 6-1 is an example of an intensive experimental case study of the ABAB type. At one level, it is a way of putting objective data into a visual display that is associated with time.

The visual display itself suggests that something happened to the dependent variable, range of motion, when the independent treatment variable, mobilization, was introduced. In the figure, time is represented on the horizontal and the measurement of the dependent variable on the vertical. The dependent variable was measured daily; the treatment was initiated after measurement on day 6 and continued through day 12, when it was discontinued. Treatment was reinstituted on day 18 after measurement and continued through day 24. Phases A are called *baseline periods* and phases B are called *treatment periods*. The second Phase A may also be called the *reversal* or *withdrawal zone* because of how the independent variable is manipulated during that phase of the experiment.

There are several common variations on the basic design. The AB design (Figure 6-2) is seldom used because of its inherent weakness. With this design, it

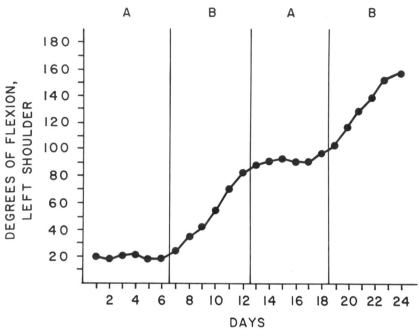
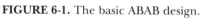

FIGURE 6-1. The basic ABAB design.

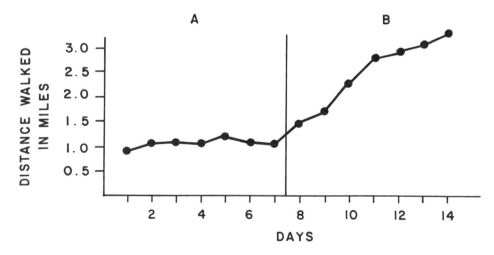

FIGURE 6-2. The AB design.

A   B   A

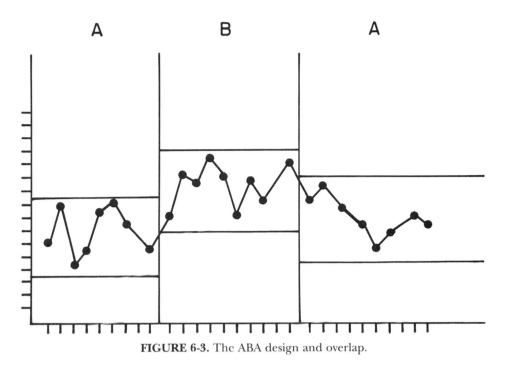

FIGURE 6-3. The ABA design and overlap.

would be very difficult to defend against the possibility that some uncontrolled variable accounted for any change observed in the dependent variable. For example, a change in the weather coincident to the initiation of treatment might have caused the observed (or self-reported) change in walking.

The ABA design (Figure 6-3) is stronger because the dependent variable is clearly associated with the initiation and withdrawal of treatment. The ABAB design (Figure 6-1), however, is still stronger; as Hersen and Barlow point out, "Unless the natural history of the behavior under study were to follow identical fluctuations in trends, it is most improbable that observed changes are due to any influence (e.g., some correlated or uncontrolled variable) other than the treatment variable that is systematically changed"[2] (p. 176).

There are two problems associated with withdrawal designs (ABA, ABAB). The first potential concern is that some behaviors, by their nature or because of the subject's response, do not revert to the initial baseline once gains have been made. For example, in Figure 6-1 the second Phase A did not revert to the original measurement but the trend did level off. Whether this is a real problem or not must be analyzed rationally in each experiment. Learning, especially motor learning, is an example of a variable that is not likely to revert to an original baseline in a short period of time.

The second concern is the ethics of withdrawing a treatment that appears to be effective. One may argue that a period of withdrawal may legitimately be made in the cause of avoiding false positive initial results that could lead to the continua-

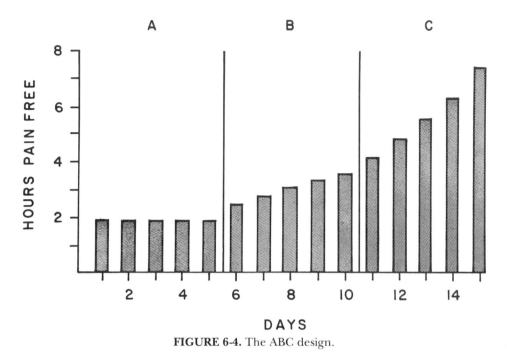

FIGURE 6-4. The ABC design.

tion of ineffective treatment. The speed and efficacy of treatment may ultimately be served by this temporary (in the ABAB case) test of the treatment. A variant design is BAB, wherein there are two treatment phases with one interspersed withdrawal phase to test the treatment.[5]

The ABC design (Figure 6-4) allows the introduction of a second independent variable in the treatment of a single subject. Thus one may study the cumulative effects of combined treatments. This design can be enhanced by withdrawing and reinstating either or both of the independent variables, for example, A-B-C-A-B-C, A-B-C-B-C, A-BC (B and C together), and so forth. Theoretically, one could become quite inventive with these arrangements, practicality and ethics aside. This design does not partial out the effects of the two treatments, but their interactive as well as their cumulative effects may be documented.

Barlow and Hersen point out that care must be taken in the design and interpretation of studies where more than one independent variable is operating, or false impressions may be generated[5] (pp. 80–87). They cite the work of Edgington, who described a variation of the ABC design calling it *response-guided experimentation*. This process permits the experimental analysis of behavior in applied research through either a manipulated or unmanipulated treatment plan involving more than one modality. (Note also that Figure 6-4 illustrates the use of a bar graph rather than a line graph to report the data.)

Goodisman describes a variation on the ABC design that is manipulation-free, eliminates the baseline problem, and permits the study of the effects of a typical

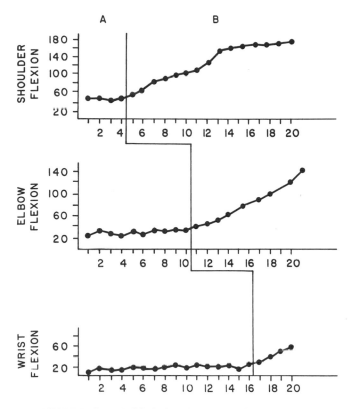

FIGURE 6-5. Multiple baseline across behaviors.

treatment program which consists of several modalities and experiences.[8] In Goodisman's example, four potentially therapeutic activities were provided to the subject in a naturalistic setting and manner; walking stability was assessed quite independently of all therapeutic activities. The analysis of this data is discussed under statistical analysis in this chapter.

When withdrawal of treatment in the ABA and ABAB designs creates a practical or ethical problem, multiple baseline designs, which do not require withdrawal, may be used. There are three common variations on the multiple baseline design, involving multiple baselines across behaviors, settings, and subjects. The first two involve single subjects. In Figure 6-5 three behaviors are examined in one subject (note that this is a variation on the problem illustrated in Figure 6-1). The hypothetical patient has limitations in shoulder, elbow, and wrist. The active exercise routine is initiated at all three joints on day 1. After the baselines are established, mobilization is initiated on the shoulder on day 5, on the elbow on day 10, and on the wrist on day 15. Withdrawal would not be necessary in this case to argue powerfully in favor of mobilization. Using a graph similar to Figure 6-5, multiple baselines may be established across settings or situations. For example, after control is achieved under supervision in the clinic, as is indicated by a steady state in Phase B of the upper graph, the technique is used in the office; when control has been achieved there, it is instituted in the home.

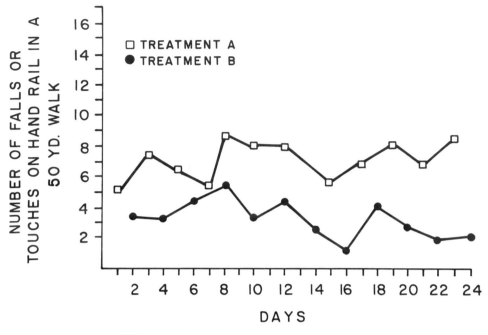

FIGURE 6-6. An alternating treatments design.

Up to this point, all examples have involved the experimental study of one "unit." A unit may be one person, one clinic, one classroom, or one hospital. Now consider a multiple baseline design involving more than one subject. Again, using a graphing format similar to Figure 6-5, one therapeutic intervention is applied to three subjects after different lengths of time have passed in the first Baseline A. When other significant variables are controlled, multiple baseline graphs argue rather forcefully for the effect of the independent variable on the dependent variable as measured. More complex variations in these basic designs may be found in Kratochwill[9] and in chapter 2 of Glass, Willson, and Gottman.[10] A follow-up "baseline" may be added to any of the designs several weeks after the termination of the last treatment phase, to document long-term effects of the intervention; examples may be found in chapter 7 of Barlow and Hersen.[5]

The *alternating treatments design* is a development of the past decade and is discussed at length in chapter 8 of Barlow and Hersen.[5] This design shares some of the characteristics of sequential clinical trials, discussed at the end of this chapter. In a typical example, the subject receives alternating treatments, A and B, on alternate treatment days or times. The subject thus serves as his own control. Both treatments are graphed on the same form so that the effects of the two treatments can be compared. An example is given in Figure 6-6. Here both A and B represent treatments, and there is no baseline. The target behavior for this design would need to be resistant to easy learning, such as head control in cerebral palsy, so that daily fluctuations in behavior would be demonstrated on the graph if the treatments made a difference. Due thought must be given to the possibilities of inter-action effects between the two treatments, interference in one treatment by the other, and carry-over effects.

Method

Much of the method involved in doing experimental research on single cases or units is implicit in the discussion of designs above. An alternate hypothesis of interest is identified: for example, in Figure 6-1 the hypothesis would be that "mobilization given prior to an active exercise routine will have a greater effect on active range of motion in shoulder flexion than will the exercise routine alone." Thus active flexion of the left shoulder is the behavior you want to control through mobilization; the target behavior is both observable and measurable. As in any research, all relevant terms should be given operational definitions. The reliability and validity of the measurement must be demonstrated. A plan that specifies the sequence of events in data collection should be written clearly. A graph for the recording of measured data is then drawn. In the Figure 6-1 example, the space between day 1 and day 2 should be approximately the same as the space between 10 degrees and 20 degrees, so that later visual analysis of the data does not create false impressions. The scale on the vertical should be complete, 0 to 180 degrees in this case. If the scale in Figure 6-1 were only 0 to 60 degrees, the unwary reader might be led to inaccurate conclusions by visual inspection of the resulting graph.

After the sampling time unit is defined (hourly, every morning at 9 a.m., etc.), baseline data collection may begin. Repeated measures are taken until a stable baseline is established. A stable baseline is essential for unequivocal interpre-tation. The therapeutic intervention is then introduced and measurement of the dependent variable continues at the same rate. Once change (or lack thereof) has been clearly established, the mobilization intervention may be discontinued to see if a second baseline can be established. In the case of Figure 6-1, it would not be necessary to return to the original baseline because it would be reasonable to expect that the patient might retain the gains achieved during days 8 to 16 (although a downward drift is a possibility). After the second baseline trend is established, mobilization may be reinstituted and recorded in the second Phase B. For this example, data collection is now completed. The modification of this basic methodology for the other designs is straightforward.

Interpretation

The most common form of analysis of single-case designs is visual inspection of the graphed measurements of the dependent variable.[3] In doing this, certain common problems arise. Consider three possible responses to a baseline that shows an upward trend. First, the trend may continue, in which case it would be difficult to argue for a demonstrable effect from treatment; continuation of an upward trend may demonstrate the effect of maturation or the passing of time. Second, the upward trend may become a steady state, which argues for a stabilizing effect from treatment. Third, the upward trend may be reversed, which suggests a negative

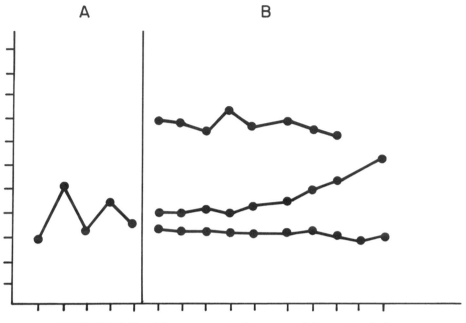

FIGURE 6-7. Possible outcomes in interrupted time-series designs.

effect from the treatment on the measured variable. The same responses could be given to a negative trend in the baseline. The ideal baseline is either stable or moving in the direction opposite to the hypothesized direction of change to be produced by the treatment variable.

The lowest line in Phase B of Figure 6-7 illustrates a possible stabilizing influence of the treatment on an unstable baseline. If one line of best fit were interpolated into the baseline data, a steady mean state could be implied in this baseline, with variability about that mean as visualized in the graph.

The middle line in Phase B of Figure 6-7 illustrates a delayed response to the therapeutic intervention. The upper line represents an abrupt change in level. With the introduction of the independent variable, the level of the dependent variable may change levels abruptly up or down. It may remain unchanged for some time and then change in either direction, either abruptly or gradually. Only some of the possibilities are graphed in Figure 6-7. A temporary effect of the treatment is characterized by a Phase B line that moves upward and then returns to baseline while still in Phase B.

In summary, it is important to look at the stability of the data in both baseline and treatment phases, the variability of the data in all phases, and changes in level and trends within and between phases. There should be enough data points within each zone to permit the demonstration of stability, trends, levels, and variability. Too much variability within phases may threaten the internal validity of the experiment.[11]

Glass et al. claim that the time-series design is "a sensitive tool for the investigation of causal claims in the behavioral and social sciences"[10] (p. 2). Users of these designs are not looking only for the final effect of their treatment at harvest time, as Fisher was when he invented the t-test. Rather, as Glass et al. explain, such users are interested in whether the effect is immediate or delayed, "whether it increases or decays, whether it is only temporarily or constantly superior to the effects of alternative interventions. The time-series design provides a methodology appropriate to the complexity of the effects of interventions into social organizations or with human beings"[10] (p. 5). In other words, users of the time-series design are interested in the unique *patterns* of response to treatment over time; this certainly applies in physical therapy. The time-series graph permits the analysis of concomitant variation where little experimental control is possible.

A causal hypothesis is based on rejecting less likely explanations of the data. Statements of causality are based on the trends demonstrated in the data in response to time and to the introduction of the independent variable and its subsequent manipulation through withdrawal or multiple baseline mechanisms. One expects the manipulation of the independent variable to have a reliable effect on the trends, levels, stability, and variability of the data. The evidence from replication in a situation where the subject has served as his or her own control contributes to the believability of the data.[11] One can conclude that the treatment has been effective if variation is minimal within the experimental phases, if level or trend or both change in response to treatment, and if the withdrawal and second treatment phases mimic the initial AB phases.[11]

Interpretation is dependent upon internal and external validity and reliability. Interrater reliability is of great importance if more than one person is collecting data.[12] Internal validity means that the changes in trends, levels, variability, and stability are consistent with the introduction and withdrawal of treatment and can logically be attributed to the treatment. Threats to internal validity include history, random uncontrolled events, inconsistent experimental methodology, patient selection bias, and interactive effects of multiple interventions.[6,11] External validity means that the results are generalizable across subjects, settings, or behaviors. External validity is demonstrated by replication of the experiment to other appropriate samples.[5]

Example from the Literature

Ostendorf and Wolf used an ABA design to study the effect of forcing a hemiplegic patient to use the affected upper extremity by restricting the use of the intact arm.[13] Each phase lasted seven days; during phase B, the patient's intact upper extremity was restrained from upon awakening to retiring. During all three phases, at three specific time periods each day, the patient kept a diary of 17 activities of daily living (ADL). Video records of some of these activity periods were randomly made to check the reliability of the self-reports. The frequency of occurrence of each task was graphed for each day, based on the patient's self-observations. The composite graph is presented here as Figure 6-8. Ostendorf and Wolf also performed studies of the quality and efficiency of the functional behaviors, and those data were reported descriptively.

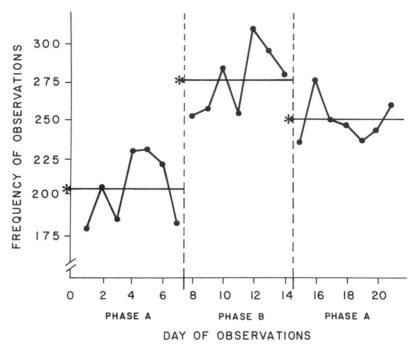

FIGURE 6-8. Daily totals for all seventeen purposeful behaviors observed during these observation periods for each phase of the investigation. Phase A, days 1 to 7, initial baseline period. Phase B, days 8 to 14, experimental phase. Phase A, days 15 to 21, second baseline period. The * indicates mean frequency in each phase. (From Ostendorf, C.G., and Wolf, S.L., Effect of forced use of the upper extremity of a hemiplegic patient on changes in function. Reprinted from *Physical Therapy* 61:1022–1028, 1981, with the permission of the American Physical Therapy Association.)

Statistical Analysis

The use of statistical tests in the analysis of replication data in single cases is highly controversial, as most writers attest.[5,9–11] In the early stages of the development of single-case designs, some researchers used conventional *t*-tests and ANOVA (analysis of variance) to analyze the repeated measures data. This is now considered unacceptable by many writers. Wollery and Harris[11] and Glass et al.,[10] among others, state that repeated measures are usually autocorrelated or series-dependent, and when this is the case, traditional *t*-tests and ANOVA are inappropriate (autocorrelation refers to correlations among successive data points in repeated measures). The visual methods of analysis described above are preferred by many writers and are considered statistical in nature by Kratochwill.[9] Mathematical approaches vary from fairly simple to very complex inferential designs. The more overlap there is between baseline and experimental phases, the greater the need for statistical treatment of the data. Overlap is illustrated in Figure 6-3. As can be seen in the figure, the *range* of the variability moved upward during the treatment phase, yet most of the range of the treatment phase is within the same range of measures as the two A phases. In this case, a statistical approach might help clarify the effect of the treatment.

The reader is undoubtedly familiar with the discussion of the relative merits of statistical versus clinical significance. It may be argued that in a practice discipline such as physical therapy, differences so small that they only show up through mathematical treatment are of minimal significance in practice. By contrast, differences large enough to be seen on a repeated-measures graph are likely to be of clinical significance. Kratochwill argues that the insensitivity of graphic analysis to subtle differences is one of the strengths of the process and that Type I errors are less likely with visual analysis; correspondingly, the likelihood of Type II errors is greater. Differences so subtle that they can only be detected by laboratory instruments or mathematical means are likely to remain in the laboratory. Variables of clinical significance are generally more robust. As Kratochwill points out:

> The preceding argument leads to the conclusion that the less sensitive measurement technique has been advantageous in the development of a functional analysis of behavior, in that it has a built-in bias against the selection of weak and unstable variables. As a result, the basic and fundamental variables of behavior are those possessing sufficient power and generality to be seen through graphic analysis.[9] (p. 113)

Even given the reasonableness of that argument, Kratochwill contended that statistically significant differences may be important for the guidance of future research and for the study of interactive effects of combined treatments.[9]

There are several ways, of varying sophistication, to quantify trends or create trend lines that are statistical in nature yet do not lead to statements of statistical significance. These include the freehand method, the semiaverage method, the method of least squares, ratio charts,[3] the median slope procedure, and the split-middle procedure.[11] The least squares and median slope procedures are complex; Wollery and Harris describe the split-middle technique in seven easy steps.[11]

Goodisman's design, described above, is a procedure wherein the dependent variable is as free of the treatment(s) as possible, for example, an ADL test in which none of the treatment modalities is a functional activity.[8] Analysis included an ANOVA model and lag sequential analysis, both of which to some extent partialed out the main effects of the four treatment variables and controlled for maturation. Goodisman gives only the results of the analyses and refers to the statistical literature for the methodology.

Wollery and Harris briefly describe the Rn statistic for the analysis of multiple (at least four) baseline designs.[11] Both level and trend in the treatment phases and stability in the nontreatment phases are considered in the analysis. A split-middle line of trend estimation is calculated for each phase; these are ranked, and a sum of ranks is compared to a statistical table for significance.

According to chapter 5 in Glass et al., the inferential analysis of intervention effects in interrupted time-series designs is a variation on the schema for the analysis of continuous variables. They call the general model the ARIMA (Auto-Regressive-Integrated-Moving-Average) model. It deals specifically with the expectation that two data points in a series of repeated measures on the same subject are correlated (autocorrelation) and that one point will tend to predict the next point (autoregression). The concept of moving averages refers to the effects of random, uncontrolled variables. Glass et al. present a number of statistical models, based on these general concepts, that are designed to deal with different experimental conditions. These models are generally referred to as *time-series analyses*. These analyses are very complex; computer programs are desirable and available. The interested reader is referred to the textbook sources.[5,10] Statistical issues in the analysis of single cases are frequently discussed in the *Journal of Experimental Analysis of Behavior* and the *Journal of Applied Behavioral Analysis*.

Kazdin recommends the randomization test for the analysis of the alternating treatments design.[14] The number of times each treatment is applied must be specified, after which treatments are randomly assigned to specified times. As Kazdin explains, "To test the null hypothesis, a sampling distribution of the differences between the conditions under every equally likely assignment of the same response measures to occasions of A and B is computed. From this distribution, one can determine the probability of obtaining a difference between treatments as large as the one that was actually obtained" (p. 303).

SEQUENTIAL MEDICAL TRIALS

Also called *sequential clinical trials*, this design (or family of designs) is ideal for use under either of two circumstances: (1) when you expect to have to recruit subjects over a long period of time (months or years); or (2) when you want to stop the experiment and reach a therapeutic decision as soon as possible. In the first instance, one avoids some of the difficult assumptions of conventional statistical designs concerning the simultaneous selection of a fixed number of subjects and their assignment to treatment and control groups. Sequential designs allow the clinician to admit patients to a study as they appear sequentially in clinical practice. In the second instance, sequential designs allow the therapist to stop the experiment as soon as the null hypothesis has been either rejected or accepted. If it is rejected, then all subsequent patients can be placed on the better regimen. Classical designs have fixed sample sizes; sequential designs permit variable sample sizes, the exact size depending on the strength of the difference between the two treatments. There are several models and statistical designs within this class of experimental designs;[15,16] however, the busy clinical scientist may well find the Bross model highly attractive.[17]

Sequential clinical trials are most often used to compare two treatments, for example, a new or innovative program versus the traditional treatment for a given problem. Thus the question would be, Is the new treatment an improvement over the conventional one?[15] There are a number of steps in planning a sequential clinical study. The first is to establish criteria for selection of subjects. The purpose of this step is to control confounding variables and introduce some necessary homogeneity into the sample, so that any change noted can be attributed to the treatment and not to extraneous factors. The second and third steps are to define carefully treatment A and treatment B and to establish standards for their administration so that subjects in each group have the same therapeutic experiences. The fourth step is to define (1) a dependent variable that is a fair measure of the target behavior and (2) the measurement tool that will provide a valid and reliable measure of that dependent variable. The fifth step is to decide how much of a difference must exist between two measures of the dependent variable (one for each treatment) before you would decide in favor of one of the treatments. The sixth step is carefully to specify methods for random assignment of selected subjects to treatments and to establish defenses against bias, for example, single- or double-blind assignments. Whitehead discusses at length processes for stratifying the sample on critical variables such as age or sex.[15] The final step is to select a statistical model for the analysis of the data.

In the typical sequential medical trial, the null hypothesis is that two treatments are of equal merit. Both one-tailed and two-tailed alternate hypotheses are possible. Comparison of three or more treatments is also described by Whitehead.[15]

Sequential designs may be used for both within-group and between-group comparisons. In within-group studies, the order of presentation of treatments A or B is presumed to be unimportant, and it is essential that there be no interactive effects of one treatment on the other. An example might be a crossover design for two symptomatic treatments for pain relief; similarities between this approach and the alternating treatments design (described above) may be seen. Matching of groups is also possible in sequential analyses, but it presents the usual problems.

Figure 6-9 is a hypothetical example of a sequential clinical trial using the Bross model for a .05 level of significance.[17] Let's say that for years your clinic has used a heat-and-exercise approach to low back pain; this becomes treatment A. A new therapist who has been trained in mobilization joins your staff and advocates the addition of that modality to the heat and exercise; this becomes treatment B. You go through the first six steps listed above. Pain will be the target behavior, and one cm difference on a 10 cm analog scale will be the decision criterion. The Bross model was chosen in step 7.

If the sample is not to be stratified, the first patient admitted to the study is randomly assigned to one of the treatments; the second is assigned to the other treatment. The two subjects form a "little pair" on which a decision will be made. A decision is reached at the preselected time, by the criteria in step 5, as to which treatment was better in this pair of subjects. The decision is graphed on the Bross form, upward one step for a decision in favor of treatment A, right one step for treatment B. If the criterion for decision is not met for any pair, the data on that pair are discarded. In Figure 6-9 the lower boundary is crossed with the decision on pair 20 (4 up, 16 right). A decision has been reached in favor of treatment B at the .05 level of significance with the power of the test fixed at 0.7.

The beauty of the Bross design is that all the statistical calculations are contained in the form itself. If the upper or lower boundary is crossed at any point, a decision has been made for that treatment at the .05 significance level. If the central borders are crossed, the null hypothesis is not rejected. On the Bross .05 form, a decision can be reached in as few as 8 pairs or as many as 58, depending on the strength of the better treatment in comparison to the other. An example of this format in the physical therapy literature may be found in Light et al.[18]

The formation of "little pairs," as was done above, is the most common approach to the use of sequential designs.[16] These pairs can be used to impose

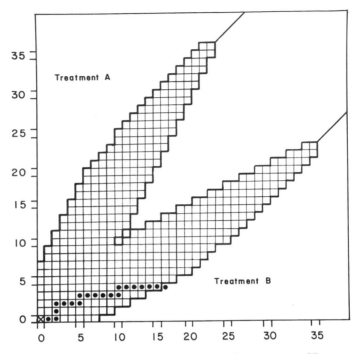

FIGURE 6-9. A sequential trials model with significance set at .05, power at 0.7.

stratification on the sample when that is considered necessary; for example, if a woman is randomly assigned to treatment A, the next woman admitted to the study is assigned to treatment B. The use of paired subjects in this manner also helps to control for changes in the environment, in concurrent therapy, or in the nature of the population, which may occur over time in a prolonged study.

In Figure 6-9, once the sample path passed pair 10 it was no longer possible for the path to turn and cross the upper limits of the chart. At this point, the researcher has to make an ethical decision as to whether to stop the experiment, declare clinically for treatment B, and start it on all patients, or to continue the study to its formal conclusion. But as Armitage contends, "Even in the least favorable situation, the sequential plan is more economical than the non-sequential proce-dure"[16] (p. 46); on the whole, the patients have benefited from the choice of designs.

Bross has provided us with two forms, at .10 or .05, with power set at 0.7. He describes how to draw other forms.[17] Armitage has provided tables that will allow us to draw plans similar to the one in Figure 6-10a. An example of this format may be found in Gault and Spyker.[19]

Using these tables, α and β can be set at any desired level, as can θ, θ being

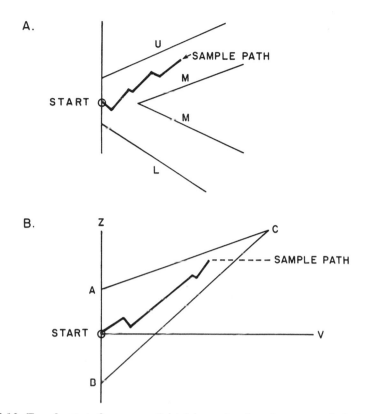

FIGURE 6-10. Two formats for sequential trials: *a.* Armitage's open-ended plot; *b* Whitehead's triangular test.

defined as the probability of deciding for either treatment A or B. The equations for this form are:

upper boundary $y = a_1 + bn$

lower boundary $y = -a_1 - bn$

upper middle $y = -a_2 + bn$

lower middle $y = a_2 - bn$

where a_1, a_2, $-a_1$, and $-a_2$ are tabled constants of the boundary intercepts on the y axis, and b and $-b$ are tabled values of the slopes of the lines. The quantity n is the number of pairs at each point.[16] Armitage's tables also provide the *average* number of preferences for A or B that are required over an imaginary series of pairs in order to reach significance.

Whitehead takes a considerably more complex mathematical approach to the statistical analysis of sequential clinical trials.[15] Simply stated, his triangular test requires the plotting of two statistics, Z and V. The basic formulas are:

$$Z = \frac{nS_m - mT_n}{m + n}$$

$$V = \frac{mn(S_m + T_n)\ [(m - S_m) + (n - T_n)]}{(m + n)^3}$$

where m is the number of patients receiving treatment A, n is the number of patients receiving treatment B, S_m is the number of successes for treatment A, and T_n is the number of successes for treatment B. These formulas are plotted on a graph like the one in Figure 6-10b. Significance levels or confidence intervals may be calculated, and provisions may be made for nominal, ordinal, or metric data.

REFERENCES

1. Gonnella, C. Designs for clinical research. *Physical Therapy* 53:1276–1283, 1973.
2. Hersen, M. and Barlow, D.H. *Single case experimental designs.* New York: Pergamon, 1976.
3. Parsonson, B.S. and Baer, D.M. The analysis and presentation of graphic data. In Kratochwill, T.R., *Single subject research.* New York: Academic Press, 1978, pp. 101–166.
4. Agnew, N.M. and Pyke, S.W. *The science game,* 3rd ed. Englewood Cliffs, NJ: Prentice-Hall, 1982.
5. Barlow, D.H. and Hersen, M. *Single case experimental designs,* 2nd ed. New York: Pergamon, 1984.
6. Campbell, D.T. and Stanley, J.C. *Experimental and quasi-experimental designs for research.* Chicago: Rand McNally, 1966.
7. Martin, J.E. and Epstein, L.H. Evaluating treatment effectiveness in cerebral palsy: Single subject designs. *Physical Therapy* 56:285–294, 1976.
8. Goodisman, L.D. A manipulation-free design for single-subject cerebral palsy research. *Physical Therapy* 62:284–289, 1982.
9. Kratochwill, T.R. Foundations of time-series research. In Kratochwill, T.R., *Single subject research.* New York: Academic Press, 1978, pp. 1–100.
10. Glass, G.V., Willson, V.L., and Gottman, J.M. *Design and analysis of time-series experiments.* Boulder: Colorado Associated University Press, 1975.
11. Wollery, M. and Harris, S.R. Interpreting results of single-subject designs. *Physical Therapy* 61:445–452, 1982.
12. Kazdin, A.E. *Single-case research designs.* New York: Oxford University Press, 1982.
13. Ostendorf, C.G. and Wolf, S.L. Effect of forced use of the upper extremity of a hemiplegic patient on changes in function. *Physical Therapy* 61:1022–1028, 1981.
14. Kazdin, A.E. Statistical analyses for single-case experimental designs. In Barlow, D.H. and Hersen, M., *Single case experimental designs,* 2nd ed. New York: Pergamon, 1984.
15. Whitehead, J. *The design and analysis of sequential clinical trials.* New York: Halsted, 1983.
16. Armitage, P. *Sequential medical trials,* 2nd ed. New York: John Wiley & Sons, 1975.
17. Bross, I. Sequential medical plans. *Biometrics* 8:188–205, 1952.
18. Light, K.E., Nuzik, S., Personius, W.P., and Barstrom, A. Low-load prolonged stretch vs. high-load brief stretch in treating knee contractures. *Physical Therapy* 64:330–333, 1984.
19. Gault, S.J. and Spyker, J.M. Beneficial effect of immobilization of joints in rheumatoid and related arthritides: A splint study using sequential analysis. *Arthritis and Rheumatism* 12:34–44, 1969.

7

PREEXPERIMENTAL, EXPERIMENTAL, AND QUASI-EXPERIMENTAL RESEARCH DESIGNS

Mark W. Cornwall and Paulette Murrell

INTRODUCTION

All of us formulate questions and seek to answer them. For example, we might consider an alternate route to work in order to save time. As physical therapists, we constantly ask questions regarding patient care. As with all questions, answers are sought, and because we believe the answers to our questions are important, we try to find correct ones. Any number of methods can be used to find the answers. We might utilize intuition, beliefs, colleague opinion, or previous experience and education. This chapter discusses the use of the scientific method in answering questions. It is not always necessary to use the scientific method. Often our common sense is correct. Unfortunately, this is not always the case, however. When mistakes occur (in patient care, in this case), our behavior is not always effective or efficient. The scientific method is not infallible, but, when used properly, it can eliminate the bias caused by personal opinions.

Before we can effectively apply the scientific method to our questions, we need a plan. This plan is called the *design*. Any research design has two primary purposes: (1) to answer the question, and (2) to control for any rival theories that might explain the results.[1] Research designs accomplish the second purpose through a series of maneuvers that minimize errors and maximize the validity of the experiment.[2] In addition to these two purposes, a research design provides organization and structure and enumerates the procedures and methods to be used. In this way, the design establishes the purpose of the study.

It is our intent to provide the reader with the basic design tools for proper scientific inquiry. These tools include an understanding of the principles of causation, control, and validity. Only after a thorough presentation of these concepts can a worthwhile discussion of specific research designs be considered.

CAUSATION

In general, the objective of any experiment is to demonstrate a "cause-and-effect" relationship between two or more variables or conditions. Let us consider a previous example. A person wishes to alter the route to and from work in order to save time. Such an experiment might involve a "test." The individual would test whether a particular route is faster than another. Based on the results of the test, the individual would either accept or reject the alternate route to work. Regardless of the outcome, the researcher in our example has assumed that there is a causal relationship between the route taken and the time required to get to work. This cause-and-effect relationship is central to experimentation. If there were no reason to think that there was a better route, the experiment would not have been attempted. Without the existence of a causal relationship, there can be no confidence in the results. A lack of confidence will negate any possibility of finding the correct answer.

Over the centuries, philosophers have debated the terms *cause* and *causality*. It is not our intent to present a lengthy discussion of the philosophical issues involved; they can be found elsewhere.[2] A brief outline of the principal tenets, however, is useful.

Neale and Liebert[3] identified four general types of causal relationships. The first is termed *necessary and sufficient*. In this situation, some factor or condition, X, is required to produce the effect, Y. In addition, the presence of X is adequate to produce Y. An example of this relationship is the presence of a specific chromosome that causes a particular eye color. The chromosome is both required and sufficient to produce the resulting eye color. When working in the behavioral sciences it is often difficult to find causal relationships that are both necessary and sufficient, because individuals vary in such things as their perception and interpretation of stimuli. Psychological and emotional factors such as motivation, level of arousal, anxiety, and fear may also differ among as well as between individuals. These elements also may interact with one another, thus further complicating the situation. This constant lack of uniformity causes a great deal of uncertainty when we try to draw conclusions concerning the cause of an observed response.

The second relationship is where X is *necessary but not sufficient* to produce Y. For example, it is necessary to prescribe exercises for muscle weaknesses, but the prescription alone is not enough for strength to improve. This relationship is frequently found in behavioral research when several factors work in concert to produce the effect.

Sufficient but not necessary is the third type of causal relationship. In this association X is only one of many causes of Y. Financial security may be a sufficient reason to recover following an injury, but it is not required. A great number of other factors will motivate individuals to accomplish the same task.

The final relationship is *contributory*. In this instance X is not necessary, and it is not sufficient to cause Y. X does, however, contribute to (or alters the likelihood of) the occurrence of Y. For example, poor nutrition is not required for, nor is it enough to cause, pressure sores. Poor nutrition does, however, increase the chance of acquiring a sore.

Scholars are not in total agreement about the exact nature of cause and effect when it is outside the realm of a well-controlled laboratory. Despite this lack of consensus, four common criteria for inferring cause have emerged: (1) the precedence of cause before the effect; (2) the use of a control group; (3) the concept of falsification; and (4) the need for replication. It is standard practice in scientific research first to administer the treatment and then to observe for any effect. Most agree that such a time sequence is a logical requirement for the demonstration of cause. In addition, a control group is considered essential if alternative interpretations of the results are to be eliminated. As is discussed later, the control group provides a standard against which the treatment effect can be compared. The third criterion is that cause is established not by confirming theories but by seeking to falsify them. At first, this statement may sound as if it is reversed, but it is not. It is simply easier to demonstrate that something is false than to show it is true. The principle of falsification is central to statistical hypothesis testing. Finally, cause-and-effect relationships should never be accepted on the basis of a single test. They should be determined by many tests. Replication of research is not only useful but essential to scientific inquiry. As is discussed later, these elements are prevalent in the more powerful research designs.

Explanations of cause may also vary according to the level of specificity. A cause established at one level may not prove sufficient at a more specific level. Consider the statement that "superficial heat causes the healing of contusions." More specifically, however, the physiological reactions created by the heat account for the healing. Each statement is correct, but at different levels of specificity. Usually, there are multiple levels at which cause can be established. The ultimate goal of research is to identify a phenomenon's cause at its lowest possible level, that is, with the most specificity.

CONTROL

Suppose a therapist is interested in the effect of a new exercise program on cardiovascular endurance. The researcher supposes that the observed change in the dependent variable (cardiovascular endurance) is the result of the independent variable (exercise). Although this causal relationship is assumed, how can the researcher be sure? Are there other factors that would produce the same result? A poorly designed experiment will fail to eliminate or correct for these rival explanations. By contrast, a well-designed study can establish that the proposed cause is the only possible explanation. This brings us to the concept of control.

Control in a research setting involves several different concepts. Cook and Campbell[2] identified three uses of the word *control*. The first concerns manipulating the experiment to rule out extraneous elements. Usually this means controlling the environment in which the study is conducted (test tubes, climate-controlled rooms, etc.). The amount of control is the significant issue, not whether there is control. All experimental designs employ control over the setting. It is the amount of control, however, that determines the strength of the causal relationship.

The second aspect of control that Cook and Campbell identify is direction over the administration of the experimental treatment. The researcher decides which subjects receive a particular treatment and when the treatment is received. Certainly, random assignment of treatments is one form of control. With random assignment of treatments, the researcher allows control to be determined by chance. For example, suppose that a person's motivational level influences compliance with a set of treatment conditions. In this case the researcher may elect to assign subjects randomly to each treatment condition. By randomly assigning the treatments, the groups can be assumed to be equivalent with respect to a number of factors, including motivation. Although random assignment is usually considered preferable, there are times when it is not possible. Treatment assignment is then determined completely by the investigator. Measurement of each subject for a particular trait or characteristic can be performed and assignment to treatment conditions based on this information. As we discuss later, causal inference can also be strengthened in such cases by utilizing a degree of control over the other aspects of the experiment. Regardless of the method used, control over treatment assignment helps to separate the effects as a result of the treatment from extraneous effects in the experiment.

The final situation in which control is used involves eliminating or ruling out threats to inference. This requires identifying a specific threat and then eliminating its influence on the dependent variable. The actual way in which the influence of the threat can be removed takes two different forms. The first involves considering how the procedures of the study are designed and subsequently implemented. A typical example might be to control for the effects of learning by having the subjects first participate in a practice session. The second form involves measuring the potential threat and then, during later data analysis, controlling its influence. An example of this procedure is the use of analysis of covariance (ANCOVA) to compensate for an extraneous variable such as subject age, weight, or pretest score. Statistical methods, however, are generally not effective in compensating for weaknesses in the experimental design. They should not be substituted for more stringent and effective methods such as randomization.[2]

In any discussion of control the concept of a control group should be addressed. In a control group the values of the independent variable are held at a base, or comparative, level.[4] Frequently a control group is thought of as receiving no treatments. This can be true, but a control group could equally consist of any baseline condition. A good example of the latter type of control group appears in the investigation of a new treatment program for stasis ulcers. In this study the investigator may elect to compare the new treatment to one that is already accepted as being reasonably effective. This allows comparison of the new treatment without compromising patient care by refusing treatment to a portion of the subjects.

In summary, control is the extent to which a researcher has freedom to manipulate the experiment. Control involves manipulating the research environment, the independent variables, and any extraneous variables that might offer alternate hypotheses. Control can also consist of holding constant the variables that are not of direct interest in the experiment, for example, a researcher may choose to study only subjects between the ages of 18 and 40 years. This is done not out of convenience but to eliminate the confounding effect that extreme age has on the dependent variable. Although holding independent variables constant provides an effective means of control, it limits the study's generalizability. The results cannot be applied to other conditions, populations, and so forth.

Another common method is to systematically vary a particular variable or set of variables. For example, speed of muscle contraction is known to influence peak muscle force. In this case a researcher may wish to control for speed of contraction in one of two ways. The study could be restricted to a single speed, or several discrete speeds could be selected. Either method has the effect of removing the variable's influence or allowing its comparison with other conditions.

It should be emphasized, again, that all research designs employ control. The element that distinguishes the various types of designs is the *amount* of control. As we will discuss later, the more control used, the more valid the inferences that can be made.

VALIDITY

Validity from a research design point of view is closely related to our discussion of cause and effect. In scientific research we can never know the truth; we can only know that which has not been ruled out as false. This brings us to the need for validity in the design of our experiment. Campbell and Stanley[5] propose that research design validity consists of two types: internal and external validity. Additional subdivisions for design validity have been proposed by Cook and Campbell.[2] For the purposes of this chapter, our discussion centers on the original definitions of Campbell and Stanley.[5]

Internal Validity

Internal validity asks the question, Did the treatment administered in this instance make a difference? Internal validity, therefore, relates to the amount of control imposed by the researcher. A study that controls the extraneous factors will invariably possess internal validity. Experiments with good internal validity successfully prevent the relationship between the independent and dependent variables from being confused or confounded.[6]

As a means of judging experimental designs, Campbell and Stanley[5] identify eight potential sources of internal invalidity, termed *threats*.

History

This threat arises from events (other than the treatment) that occur between successive measurements of the dependent variable. Obviously, the greater the length of time between measurements, the greater the chance that extraneous events will occur. Confounding events typically include alterations in the subject's environment.

For example, suppose a person wished to investigate the impact of an educational module on the physical therapist's knowledge of sexual dysfunction as a result of a spinal cord injury. History would become a threat to the study's internal validity if a portion of the subjects happen to have seen a television program on the topic between the pretest and posttest.

Maturation

This situation exists when the subjects themselves change. The threat is a function of the passage of time. The subjects may become hungrier, more tired, or even older. All of these threats can offer explanations of the results other than the administered treatment.

An example of this would occur if subjects in a strength development study participated in some form of physical exercise in addition to the treatment. In this case it would be impossible to determine if the observed strength gains were the result of the treatment or the extra physical activity.

Testing

The third threat to internal validity involves testing methods. It is entirely possible that the way in which the investigator tests for alterations in the dependent variable can bias the results. This situation should always be considered when the design involves a test-retest protocol.

Consider a study designed to demonstrate improvement in a physical skill after some form of treatment. Depending on the level of skill required, if a pretest-posttest methodology is used, all learning may occur with the first test, regardless of any treatment. In this situation the initial test could easily be the explanation for the improved scores.

Instrumentation

Changes in the measurement of the dependent variable can also influence the results. This threat can take the form of changes in calibration or sensitivity of the instrument. Changes in specific attributes of the testers can have a similar influence. Chapter 3 has extensively addressed measurement validity and reliability. It should be emphasized that unless the instrument used is reliable, it can offer an alternate explanation for the results.

Statistical Regression

Almost all measurements are imperfect. A single measurement on a subject will fluctuate around the individual's "true" score. This fluctuation is the result of such things as the person's mood, motivation, or fatigue. If a subsequent test is given, there is a high probability that the score will be less extreme (more toward the mean) than the previous measurement. Although this phenomenon is active with all subjects, the error in a single measurement tends to be in the direction of the extremity when an extreme group is used.[7] The tendency for individuals who score extremely high or low on a test to score closer to the average on subsequent administrations of the test is due to statistical regression. This principle applies specifically to research involving experimental groups selected on the basis of extreme scores. In such a situation the causal relationship between the independent and dependent variable is in doubt.

Let us consider an example of statistical regression. Suppose an investigator tests a large number of people in the ability to throw a ball and hit a target. Individuals who score in the bottom 10% are selected as subjects for a subsequent study. Following the administration of the treatment, the test is given again, and the subjects' scores have improved. The principle of statistical regression states that extreme scores will move (regress) toward the average of the whole group upon retesting. In the example, improvement would therefore be observed with or without the administration of the treatment.

Selection

Bias may be inadvertently introduced into an experiment during the selection of subjects. Consider subjects chosen for a study of stroke rehabilitation. Unless careful consideration is given to how the subjects are chosen, the groups may be different from the start. It is possible that the groups will differ from one another in age, diagnosis, motivation, and muscle tone. All of these factors have the potential of offering alternate explanations for the experimental outcome.

Mortality

Experimental mortality becomes a source of invalidity when subjects withdraw from the study. Although the comparison groups may have been equivalent at the start, they may not be at the conclusion of the study. Because of attrition, a situation can exist similar to that observed with improper subject selection. The groups are no longer equivalent. Experimental mortality results from voluntary withdrawal, disqualification, or death.

Interaction Among Factors

The final threat to internal validity is the interaction of two or more of the above threats. The resulting combination of multiple threats can effect a change in the dependent variable. This could then be mistaken as the treatment effect. This threat to internal validity constitutes an entire class of possible pitfalls in research design. As we discuss later, this type of threat is more prevalent in the multiple-group, quasi-experimental designs

Consider the situation in which a physical therapist wants to investigate a new cardiac rehabilitation protocol. The therapist selects two different hospitals in the area, and the program is initiated. If selection of the test site is not performed carefully, the selected individuals will differ in several aspects, such as age, diagnosis, other medical problems, and motivation. If the exercise program is lengthy and rather involved, subject motivation may be crucial. Those subjects with low motivation may have a strong tendency for noncompliance with the research protocol. If these subjects constitute the control group, a false positive effect will be shown because their lack of compliance will make the control group protocol appear less effective than it is. If they are in the experimental group, then a false negative effect would result because the experimental protocol will appear less effective than it is. In either case, the conclusions are biased. As demonstrated in this example, experimental compliance and selection can interact with each other, resulting in a mistaken treatment effect.

In theory, any of the previous seven threats can combine to confound the results of the study. Practically speaking, however, the only interaction that occurs frequently is between selection and maturation.[7]

External Validity

Now let us turn our attention to external validity, which involves the idea of generalizability. It asks the question, Can the results of this experiment be generalized to other populations, settings, treatments, or measurement variables?[1] Studies that possess good external validity can extrapolate the results beyond the limits set by the experiment. These studies successfully bridge the gap between the laboratory and the "real world." Clinical research strives for this quality. Campbell and Stanley[3] specifically identify four threats to external validity: (1) interaction of testing and treatment; (2) interaction of selection and treatment; (3) reactive effects of experimental arrangements; and (4) multiple treatment interference.

Interaction of Testing and Treatment

We have already discussed how testing can affect a study's internal validity. Testing methods can also jeopardize our ability to generalize the results. In this situation the testing procedure (usually a pretest) sensitizes the subjects to the particular treatment. The test might, therefore, increase or decrease the subject's performance on subsequent tests. In this way the results of the study could only be generalized to those situations where a pretest was given.

Such a situation might exist in a study of isokinetic strength. The measurement of a person's muscular strength is dependent upon the subject's familiarity with the equipment and whether practice trials are allowed prior to testing. If a novice were not allowed initial practice, the results could not be generalized to situations where practice had been given.

Interaction of Selection and Treatment

Just as the selection of subjects for the comparison groups can influence a study's internal validity, it can also affect external validity. If, for some reason, the subjects selected were unusually susceptible to the experimental treatment, the results obtained could not be extrapolated to a larger population.

For example, a study is designed to investigate attitudes toward individuals with disabilities. If, in the process of selecting respondents, it was found that a majority were health care professionals, the results of the study could not realistically be generalized to a broader group of people. Although the selection process did not limit the study's internal validity, its generalizability (external validity) is restricted. Thus it is possible for an investigation to be valid only within the confines of that study.

Reactive Effects of Experimental Arrangements

This threat involves the setting or environment used to conduct the experiment. A particular environment can influence the ability to generalize to other situations, settings, or conditions. Most individuals would agree that results obtained in a strictly controlled laboratory setting may not apply outside that laboratory; what is true in a laboratory is not necessarily the case in real life. The most dramatic example of this problem is found in animal research. Treatments found to be effective in mice or rabbits may or may not prove to be effective in humans.

Similar examples are found in physical therapy research. Therapeutic procedures that have been validated using predominantly young, healthy college students may not apply to other populations. This is certainly the case if the results are to be generalized to individuals who are sick or injured. A fairly good example would be the use of electromyography (EMG) to study the benefits of spinal traction for relaxation of muscle spasm. Despite the fact that EMG activity may decrease in normal, healthy subjects, similar results may not be obtained with a patient population.

Multiple Treatment Interactions

The final threat to external validity arises when several treatments are administered sequentially to the same subjects. In such a case early treatments may interact with subsequent ones to alter the subject's response. For example, patients might receive three different treatment procedures, the first being biofeedback; the second, exercise in the cardinal planes; and, finally, proprioceptive neuromuscular facilitation (PNF). It is conceivable that any benefit derived from one procedure would carry over to the next, thus confusing the issue of cause. It would be difficult to separate the effects of PNF from biofeedback, or the conventional exercise from biofeedback, and so on.

In addition to the four threats identified by Campbell and Stanley, other threats need to be considered. The principal ones to be considered are: (1) Hawthorne effect, (2) Rosenthal effect, (3) placebo effect, and (4) inadequate dependent variable selection.

Hawthorne Effect

This threat occurs when the effects of a treatment are either accounted for or confounded by the subject's knowledge of participation in the study.[1] Simply stated, if people are singled out and given special attention, they respond. Any perceived change in the experimental situation, any extra attention, or even the absence of treatment can therefore be sufficient to cause a change in the behavior of the subject.[8] The easiest way to avoid these threats is to "blind" the researcher, the subjects, or both as to what treatments are administered, as well as to when they are administered.

Rosenthal Effect

This threat exists when the researcher influences or modifies the subject's behavior through verbal and nonverbal cues or behaviors.[1] In addition, the researcher may have certain expectations about the outcome of the study. When such an influence exists, the research hypothesis becomes a "self-fulfilling prophecy." As previously stated, one way to control for this threat is to blind the subjects and the researcher concerning the experimental situations. Other techniques suggested to minimize this threat to external validity include replication either in another setting or with another researcher.

Placebo Effect

This threat often exists when a control condition is used and subjects are unaware that they are not receiving a treatment. In this situation it is possible for subjects to improve not because a treatment was administered but because they felt a treatment was administered and improvement would be the natural consequence. It is also possible for this effect to exist for any subject who is part of a treatment group. Again, the subject responds because he or she feels it is appropriate, not as a result of the treatment.

Inadequate Dependent Variable Selection

The final threat to external validity that we discuss here relates to the improper selection of the dependent variables. If the researcher selects a dependent variable that has little or no relevance to the real world, the results of the study will have no application, regardless of the outcome.

A good example might be a study that uses EMG biofeedback to improve ankle dorsiflexion in seated stroke patients. The researcher's overall intention is to use the protocol as a gait-training technique. Even if the treatment proved to be effective, the lack of a functional relationship between dorsiflexion while seated and during walking severely limits the extrapolation of the results to a clinical setting.

It should be emphasized at this point that the researcher should always strive for internal as well as external validity. This is true despite the fact that internal and external validity frequently disagree. An increase in one type of validity may jeopardize the other. Although both types of validity are sought, internal validity is considered to be the minimum. If a study does not have internal validity, the results of the experiment are uninterpretable.[1,5] Remember also that just because a design may have good internal validity, there is no guarantee that it will have external validity.[7] The two can be mutually exclusive.

NOTATION

The remainder of this chapter discusses three types of research designs. The specific strengths and weaknesses of each design will be presented. We have adopted a notation scheme similar to Campbell and Stanley[5] to represent each design. The symbol X is used to denote that a treatment has been administered; this could be an exercise program, a treatment modality, or an educational unit, among others. The symbol O represents an observation (measurement) of the experimental unit (subject) on the dependent variable(s). The sequence of events is designated to occur from left to right. For example, if subjects received a specific treatment and then are measured on the dependent variable, our notation would look like this:

X   O

In situations where the subjects are observed more than once, each observation will be represented by subscripts. Therefore, if two observations were made, the notation would be O_1 and O_2. For designs that employ more than one group of subjects, it is necessary to distinguish whether the groups are equivalent or nonequivalent. The symbol R is used to show that the subjects were randomly assigned to the particular group. If subjects are matched on a particular characteristic or set of characteristics, then the symbol M is used. In either situation, groups are assumed to be equivalent. The following example illustrates two equivalent groups, one of which received the treatment prior to observation:

R   X   O
R   O

Nonequivalent groups are illustrated by a horizontal dashed line. For example, the first situation, with nonequivalent groups, would look like this:

$$X \quad O$$
$$----------$$
$$O$$

It is now appropriate to introduce the various types of research designs. Again, we have decided to use the terminology of Campbell and Stanley[5] because of its universal acceptance. There are three basic types of designs: preexperimental, experimental, and quasi-experimental. The basic difference between the categories involves the amount of control each utilizes. This section presents and discusses specific research designs from each of the three types. In assessing a particular design, the primary consideration should be validity. If the design lacks validity, the results are automatically suspect, and little if any inference can be made about the results.

PREEXPERIMENTAL DESIGNS

Preexperimental designs are so named because they contain pieces of true experimental designs. These designs contain no built-in (satisfactory) controls and no random assignment of subjects. As a result, preexperimental designs contain numerous and serious threats to internal validity.[2] The preexperimental designs are not generally recommended, and, if used, a cautious use of the results is necessary, because there may be additional explanations for the observed results than the administered treatment. The designs do, however, provide a quick and easy method of data collection and may provide useful insights that can be incorporated into other designs. They are also worthy of discussion because of their frequent, as well as erroneous, use.

We will discuss three basic designs that fall under the heading of preexperimental design: the one-shot case study, the one-group pretest-posttest design, and the static-group comparison design.

One-Shot Case Study

In this design a treatment (X) is administered to a single subject or to a group of subjects, followed by an observation (O). A schematic representation would look like this:

X   O

For example, suppose an investigator wanted to study the effectiveness of an eccentric training program in decreasing the occurrence of hamstring muscle strains. First, the investigator might select a group of high school athletes for study. Each subject would then participate in a standardized training program, emphasizing eccentric muscle contraction. At the conclusion of the training period, the athletes would be observed during the course of their sports participation. The frequency of hamstring strains would then be used as the dependent variable. In this type of design there is no control group, and the design has almost a total absence of control over the threats to internal validity (Table 7-1). In our example there is no control over what happens to the subjects between the time the training period stops and when the athlete either is injured or completes the season. The type of sport or position played by the subject, as well as the frequency of participation in the sport, could alter the expected result. In addition, the subjects may change (e.g., in altered flexibility). These changes may also confound the results. Because there are many other explanations for the results, it is almost impossible to conclude that X caused O. The one-shot case study design might be useful during the pilot stage of an investigation but should never be used when the establishment or demonstration of a cause-and-effect relationship is desired.

One-Group Pretest-Posttest Design

In this design a group of subjects is administered a pretest (O_1). Then the treatment or event occurs. Finally, a posttest (O_2) is administered. The treatment effect is determined by the change in the pretest and posttest scores. The following is a schematic representation of the design:

O_1 X O_2

To illustrate the strengths and weaknesses of this design, suppose you want to know if occlusive dressings accelerate wound healing. A sample of all patients admitted for wound care to a local hospital during a specific period of time would be selected as subjects. As subjects are selected, the size of each patient's wound would be measured. The wound would then be treated using an occlusive dressing. Finally, at the end of the treatment period, the size of the wound would again be measured and compared to the initial value.

Because this design has no control group, it is subject to numerous threats to internal and external validity (Table 7-1). Problems similar to those of the one-shot case study exist relative to subject variation and to events or conditions present between wound measurements. Influences such as age or the general nutrition of the patients, as well as the presence of infection, are not controlled. Any of these, as well as numerous other variables, could provide plausible counter-interpretation of the results. Although this design is better than the one-shot case study, it is still considered a weak design and should not be used to demonstrate cause.

Static-Group Comparison Design

In this design a group that has received the treatment is compared to one that has not. At the end of the study, both groups are observed to assess the effect of the treatment. The following schematic illustrates this design.

X   O

O

TABLE 7-1. Control for Threats to Internal and External Validity

Preexperimental Designs

	Internal Validity								External Validity			
	History	Maturation	Testing	Instrumentation	Regression	Selection	Mortality	Interaction	Interaction of Testing and Treatment	Interaction of Selection and Treatment	Reactive Arrangements	Multiple Treatment Interactions
One-Shot Case Study	No	No				No	No				No	
One-Group Pretest-Posttest Design	No	No	No	No	?	Yes	Yes	No	No	No		?
Static-Group Comparison Design	Yes	?	Yes	Yes	Yes	No	No	No			No	

(Adapted from Campbell, D.T. and Stanley, J.C., *Experimental and Quasi-Experimental Designs for Research* [Boston: Houghton Mifflin Company, 1963]. Used with permission.)

The horizontal dashed line indicates that subjects were not randomly assigned. In this situation the groups cannot be assumed to be equivalent. Because of the similarities between the two designs, we illustrate this design with the same research question used in the one-shot case study: a therapist wishes to investigate the effectiveness of an eccentric training program on the occurrence of hamstring strain. In a static-group comparison design, two groups of subjects are selected for the study. One group undergoes the eccentric training while the other group does not. At the end of the study, the occurrence of muscle strains in each group is compared. An important element to remember is that no attempt is made by the investigator to ensure the two groups are equivalent. Subjects are not randomly assigned to the groups, nor are they matched on specific criteria.

The static-group comparison design corrects many of the deficiencies found in the one-shot case study. However, with no random assignment and no pretest to determine group equivalence, there are numerous threats to internal and external validity (Table 7-1). When the groups are not equivalent, it is highly likely that one group differs from the other. This difference may prevent a conclusion that the treatment caused the result. In our example, the flexibility of one group might have been superior to that of the other before the study began. The groups may also differ as to their skill or participation level. Any of these inequalities could ultimately confound the results.

Although not in widespread use, the static-group comparison is frequently employed in research where it is impossible or unethical to expose subjects to a risk. Examples include studies involving smoking or hazardous waste. It is important to remember, however, that the results of such studies do not establish a cause-and-effect relationship.

In summary, it is not possible with any of the preexperimental designs to ensure that the results can be attributed exclusively to the treatment. There are numerous rival and plausible explanations for the observed differences. For this reason, preexperimental designs should only be used in limited situations and certainly not to demonstrate cause.

EXPERIMENTAL DESIGNS

The preexperimental designs offer no certainty that the treatment is the true explanation for the observed results. Each of the preexperimental designs has numerous uncontrolled threats to internal validity.

In this section we present the *true* experimental designs. Such designs have built-in controls for threats to internal validity, thus providing sufficient evidence that the independent variables (treatment) were responsible for the observed differences in the dependent variable. Concepts important in this regard are (1) the selection of subjects, and (2) the assignment of subjects to groups.

Experimental designs are distinguished from other types of designs by three characteristics. First, all experimental designs involve one or more control groups, as well as one or more experimental groups. Second, experimental designs involve the random assignment of subjects (from the same initial population of interest) to the control and experimental group(s). As previously discussed, random assignment refers to any method in which every subject in the study has an equal chance of being assigned to any of the experimental groups. Finally, in an experimental design the variables of interest can be directly manipulated. These features, as well as appropriate instrumentation and procedures, permit the inference that the differences between the groups after the completion of the study were actually due to the treatment. In other words, these designs help rule out all, or almost all, rival explanations for the differences in the results.

There are three true experimental designs that we will examine: the *pretest-posttest control group design*, the *posttest-only control group design*, and the *Solomon four-group design*.

Pretest-Posttest Control Group Design

In this basic design two groups of subjects are compared relative to some measurement or observation (O). Both groups are measured twice, using a pretest and a posttest. The groups differ regarding what happens to the subjects between the pretest and the posttest: one group (experimental) receives a treatment, whereas the other group (control) does not. Actually, this design is of two types, each used for a particular reason. In the first, type A, subjects are randomly assigned to one of two groups, and both groups are administered a pretest. The experimental group receives the treatment, and after an equal amount of time both groups are administered the posttest. The following schematic depicts this type of design.

Type A: R   O   X   O
               R   O   O
                    Time →

In the second, type B, subjects are first pretested and subsequently matched and assigned randomly to either the experimental or the control group. The matching process can be done either with the observational (dependent) variable or with some other variable of interest. This allows a check on the adequacy of the randomization but does not necessarily guarantee group equivalence. As in type A, the experimental group receives the treatment and then both groups are administered the posttest after an equal period of time. The schematic below depicts this second type.

Type B: O   M   R   X   O
               O   M   R   O
                    Time →

Let us consider a study designed to determine the effectiveness of selected amino acids on the pain threshold of normal subjects. The subjects are randomly assigned to a treatment or a control group. The pain threshold level of each subject is initially determined (pretest). The treatment group subsequently receives the amino acid supplements for a specified time period. The control group is given a placebo during the same time period. After the treatment regimen has ended, the subjects are again measured for pain threshold level (posttest). The means from the two posttests are then used to determine what effect, if any, the amino acid supplements have on pain threshold.

Now consider the same study using design type B rather than type A. The subject's pain threshold or some other variable, such as age or body weight, would first be recorded. Subjects would then be grouped in pairs based on this pretest. Following this matching procedure, a subject in each pair would be randomly assigned to either the experimental or control group. The study would then proceed in the same manner as the type A design.

As can be seen by the chart in Table 7-2, both forms of the pretest-posttest control group design are effective and provide controls for most threats to internal validity.

Statistical Analysis

There are both correct and incorrect statistical procedures used with the pretest-posttest designs. For example, one correct method is the use of gain scores obtained by subtracting, for each subject, the pretest from the posttest. A mean gain score is then calculated for the experimental and control groups. The differences between the mean gain scores can then be properly tested using either

TABLE 7-2. Control for Threats to Internal and External Validity

Experimental Designs

	Internal Validity								External Validity			
	History	Maturation	Testing	Instrumentation	Regression	Selection	Mortality	Interaction	Interaction of Testing and Treatment	Interaction of Selection and Treatment	Reactive Arrangements	Multiple Treatment Interactions
Pretest-Posttest Control Group Design	Yes	Yes	Yes	Yes	Yes	Yes	Yes	Yes	No	?	?	
Posttest-Only Control Group Design	Yes	Yes	Yes	Yes	Yes	Yes	Yes	Yes	Yes	?	?	
Solomon Four-Group Design	Yes	Yes	Yes	Yes	Yes	Yes	Yes	Yes	Yes	?	?	

(Adapted from Campbell, D.T. and Stanley, J.C., *Experimental and Quasi-Experimental Designs for Research* [Boston: Houghton Mifflin Company, 1963]. Used with permission.)

a *t*-test for independent measures or a Mann-Whitney U test. If more than two groups are involved, then the procedure of choice becomes an analysis of variance (ANOVA). Another acceptable procedure is the use of analysis of covariance (ANCOVA), using the pretest scores as the covariate. According to Cook and Campbell,[2] if the subjects are randomly assigned, then the ANCOVA procedure provides a more precise test of the hypothesis. The greater precision is the result of reducing the error variance by including the pretest as a predictor of posttest scores.

In contrast, it is inappropriate to use a *t*-test for correlated measures to compare the difference between the pretest and posttest means of the experimental group and then a second *t*-test for correlated measures to compare the pre- and posttest means of the control group.[1] Another inappropriate procedure is the use of one *t*-test for independent measures to compare the two pretest means and then a second *t*-test for independent measures to compare the two posttest means.

Posttest-Only Control Group Design

In this design subjects are randomly assigned to a control group or an experimental group. No pretest is administered before the treatment, and both groups receive identical posttests. The following schematic illustrates this design.

```
R    X    O
R         O
     Time →
```

Consider a study designed to measure the effectiveness of a specific therapeutic intervention on the neuromotor development of mentally retarded children. The subjects are randomly assigned to an experimental group and a control group and are matched on particular criteria, such as gender and IQ. The experimental group then participates in the specified plan of intervention, and both groups are tested to determine the level of neuromotor development. Mean posttest scores are then used to determine if the therapeutic intervention program had any effect on neuromotor development. As can be seen in Table 7-2, the posttest-only control group design is effective in controlling for all threats to internal validity.

Statistical Analysis

The most widely used parametric statistical analysis is the *t*-test for independent measures to compare the mean posttest scores of the experimental and control groups. The nonparametric Mann-Whitney U test can also be used. As in all cases where more than two group means are to be compared, ANOVA procedures should be used. The use of ANCOVA with this design would not be appropriate.

Comparison of Designs with and Without a Pretest

The pretest-posttest control group design is used more frequently than the posttest-only control group design in many research areas, presumably because of certain advantages of the pretest. More specifically, a pretest is frequently used to test for group equivalence, and it permits a check on the randomization process.[3]

In addition, the pretest is used if the research situation requires the subject to possess some attribute crucial to the experiment and treatment conditions. Hence the pretest is administered before the experiment begins to provide necessary information about the subjects.

In other situations the posttest-only control group design is superior because of certain disadvantages of a pretest. As previously discussed, the testing condition (pretest) may sensitize the subjects and alter performance on subsequent testing. Such reactive and interaction effects can jeopardize the generalizability of the results beyond the immediate experimental situation.

Solomon Four-Group Design

This design, by allowing the effects of the pretest and the treatment to be determined separately, provides an effective method of managing the pretest problem. In this design subjects are randomly assigned to one of four different groups, two of which receive the treatment. One of the experimental groups and one of the control groups are pretested. All four groups are then posttested after the treatment is administered. This configuration can be visualized as a combination of the pretest-posttest and posttest-only control group designs. The schematic representation looks like this:

```
R    O    X    O
R    O         O
R         X    O
R              O
     Time →
```

To illustrate this design we use the previous example concerning therapeutic intervention and the neuromotor development of mentally retarded children. Subjects are randomly assigned to one of four different groups. Two of the groups are administered a pretest to determine the level of neuromotor development. One of these groups, along with a group that was not administered a pretest, participates in the specified therapeutic intervention. When the treatment sessions have been completed, all four groups are administered a posttest to measure the level of neuromotor development. Comparison of the means from each of the groups is made to determine exactly what effect the treatment and the pretest had on the posttest scores. The researcher is not only interested in the two treatment effects but also in the possible pretest interaction, which might influence the results. As can be seen in Table 7-2, this design is very effective in controlling all threats to internal validity.

The primary advantage of the Solomon four-group design is its ability to control for testing and its interaction with other threats. By controlling for reactive or interaction effects of testing, this design controls for one of the threats to external validity.

Statistical Analysis

The most widely used statistical analysis for the Solomon four-group design is a two-way ANOVA. Means for each of the four groups can then be simultaneously compared. Figure 7-1 shows how the design may be represented as a 2 × 2 table. The use of a two-way ANOVA allows the investigator to make three major comparisons. First, did the treatment (X) have an effect? Second, is there a difference between those subjects who received a pretest and those who did not? Finally, did the use of a pretest interact with the treatment? Not only is this efficient but an interaction effect could never be determined with a series of t-tests.

The Solomon four-group design points to a frequently used tactic of scientific research, the inclusion of two or more simultaneous independent variables in the study. Consider the hypothetical example of the effect of moist heat and massage on increasing blood flow to a limb. In this situation the researcher may have reason to believe that the duration of the treatment also affects blood flow. Instead of conducting two separate studies, the researcher expands the number of subjects in the study and tests the theory all at once. One way to accomplish this goal is to give half of the subjects either moist heat or massage for 10 minutes while the other half

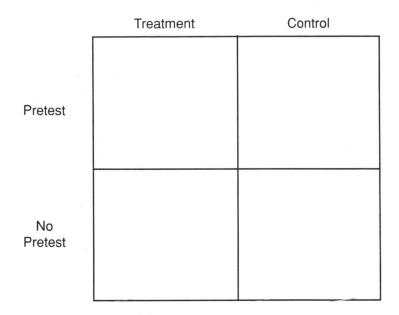

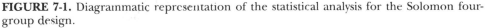

FIGURE 7-1. Diagrammatic representation of the statistical analysis for the Solomon four-group design.

receives the two treatments for 20 minutes. It is possible that blood flow is greater with moist heat for 10 minutes but that after 20 minutes the two treatments show similar results. Such a relationship would have remained hidden had the investigator not used the multiple variable approach.

QUASI-EXPERIMENTAL DESIGNS

Quasi-experimental designs also have one or more manipulated independent variables (treatments), outcome measures, and experimental units. In a quasi-experimental design, however, subjects are not randomly assigned to the different treatments or conditions. Quasi-experimentation evolved as a result of the reduced possibility for control in field settings and an unwillingness to continue to conduct tests in strictly controlled settings that were irrelevant to current practice. In addition, the alternatives to true experimental designs were very limited in their ability to infer causation.[2]

Without the benefit of random selection and assignment, threats to validity are increased in quasi-experimental designs. Without random assignment, these designs do, however, become more feasible for applied or field settings where randomization is impractical, impossible, or unethical. This is often the situation when doing clinical research. It would not be ethical to randomly assign patients to a control group where treatment would purposely be withheld. Quasi-experimental designs are also commonly used when subjects have already been formed into groups for social, educational, or economic purposes. For example, suppose you wanted to investigate the length of hospital stay following hip arthroplasty. Predetermined groups could be used by selecting patients based on diagnosis, sex, or the attending physician. Membership in these groups could not be randomly determined yet could still be compared using a quasi-experimental design.

Although the lack of random assignment makes the quasi-experimental design more feasible, it also makes it a weaker tool than true experimental designs for formulating solid causal inferences, because comparisons are based on "nonequivalent" groups. The groups differ in numerous ways other than the effects being measured. Cook and Campbell stated that the problem then becomes "interpreting the results and separating the effects of treatment from those due to the initial incomparability between the average units in each treatment group."[2] To solve this problem, the researcher must analyze the threats to validity that random assignment would have controlled and then take steps to correct them. The degree to which this happens, to a great extent, determines the inferences that can be drawn from the study.

There are two broad types of quasi-experimental designs: *pretest-posttest group designs* and *interrupted time-series designs*. In the pretest-posttest group design the subjects are typically those in whom responses of a treatment group and a comparison group are measured before and after a treatment. These designs involve an actual or simulated "between-subjects" comparison. For example, a comparison would be made between subjects who had received two different types of treatments. A comparison could also be made before and after the administration of some treatment. In this way the researcher controls when the subjects are observed and which subjects are administered the treatment.

Interrupted time-series designs involve successive observations of the subjects at various time intervals, before and after a treatment. This would be the case, for example, when several measurements are recorded during the course of a treatment program. Such designs involve "within-subject" comparisons, that is, repeated measurements of the subjects with the introduction of a treatment or treatments between measurements.

Our discussion of quasi-experimentation begins with the pretest-posttest group designs.

Nonequivalent Control Group Design

The design of the nonequivalent control group is similar to the true pretest-posttest control group design. The schematic representation of the design looks like this:

$$
\begin{array}{ccc}
O & X & O \\
\hline
O & & O
\end{array}
$$

The use of a horizontal dashed line denotes that the two groups of subjects are *not* equivalent; specifically, the subjects in each group have not been randomly assigned from a common population. This lack of randomization effectively distinguishes this design from the true pretest-posttest control group design. The non-equivalent control group design is frequently used in natural or field settings because it does not have the restrictions imposed by randomization.

Suppose a researcher wished to assess the effectiveness of a new exercise program for ataxic patients. The dependent (outcome) variable is the amount of time needed to move the patient's involved right arm from one position to another. Using the nonequivalent control group design, ataxic patients from a local clinic are assigned to one of two groups. The first group's movement time (MT) is tested, and then the group participates in the prescribed exercise program. The patients' MT is again measured at the conclusion of the treatment. The second group also receives a pretest and posttest of their speed of movement, but it does not receive the exercise program.

As can be seen from Table 7-3, the design is able to control most threats to internal validity. Although the potential for control exists with this design, the researcher must be very careful that selection, maturation, history, and regression do not confound the results. The most common threat is selection and its interaction with the other possible threats. The selection process creates two or more nonequivalent groups (they differ in more than one respect). Selection can interact with any of a number of other threats to preclude causal inference. The nonequivalent control group design is used frequently in social science research, and if it is applied with care, it yields satisfactory results.[2]

In an attempt to determine the degree of selection bias on causal inference, the pattern of results should be examined.[2,3] Figure 7-2 illustrates three possible outcome patterns when using nonequivalent control group designs. If the pretest scores of the treatment group are higher than those of the control group (Figure 7-2a), the experiment is seriously threatened by a selection-maturation interaction. As this applies to our example, it is possible that, compared to the subjects in the control group, the subjects in the treatment group were less involved and therefore may be progressing at a more rapid rate. As a result of this inequality, the result of the posttest might be explained by the differences in pretest scores rather than by any superiority of the new exercise program. Figure 7-2b illustrates a case where the two groups begin with virtually identical pretest values. This case is much more favorable to an unambiguous interpretation because there is reduced plausibility that the posttest differences occurred as a result of initial differences. The least ambiguous interpretation would be when the treatment group scored lower than the control group (Figure 7-2c). For example, if the new exercise group began with slower MT values than the control group, it would be highly unlikely that they had an advantage or were maturing at a faster rate.

Statistical Analysis

A number of statistical methods are available to analyze nonequivalent control group designs. Regardless of the analysis chosen, the greatest problem is in separating the treatment effect from the effect of selection differences. Because the groups are assumed to be nonequivalent, the chosen analysis must properly control for these initial differences. The four most common and simple methods of

TABLE 7-3. Control for Threats to Internal and External Validity

Quasi-experimental Designs

	History	Maturation	Testing	Instrumentation	Regression	Selection	Mortality	Interaction	Interaction of Testing and Treatment	Interaction of Selection and Treatment	Reactive Arrangements	Multiple Treatment Interactions
	Internal Validity								*External Validity*			
Nonequivalent Control Group Design	Yes	Yes	Yes	Yes	?	Yes	Yes	No	No	?	?	
Separate-Sample Pretest-Posttest Design	No	No	Yes	?	Yes	Yes	No	No	Yes	Yes	Yes	
Simple Interrupted Time-Series Design	No	Yes	Yes	?	Yes	Yes	Yes	Yes	No	?	?	
Interrupted Time-Series with a Nonequivalent Control Group Design	Yes	Yes	Yes	Yes	Yes	Yes	Yes	Yes	No	No	?	
Interrupted Time-Series with Removal Design	Yes	Yes	Yes	Yes	Yes	Yes	Yes	Yes	No	?	No	No
Interrupted Time-Series with Multiple Replications Design	Yes	Yes	Yes	Yes	Yes	Yes	Yes	Yes	No	?	No	No

(Adapted from Campbell, D.T. and Stanley, J.C., *Experimental and Quasi-Experimental Designs for Research* [Boston: Houghton Mifflin Company, 1963]. Used with permission.)

analysis in this regard are (1) elementary ANOVA, (2) ANCOVA, (3) ANOVA with blocking or matching, and (4) ANOVA with gain scores. In most cases a *t*-test for independent measures or Mann-Whitney U test may be substituted for the ANOVA when only two means are to be compared. Again, it is not proper to use multiple *t*-tests for correlated measures to compare the pretest and posttest means for each group, or to use one *t*-test for independent measures to compare the two pretest means and a second *t*-test for independent measures to compare the post-test means.[1]

Although each of the four statistical tests is considered correct, each has specific strengths and weaknesses. Any of the procedures can be biased under different circumstances. It is beyond the scope of this discussion to present the various biases of each analysis method. The reader is encouraged to consult the excellent review by Cook and Campbell[2] for additional information. Suffice it

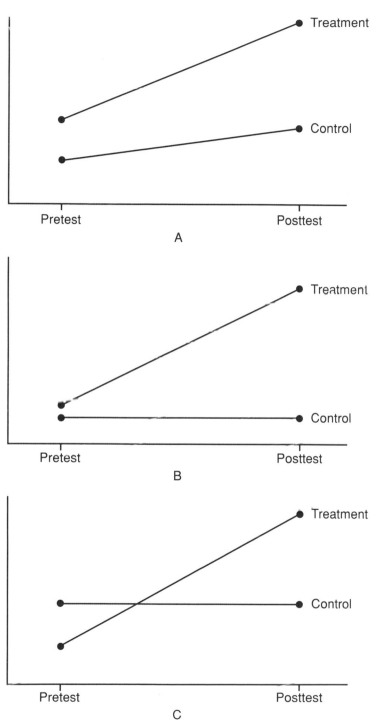

FIGURE 7-2. Three hypothetical results of a pretest-posttest nonequivalent control group design. (Adapted from Neale, J.M., and Liebert, R.M., *Science and Behavior: An Introduction to Methods of Research*, 3rd ed. [Englewood Cliffs, NJ: Prentice-Hall, 1986].)

to say that no analysis can be applied automatically and blindly to any design. The characteristics and likely biases of each method should be considered prior to interpretation of the results.

Separate-Sample Pretest-Posttest Design

This type of design category is frequently utilized in situations where randomization of individual subjects cannot be easily obtained. It is therefore useful in studying large, discrete populations, such as cities, schools, factories, or hospitals. The cities, schools, factories, or hospitals are randomly selected, rather than the individuals, thus becoming the experimental unit.

The schematic representation for this design would look like this:

R   O   X
R   X   O

Notice that the groups are considered equivalent since random assignment is used. Although each group receives the treatment, the timing will vary. Because the first group is exposed to the treatment after being observed, it is irrelevant to the research question.

An example may help to illustrate this design. Suppose a researcher wanted to assess physical therapists' attitudes toward the professional code of ethics. The hypothesis also involves the use of a special educational videotape. To circumvent the need for all therapists to answer a lengthy questionnaire twice or become sensitized by a pretest, two subgroups of therapists are randomly selected. One of these equivalent groups completes the questionnaire a week before viewing the videotape. The second group fills out the questionnaire a week after viewing the videotape. By using this design, the researcher is able to assess whether the videotape altered the therapists' attitudes concerning the professional code of ethics.

Table 7-3 shows that the design adequately controls for such threats to internal validity as testing, regression, and selection. Its greatest weaknesses, however, are in the areas of history, maturation, and mortality. Each of these threats involves extraneous events that occur prior to viewing the videotape and can account for observed changes in attitude. Changes in therapist attitudes might be influenced by a highly publicized medical malpractice suit just prior to viewing the video or during the time the posttest was administered. This design also fails to control adequately for subject mortality. If a considerable number of therapists drop out of the study or are not posttested, the results will be confounded. The longer the time interval between the various stages of the study, the greater this threat becomes.

As we mentioned, the various groups were randomly selected and therefore equivalent. If randomization had not been used, the threats discussed for nonequivalent group designs would also exist. The separate-sample pretest-posttest design has very good external validity, because fewer demands are made on subjects in a natural setting than would be made in a laboratory. The trade-off for this generalizability, however, is the design's weak internal validity. Additional variations of this particular design exist, and those interested should consult Campbell and Stanley.[5]

Statistical Analysis

This type of quasi-experimental design can be appropriately analyzed using either the nonparametric Mann-Whitney U test or the parametric *t*-test for independent measures. An appropriate ANOVA design should obviously be used when the study involves comparison of more than two groups.

Interrupted Time-Series Designs

We now focus on specific examples of interrupted time-series designs. There are several designs grouped in this classification. We present and discuss four of the more common ones in this chapter: (1) *simple interrupted time-series*, (2) *interrupted time-series with a nonequivalent control group*, (3) *interrupted time-series with removal*, and (4) *interrupted time-series with multiple replications*. As with any of the interrupted time-series designs, the central feature is that the ongoing flow of events, including observations, is interrupted by the introduction of a treatment at a specific point in time.[3] Although our schematic representations of these designs show a discrete number of observations either before or after the treatment is introduced, any number may be employed. In addition, the treatments may be temporary (introduced briefly and then removed), or they may be continuous (remain in effect during subsequent observations). For most of our discussion, we assume that the treatment is continuous. All of these designs may be used with small or large groups, as well as with single subjects, because the logic is the same. Our discussions, however, will concern only groups of subjects. Single subject designs present unique problems and the reader is encouraged to consult chapter 6 in this text.

Simple Interrupted Time-Series Design

We saw the simplest form of an interrupted time-series design earlier in the chapter when we discussed the one-group pretest-posttest design. As we discussed, that design is weak and has little causal value. A major improvement to the design, however, is the simple interrupted time-series design. Campbell and Stanley[5] refer to this as the time-series design. Schematically it is represented like this:

$$O_1 O_2 O_3 \; X \; O_4 O_5 O_6$$

As you can see, a series of observations on the dependent variable is made before and after the treatment. The treatment can be introduced at any point in the series, but the design is strengthened significantly if its position is determined randomly.

Consider a hypothetical example in which a therapist wishes to investigate the effectiveness of biofeedback on resting heart rate of cardiac patients. Using a simple interrupted time-series design, each patient's resting heart rate is recorded each week for six weeks. At the conclusion of the six-week period, the subjects are placed in a biofeedback training program. Following the training period, the subjects' resting heart rates are again measured each week for six weeks. If we were to diagram this study it would look something like this:

$$O_1 \, O_2 \, O_3 \, O_4 \, O_5 \, O_6 \;\; X_{biofeedback} \;\; O_7 \, O_8 \, O_9 \, O_{10} \, O_{11} \, O_{12}$$

From Table 7-3 we observe that the greatest threats to the design's internal validity come from history and instrumentation. History is the greatest threat because it is difficult to control the events that transpire following the introduction of the treatment. In our example, it might be that a particularly stressful public event, such as a natural disaster or military conflict, occurred soon after the implementation of the biofeedback program. If the event were stressful enough, the patients' resting heart rates might increase rather than decrease as expected. The influence of history may be minimized by decreasing the timespan between the treatment and subsequent observations. Increasing the number of observations will also serve to minimize the influence of historical events on the internal validity.

Instrumentation becomes a threat to internal validity when it leads to instability of the dependent variable(s). If the variation of the dependent variable is large, then changes in the posttreatment scores will be very difficult to determine.

Interrupted Time-Series with a Nonequivalent Control Group Design

If a control group is added to the previous design, the majority of problems related to history can be controlled. The diagram for this design, which Campbell and Stanley[5] call a *multiple time-series design*, is shown below.

$$O_1 \, O_2 \, O_3 \; X \; O_4 \, O_5 \, O_6$$
$$\overline{O_1 \, O_2 \, O_3 \qquad O_4 \, O_5 \, O_6}$$

Using our previous example, a second group of patients would have their heart rates recorded for 12 weeks without participating in the biofeedback program. As in most designs, we do not receive something for nothing. Because the groups are not equivalent, the threats to validity posed by subject selection become real. The design, therefore, suffers from all of the same threats that the nonequivalent control group design did. The interrupted time-series with a nonequivalent control group design is, however, much stronger than the simple interrupted time-series design. Some researchers even consider it the strongest of the quasi-experimental designs.[1]

Interrupted Time-Series with Removal Design

This design was termed the *equivalent time-samples design* by Campbell and Stanley.[5] In this design baseline measurements are recorded and a treatment introduced. After a specified length of time, the treatment is removed and the baseline values are again measured. Graphically, the design would look like this:

$$O_1\ O_2\ O_3\ \ X\ \ O_4\ O_5\ O_6\ \ \bar{X}\ \ O_7\ O_8\ O_9$$

The X with a horizontal bar over it denotes that the treatment has been removed. The intent of this design is to demonstrate that the observational variables change with the introduction of the treatment and then return to the original values when the treatment is removed. If such a pattern exists, there is little doubt that the treatment caused the change, not chance or some uncontrolled factor.

As an example, consider a study on the influence of an ankle-foot orthosis (AFO) in the prevention of excess knee flexion during gait. A group of patients with flaccid instability of the knee joint during the stance phase of gait is first selected. The amount of knee flexion during the walking cycle of several trials is recorded. At this point, each patient is fitted with the AFO and serial measurement of knee flexion is again recorded. After this second measurement period, the AFO is removed and a third set of knee flexion measurements is performed. If the AFO is beneficial in preventing excess knee flexion during gait, we should see that pattern with the introduction of the brace. When the brace is removed, excess knee flexion should again be evident in the patient's gait cycle.

The greatest advantage of this type of design is that the threat of history is reduced because, to be relevant, the historical threat must operate in different directions and at different times.[2] As presented in Table 7-3, this design has excellent potential for controlling all types of internal validity. Threats of cyclical maturation (regular up and down cycles, regardless of a treatment) may be further minimized by randomly determining when the treatment will be introduced and removed.[2]

It should be cautioned that great care needs to be taken before adopting a design that involves the removal of a treatment. First of all, there is the question of ethics. It may be unethical to remove a treatment from a patient in order to observe what effect that will have. Second, the treatment must be introduced fairly quickly so its effects can be measured. Treatments whose application is prolonged and whose effects are not immediate are not well suited for this design. The treatment effect must also be transient so as to demonstrate the effect of its removal.

Interrupted Time-Series with Multiple Replications Design

A modification of the previous design yields this fourth and final design. This design employs multiple replications of introducing and removing the treatment. In effect, it becomes a series of interrupted time-series with removal designs. Diagrammatically it is represented as:

$$O_1\ O_2\ \ X\ \ O_3\ O_4\ \ \bar{X}\ \ O_5\ O_6\ \ X\ \ O_7\ O_8\ \ \bar{X}\ \ O_9\ O_{10}$$

Again, the horizontal bar over the X denotes that the treatment has been removed and the conditions have reverted to what they were before introducing the treatment. This design is a powerful tool for inferring cause, especially if random distribution is used to rule out cyclic maturation.

The design has two major disadvantages, however. First, the treatment effects must be expected to dissipate rapidly. If there is any persistence in the effect following treatment removal, it will be difficult to demonstrate its effect on subsequent introductions. Second, the design requires a large amount of control by the experimenter and is therefore poorly suited for settings outside of the laboratory.[2]

With respect to external validity, all of the interrupted time-series designs show significant weaknesses. It is possible that the effects demonstrated are only applicable to those subjects tested in the study. The greatest threat to generalizability, however, is the interaction of testing and treatment. This is most evident where there is a learning effect due to repeated testing. Despite these limitations, the interrupted time-series designs are very sensitive and provide a good substitute for situations where the true experimental designs are impractical or unfeasible.[1]

Statistical Analysis

The initial phase of data analysis for any of the interrupted time-series designs is to represent the data graphically. The researcher should then carefully note any abrupt change in the outcome variable(s) and their relationship to the introduction or removal of the treatment. Figure 7-3 illustrates six hypothetical outcomes of interrupted time-series designs. The results diagrammed in patterns A and B would have the greatest legitimacy for inferring cause. Case A is likely to be seen if the treatment was continuous or if its effects did not quickly decay. Pattern B is representative of a temporary treatment or one whose effect is transient. Results similar to patterns C and D are less likely to be the result of the treatment. The change in C occurred after O_4 and may or may not be a function of the treatment. Pattern D appears to show an increasing trend regardless of any treatment. This is typical of maturational effects. An extreme case of this is pattern E. The final pattern, F, shows no consistent baseline prior to or following treatment. Causal inference in such a case is totally unjustified.[5]

From the standpoint of significance testing, graphic representation of the data is not sufficient. Because of the nature of interrupted time-series designs, conventional significance tests are both inadequate and inappropriate.[2] Several researchers have advocated the use of an autoregressive integrated moving average (ARIMA) model.[1,2] A more detailed explanation of this model and its use is beyond the scope of this chapter. Readers who are interested in using interrupted time-series designs should consult the works of Cook and Campbell[2] and Box and Jenkins.[9]

SUMMARY

In this discussion of the various research designs, we have emphasized the importance of demonstrating a cause-and-effect relationship between the treat-

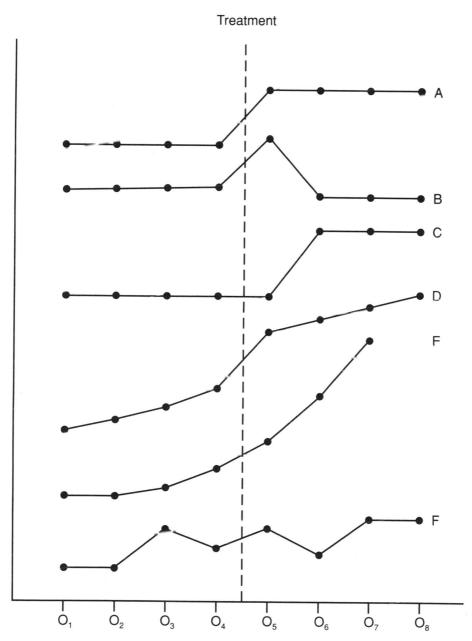

FIGURE 7-3. Six possible outcome patterns resulting from interrupted time-series designs. (Adapted from Campbell, D.T. and Stanley, J.C., *Experimental and Quasi-Experimental Designs for Research* [Chicago: Rand McNally College Publishing, 1963].)

ment and outcome variables. Because causation may be demonstrated in several different ways, the key to any research is the investigator's ability to demonstrate that the change in the dependent variable was only the result of the treatment. When an investigation is able to demonstrate this cause-and-effect relationship successfully, it is said to have *internal validity*. If the results can be inferred beyond the constraints of the study, it is said to possess *external validity*. Both types of validity are important, but unless the design first has internal validity, external validity is meaningless. Central to our discussion of causation and validity was the concept of experimental control. Several different methods of control were presented, as well as the utility and importance of a control group.

As each of the research designs was presented, the various threats to its internal and external validity were enumerated and discussed. As a general rule, preexperimental designs have the least control and lack significant internal validity.[1] Experimental designs, by contrast, have the most control. They possess good internal validity but as a group have less external validity than other designs.[1] The greatest single feature of experimental designs is the use of randomization. Given enough subjects, random assignment of subjects ensures that the average subject in each group is the same. The groups can therefore be considered equivalent and the effect of treatments more easily determined.[2]

Quasi-experimental designs employ more control than does a preexperimental design, but they do not have the strict limitations imposed by true experimental designs. Like the preexperimental designs, they generally involve nonequivalent groups. Although extraneous variables are not controlled in the same manner as experimental designs, they do exert control in three distinct ways. They control when the observations (measurements) are made, who receives the treatment, and when the treatment is administered.[1] In this way causation is enhanced. Because quasi-experimental designs do not, as a rule, randomly assign subjects, the threats that would have been controlled by randomization must be handled specifically by the researcher.[2] As a group, quasi-experimental designs have the potential for greater external than internal validity.

The final question to be asked is, Which design is the best? This is not an easy question to answer. Each design has assets and liabilities. It is, therefore, the responsibility of the investigator to make that choice based on information about the subjects to be used and the measurements to be taken. Slater put it this way:

> Given the objective of the study, the nature of the setting, subjects, measurement and the anticipated utility of the findings for future practice, it is necessary to select the experimental design which maximizes internal validity, external validity or if desired, both.[6]

REFERENCES

1. Huck, S.W., Cormier, W.H., and Bounds, W.G. *Reading statistics and research.* New York: Harper & Row, 1974.

2. Cook, T.D. and Campbell, D.T. *Quasi-experimentation: Design and analysis issues for field settings.* Boston: Houghton Mifflin, 1979.

3. Neale, J.M. and Liebert, R.M. *Science and behavior: An introduction to methods of research,* 3rd ed. Englewood Cliffs, NJ: Prentice-Hall, 1986.

4. Spector, P.E. Research designs. In Sullivan, J.L. and Niemi, R.G., eds., *Series: Quantitative applications in the social sciences.* Beverly Hills, CA: Sage Publications, 1981.

5. Campbell, D.T. and Stanley, J.C. *Experimental and quasi-experimental designs for research.* Chicago: Rand McNally College Publishing, 1963.

6. Slater, S.B. The design of clinical research. *Journal of the American Physical Therapy Association* 46(3):265–273, 1966.

7. Mason, E.J. and Bramble, W.J. *Understanding and conducting research: Applications in education and the behavioral sciences.* New York. McGraw-Hill, 1978.

8. Kerlinger, F.N *Foundations of behavioral research,* 2nd ed. New York: Holt, Rinehart and Winston, 1973.

9. Box, G.E.P. and Jenkins, G.M. *Time-series analysis: Forecasting and control.* San Francisco: Holden-Day, 1976.

8

QUESTIONNAIRE DESIGN AND USE

Katherine F. Shepard

QUESTIONNAIRES FOR A CAPTIVE AUDIENCE

INCREASING THE RETURN RATE

THE DELPHI TECHNIQUE:
CONSENSUAL DATA GATHERING BY QUESTIONNAIRE
    Advantages of the Delphi Technique

CONCLUSION

The most popular data-gathering tool used in survey research is a written questionnaire. The questionnaire is designed to gather information about people's knowledge, perceptions, attitudes, and beliefs, as well as facts such as demographic data about people or organizations.[1] The creation and effective use of a questionnaire as a data-collection tool is surprisingly difficult. There are two major problems: first, designing a reliable, valid questionnaire instrument; and second, convincing people who have no vested interest in your research to respond willingly, promptly, and honestly. The purpose of this chapter is to present ideas about when it is appropriate to use a questionnaire for data collection and how to design and use questionnaire instruments.

SURVEY RESEARCH—QUESTIONNAIRE OR
PERSONAL INTERVIEW?

There are distinct advantages and disadvantages to using both written questionnaires and person-to-person interviews to collect descriptive data. The choice of method rests upon your answer to the question, What specific information do you want to gather that will help you answer your research question? Demographic data? Knowledge? Opinions? Attitudes? Reported behaviors? Perceptions?

After you have decided what type of information you want to gather, the choice between a questionnaire and an interview is relatively simple. If you want focused, limited data, such as demographic data or opinions about certain events or phenomena, and if you can identify the possible scope of likely responses, use a questionnaire. Use an interview to acquire data if the possible scope of responses is unknown or for in-depth data concerning select individuals' knowledge, perceptions, or feelings. Thus, for example, if you were interested in sex and salary differences among physical therapists in the United States, you would probably use a questionnaire.[2] If you were interested in why it is difficult to locate and retain attendants for disabled individuals and had little idea as to the scope of reasons (lack of knowledge about disabilities? lack of training in activities of daily living [ADL] skills? low salary? emotional drain? perceived low status value of the work?), you would probably use an interview.[3]

TABLE 8-1. Advantages and Disadvantages of Mail Questionnaire and Person-to-Person Interview in Survey Research

Questionnaire	*Person-to-Person Interview*
Advantages	
1. Can secure responses from a broad spectrum of people	1. Can get considerably more and richer data from each subject
2. Lessens interviewer effect on subject Do not need to train interviewers	2. Can get more valid results by use of follow-up probe questions (results reflect respondents' view of reality, not researcher's predetermined view of reality)
3. Costs less than interview in both time and money	3. Can control response rate
4. Protects respondents' anonymity	4. Better choice than questionnaire for subjects who are young, old, minimally educated, or speak a different language
5. Can gather data from a large sample in a short period of time	5. Can observe nonverbal behaviors to guide pacing of threatening questions and to help validate candor of verbal responses
Disadvantages	
1. Little control over respondent return rate	1. Requires trained interviewers
2. Cannot ensure valid responses	2. Time-consuming and costly for interviewer and respondent
3. No possibility for follow-up to ensure respondent understood question or would have given a different response from choices posed in a closed-ended question	3. Not enough quantitative data to use analytical statistics, thus cannot generalize results to a population

There are other differences between questionnaires and interviews and other reasons why you would use a written questionnaire versus a person-to-person interview. See Table 8-1 for a compilation of advantages and disadvantages of each of these survey techniques.

You may want to consider using *both* an interview and a questionnaire to collect survey data. For example, if you are unsure what possible questions and choices should be included in a questionnaire, you may wish to interview a small, representative subsample of the population you plan to study. From this subsample data, you would select the questions and identify possible choices for answers to each question to be used in the questionnaire. To illustrate, suppose you wanted information from a broad spectrum of physical therapists and therefore were going to distribute your questionnaire to a sample of physical therapists listed in the American Physical Therapy Association Membership Directory. To define a subsample of this group to interview, you might include men and women who were both experienced and inexperienced therapists and who worked in different practice settings.

When Ballin et al. were working on their questionnaire design to determine the extent of research involvement by clinical physical therapists, they used this subsample interview technique.[4] By asking their subsample such questions as, "Why do you think clinical physical therapists should or should not be doing research?" and "What things make it difficult for you as a practicing therapist to be involved in research?" they were able to generate an extensive list of possible responses to include in their questionnaire. This strategy helps to ensure the design of a valid questionnaire (all possible responses are present for the respondents to choose from) and decreases the possibility of large data clumping under an "other" category.

Both questionnaires and interviews may be used in the same study to obtain different data most efficiently and validly from the sample under study. For example, in a study by Stapleton et al., an interview was used to collect data on coaches' perceptions of their responsibilities and abilities regarding the health care of high school athletes.[5] In individual interviews, coaches were asked, among other questions, "Describe your responsibility in providing your athletes with rehabilitation care." At the end of the interview, the coaches were asked to report specific facts by filling out a short questionnaire that included demographic variables, such as the coach's experience and education, and the type of health care personnel who were involved in treatment of injured athletes in the coach's high school.

LOCATING A QUESTIONNAIRE

Most survey research is performed one time only, that is, a survey instrument is designed for and administered during the life of one study alone. Because of this, there are few, if any, instruments already designed and validated that are available for collecting the specific information you want from the designated group of subjects from which you want it. The exception to this is standardized scales of self-reported public attitudes, perceptions, and behaviors. If you are interested in gathering data on generalized attitudes or behaviors, refer to the *Mental Measurement Yearbook,* a compilation of all currently published and available standardized scales.[6] Information on each scale includes a description of the scale content and design, any reliability and validity studies that have been performed on the scale, normative data for the scales, and where to write to obtain copies of the scale. If you are unable to find an instrument that meets your particular needs, you must assume the major task of questionnaire instrument design.

QUESTIONNAIRE DESIGN

Writing good questions entails constant revision. One of the biggest mistakes made by researchers new to survey research is to assume that questionnaire construction is a simple, straightforward process. It is no more simple or straightforward than is organizing any kind of research instrumentation that must fit the constraints of reliability and validity in order to be considered an acceptable research tool. Each question may be revised up to a dozen times before you are ready for the final printing and distribution of your questionnaire. During this winnowing process, your questions become more precise, less relevant questions are deleted, and the response categories shift in quantity and breadth.

In your questionnaire, *each* question asked must be vitally important to the purpose of your study. Remember, the longer the questionnaire, the less likely your subjects will be to respond. Each question must stand alone in relevance and clarity. The challenge you assume when creating a superb questionnaire will stretch your understanding and skills not only in the desired subject matter itself but also in the use of language, cognitive processing, and social psychology.

Content of Questions

In deciding the content of your questions, you should seek out and be responsive to as many different resources as possible: prior research findings reported in the literature, questions posed on survey instruments even dimly related to your idea, brainstorming with your colleagues, interviewing a subsample of the population you wish to study (as previously described), and pilot studies. Through this process of information gathering, reflecting, and revision, your questions will become clearer and easier to answer. This process is of critical importance because the clearer your questions are, the closer each respondent comes to interpreting your questions in the same way (internal validity).

Researchers undertaking survey research should strongly consider establishing conceptual and operational (statistical) hypotheses to guide their data collection and analysis. Conceptual hypotheses clearly define the various domains of information you wish to study. For example, suppose you wanted to know if physical therapy administrators perceived differences between clinicians with baccalaureate degrees and clinicians with entry-level master's degrees. You might decide that the following information may yield a difference in perception: the administrator's own educational background, the amount of contact the administrator has had with students from different educational backgrounds, and the amount of contact the administrator has had with clinicians from different educational backgrounds. These three factors would become three domains of information. Each of these domain factors would be turned into a conceptual hypothesis. One such hypothesis might be: "Administrators with postbaccalaureate degrees have higher expectations of master's degree-prepared physical therapists than do administrators without postbaccalaureate degrees."

From each conceptual hypothesis, one or more specific operational or statistical hypotheses can be generated. One example of a specific operational hypothesis that could be generated under the conceptual hypothesis stated above would be: "Administrators with postbaccalaureate degrees will have significantly higher expectations of competence in clinical problem solving for master's degree-prepared therapists than for baccalaureate degree-prepared therapists." A number of additional operational hypotheses regarding different areas of competence in clinical practice could be generated. Such specific, directly testable, operational hypotheses assist in defining the *specific* information you wish to gather through your survey questions. The responses generated from these questions will be the data you use to accept or reject your operational hypotheses (and ultimately your conceptual hypotheses).

See Display 8-1 for an example of the relationships between a research question, conceptual and operational hypotheses, survey questions, and proposed data analysis taken from a survey research proposal.[7] The thought process of creating this guiding framework is not a linear, step-forward process. The researcher works back and forth between the hypotheses and questionnaire items, synchronizing and clarifying the content relative to the research question, searching for a tight and relevant fit among all parts of the guiding framework. The beauty of this process is that you can both determine what questions are lacking in the questionnaire and decide which questions are superfluous and need deleting. Equally important, your operational hypotheses become the road map that will guide you in analyzing your data.

DISPLAY 8-1
EXAMPLE OF A FRAMEWORK FOR A SURVEY RESEARCH PROPOSAL:
THE RESEARCH QUESTION, EXAMPLES OF GUIDING CONCEPTUAL AND
OPERATIONAL HYPOTHESES, RELATED QUESTIONNAIRE QUESTIONS, AND
PROJECTED DATA ANALYSIS

KEY: RQ = Research Question
      CH = Conceptual Hypothesis
      OH = Operational Hypothesis
      Ques = Questionnaire items
      Data = Data Analysis

RQ: What is physician knowledge of and use of physical therapy procedures?

CH 1: Physicians will differ by specialty area in their knowledge of physical therapy procedures.

OH 1.1: Orthopedic surgeons will have significantly higher overall knowledge of physical therapy procedures than physiatrists or neurologists.

OH 1.2: Physiatrists will have significantly higher overall knowledge of physical therapy procedures than neurologists.

Ques: Twelve questions will be used to access knowledge of physical therapy procedures. The total number of correct answers will provide a knowledge score (see Display 8-3, question 3).

Data: Test by two-way ANOVA of physician specialty by knowledge score.

CH 2: Physicians' knowledge of physical therapy procedures will influence their utilization of physical therapy procedures.

Continued

DISPLAY 8-1 *(Continued)*

OH 2.1: Physicians with higher overall knowledge of physical therapy procedures will refer significantly more patients to physical therapy than physicians with lower overall knowledge of physical therapy procedures.

Ques: Knowledge score provided by 12 questions to assess knowledge of physical therapy procedures. Demographic data will be obtained on average number of new patients referred to physical therapy each week (five ordinal categories provided for respondent).

Data: Test by chi-square high and low knowledge scores with categories for average number of new patients referred to physical therapy each week.

OH 2.2: Physicians with higher knowledge scores of professionally skilled physical therapy procedures will use significantly more consultative requests than physicians with lower knowledge scores of professionally skilled physical therapy procedures.

Ques: Six of the 12 questions used to assess knowledge will assess professional skill knowledge and six questions will assess technical skill knowledge. Demographic data will be obtained on relative percentage of referrals that are specific prescriptions, general prescriptions, open referrals, and consultative requests.

Data: Test by chi-square high and low knowledge scores of professional knowledge with four categories of referral.

(Examples adapted from Uili, R., Shepard, K., and Savinar, E., Physician knowledge and utilization of physical therapy procedures, *Physical Therapy* 64:1523–1530, 1984.)

Design of Questions

The most difficult part of designing questions for a survey instrument is asking a question in such a way that everyone who answers the question will interpret it in exactly the same way. There are a number of guidelines to help in question construction.

1. Put only a single idea in each question. Be wary of using the word "and" anywhere in the question, as in, "Do you offer inpatient and outpatient services for patients with spinal cord injuries?" Obviously, this question cannot be answered yes or no if the facility offers inpatient but not outpatient services.
2. Make sure the words you use have only one meaning. More than one meaning yields more than one way for respondents to answer your question. Suppose you asked, "Do you consult with an orthotist frequently?" Respondents would answer that question differently depending on how they interpreted the meaning of "frequently." To one person, frequently might mean every day; to another, every week; and to a third, every month.
3. Ask short questions. The shorter the better. Do not ask, "How satisfied do you think you would feel working in an outpatient setting, such as a private

DISPLAY 8-2
EXAMPLE OF ONE TYPE OF FOG INDEX

FOG FORMULA BY GUNNING

1. Count 100 words in succession (W). If the piece is long, take several samples of 100 words each from throughout the selection and average the results.
2. Count the number of complete sentences. If the 100-word mark falls past the middle of a sentence, include this sentence in the count. This count becomes S in the formula below.
3. Divide the words (W) by the number of sentences (S).
4. Count the number of words having three or more syllables (A), but do not count (a) verbs ending in "ed" or "es" that make the word have a third syllable, (b) capitalized words, or (c) combinations of simple words such as "butterfly."
5. Apply the formula to calculate the grade level.

$$GL = (W/S + A) \times 0.4$$

where GL is the grade level, W is the number of words (usually 100), S is the number of sentences, and A is the number of words having three or more syllables.

(From Gunning, R., *The Technique of Clear Writing* [New York: McGraw Hill Book Company, 1968].)

practice or home health agency, with geriatric patients who have multiple health care problems due to the aging process." Instead ask, "How satisfied do you think you would feel working in an out-of-hospital setting with the frail elderly?"

4. Use a fog index to determine the reading comprehension grade level of your questions. Questionnaires used with patient respondents should have a fog index no higher than sixth grade. For health care professionals, a reading level of from 12 to 14 years is appropriate. See Display 8-2 for an example of how to calculate one type of fog index.[8]

5. Be sure your questions are grammatically correct. If appropriate, the stem (beginning) and each choice should form a complete sentence, for example: "Currently the most important element related to my job satisfaction is: *a.* salary; *b.* opportunity for professional advancement;" and so forth.

Alternatively, questions may be asked as complete sentences and followed by a selection of choices. For example: "Check *two* of the following characteristics you would most value in a clinical instructor: *a.* empathy; *b.* level of knowledge;" and so forth. Reading your questions out loud, including the stem and each response, will help you spot problems with grammar and sentence structure.

6. Avoid the use of value-laden words or implications. For example, rather than asking, "Have you attended any continuing education courses to update your professional knowledge and skills in the past five years?" you might ask, "How many continuing education courses have you attended in the past five years?" and give a checklist of responses ranging from, for example, "less than two courses" to "ten or more courses."

7. Do not make the questions difficult to answer by using words such as *always* and *never* or double negatives, for example: "How strongly do you feel that no faculty member who has not been engaged in clinical practice should receive tenure?" Subjects who feel frustrated when answering your questionnaire or feel as if they are taking a tricky examination will simply give up and not respond.

8. Decide whether to use open- or closed-ended questions. Examples of closed-ended questions are in Display 8-3 (nominal data) and Display 8-4 (ordinal data). Examples of open-ended questions are in Display 8-5. With a closed-ended question you must either determine in advance all possible responses (see Display 8-3, question 1) or determine the most popular responses and then allow for an "other" category (see Display 8-3, question 2). There are advantages and disadvantages to using either open-ended or closed-ended questions.

Open-Ended and Closed-Ended Questions

There are several advantages to using closed-ended questions. The first advantage is that data gathered is very easy to summarize and exhibit. Nominal data (Display 8-3) or ordinal data (Display 8-4) can be displayed in frequency tables or histograms. These data can also be easily cross-compared by simple, nonparametric statistics such as chi square.

The second advantage to closed-ended questions is that because the responses are forced choice, the data tends to be reliable. That is, if asked to fill out the questionnaire more than once, the respondent will likely choose the same response to the same question. (This depends somewhat on how much time has passed and what intervening experiences the respondent has had between the first and second requests to complete the questionnaire.)

For potentially embarrassing questions for which respondents might be prone to "fudge" their answers, the best choice is a closed-ended question. Embarrassing questions might include demographic information, such as educational level or income; questions that point out the respondent's lack of knowledge; or responses that may involve ethical issues, for example, about receiving professional kickbacks. Using closed-ended questions for demographic data gives the respondent an opportunity to "hide" in a category; that is, the respondent is assured that the researcher cannot tell which end of the category (e.g., 35 to 44 years old) the respondent fits into. For potentially threatening questions dealing with knowledge, opinions, or beliefs, predetermined categories that contain a wide spectrum of choices convey to the respondent that it is acceptable to think, feel, or believe as

DISPLAY 8-3
EXAMPLES OF CLOSED-ENDED QUESTIONS (nominal data).

1. What is your entry-level physical therapy degree?

☐ Baccalaureate degree
☐ Certificate
☐ Master's degree

2. Which of the following *most* influenced your present attitudes toward death? (check one)

☐ Death of someone close
☐ Specific reading
☐ Religious upbringing
☐ Introspection and meditation
☐ Ritual (e. g., funerals)
☐ TV, radio, or motion picture
☐ Longevity of my family
☐ My health or physical condition
☐ Other (Specify)_____

(From Lutticken, C., Shepard, K., and Davies, N., Attitudes of physical therapists toward death and terminal illness, *Physical Therapy* 54:226-232, 1974.)

3. Please *circle* the letter of the correct response:
Proprioceptive Neuromuscular Facilitation (PNF) is:

   a. an exercise using cardinal planes and prolonged stretch to strengthen and increase range of motion.
   b. an exercise using diagonal movement and quick stretch to strengthen and increase range of motion.
   c. not familiar to me in my practice.

(From Uili, R., Shepard, K., and Savinar, E., Physician knowledge and utilization of physical therapy procedures, *Physical Therapy* 64:1523–1530, 1984.)

they do and that others will too. That is why the category is there (see Display 8-3, question 3, answer c).

The major problem with forced-choice answers is the issue of validity. Did the question's phrasing and limited choices really capture what the respondent knew, felt, or perceived? Obviously, if the question does not yield information that reflects the reality of the respondent, the data obtained will reflect a distorted picture of the truth.

There are also advantages and confounding disadvantages to open-ended questions. The major advantage of open-ended questions is that such questions allow you to capture information from the respondent in a way that is less subject

DISPLAY 8-4
EXAMPLE OF CLOSED-ENDED QUESTIONS (ordinal data)

Please rate each item below from (1) Least Important to (4) Most Important or (0) Not Applicable as a reason why you would change jobs.

	Least Important	Somewhat Important	Very Important	Most Important	Not Applicable
Insufficient salary to meet financial needs	1	2	3	4	0
Lack of opportunity or financial resources for continuing education	1	2	3	4	0
Little feeling of accomplishment in my work	1	2	3	4	0
No opportunity for promotion	1	2	3	4	0
Lack of independence in decision making with regard to direct patient care	1	2	3	4	0
Desire to move to a new location	1	2	3	4	0
Few opportunities for personal development	1	2	3	4	0
Desire to pursue a different area of physical therapy	1	2	3	4	0

(Adapted from Harkson, D., Unterreiner, A., and Shepard, K., Factors related to job turnover in physical therapy, *Physical Therapy* 62:1465–1470, 1982.)

to your bias. Because you have not predetermined the answers from which the respondent must select, the answers are more likely to be an authentic (valid) indication of the respondent's knowledge, attitude, or beliefs. Additionally, if you do not know the possible range of responses the respondent may give or if you want to find out *why* someone thinks as they do, open-ended questions should be the format selected.

Another advantage of open-ended questions is that a broad range of numerical (metric level) data can be obtained. For example, instead of asking the respon-

DISPLAY 8-5
EXAMPLES OF OPEN-ENDED QUESTIONS

1. _____ How many times have you been hospitalized in the past year?

2. What are the three most important issues facing the profession of physical therapy today?
   a. _____
   b. _____
   c. _____

3. How would you characterize an ideal physical therapist–physician working relationship?

4. What are the two or three things you find most difficult about raising a child who has a physical disability?

5. Is there anything you want to add about your fears or concerns about working with patients who are HIV positive that has not been asked in the preceding questions?

dent to check the appropriate age category (e.g., 35 to 44 years of age), you simply ask the respondent to write in his or her age. Obtaining a range of numbers (metric level data) allows a researcher to correlate responses obtained on one question to responses obtained in another. For example, one correlation may be between the number of years a therapist has been in practice and the number of jobs held in different settings.

A third advantage of using open-ended questions is that you do not have to think through in advance what the respondent's answers might be and establish relevant and comprehensive response categories. Thus open-ended questions are easy to construct and save time.

The primary difficulty with open-ended questions is the data analysis: each response to each question must be handled separately by the researcher. If the answer is quantitative (e.g., see Display 8-5, question 1), handling the data is relatively simple, especially if you enter the data into a computer program. Each response is entered into a statistical database, and descriptive statistics such as mean, standard deviation, mode, and range are easily generated. However, if the answer is in words (e.g., Display 8-5, questions 2 through 5), the analysis is considerably more difficult. This data must also be synthesized to produce a representative and meaningful data analysis. You must first go through the raw data (answers) to determine major themes or categories. Then the raw data must be handled a second time in order to place each response into one of the established categories you created. The raw data categorization should be performed by someone who is unfamiliar with the research (unbiased). When two or more data coders are trained in how to code, an interrater reliability of 80% or more agreement between the two coders should be established before the final data categorization occurs. See Haley and Osberg for information on how to calculate a Kappa coefficient to determine the level of interrater reliability.[9]

A second potential difficulty with open-ended questions is that more leeway is given to the individual respondent to offer peripheral answers that have little to do with the question posed. For example, in response to the question, "How would you characterize an ideal physical therapist–physician relationship?" the respondent might reply, "The APTA should direct more of its resources toward a public relations campaign to enhance physician–PT relations." If you had determined that the primary coding categories for this question were mutual respect, flexibility, trust, and openness, this respondent data could not be categorized. Thus the data is unusable or "lost."

A third disadvantage to open-ended questions is that respondents may differ in their ability to express themselves in writing. Respondents may use words that have more than one meaning to convey concepts or beliefs, and it is left to the researcher to accurately interpret and code this information.

Open-ended questions also require more time and thought from the respondent. Respondents often check off their responses to closed-ended questions but skip open-ended questions. If a questionnaire is comprised predominantly of open-ended questions, the respondent may simply throw it out. This is problematic, because the lower the response rate, the less you can be assured that the data is representative of the population you have sampled. Thus the data set would have questionable external validity. To avoid this problem a questionnaire should be composed primarily of closed-ended questions with, perhaps, one or two very important open-ended questions. You must feel *certain* that the data from the open-ended questions will be worth the time and effort spent to get, collapse, and code the data, as well as worth the likelihood of a lower response rate.

Instructions to Respondents

Instructions should be clear: Check one of the following. Check all that apply. Put a check mark by the *three most important*. Check the response that *best* expresses how you feel.

Wherever possible, keep instructions the same within a single section of the questionnaire. If you must switch instructions, try to put the questions that have different instructions at the end of the section.

Order of Questions

Start the questionnaire with interesting questions. If you capture the respondent's interest immediately, he or she is more likely to fill out your questionnaire. Age, the number of years since graduation, educational level, and current job title are boring to answer. For this reason, put demographic data questions at the end of the questionnaire, where they are out of sight at first glance and can be answered in a perfunctory manner.

Think about how the people answering the questionnaire will retrieve from their memory the data you request. The more accurately you can predict the easiest way for your respondents to identify or recall the information you want, the easier the questionnaire will be for them to answer—and the more accurate the data is likely to be. One good rule of thumb is to ask questions in chronological order. Another is to ask for general information before specific information. For example, ask the question, "How many different full-time clinical internships did you have as a student?" before you ask, "When you were a student did you feel that clinical instructors who had little experience in clinical education were more or less rigorous in their grading of your clinical skills than clinical instructors who had more experience?"

Put questions together by themes that make sense. For example, in designing a questionnaire to measure job satisfaction, put together questions related to tangible benefits, such as pay, support for continuing education, and opportunity for promotion. Similarly, put intangible benefits together, such as the amount of independence for decision-making, sense of achievement, and opportunity to be creative on the job.

Be careful not to split questions or responses between pages. Putting half the question on one page and half on another makes it more difficult for the respondent to follow and increases the chance of response error.

One last rule of thumb. Resist the temptation to ask additional questions because it would be "fun to know the answer" or in order to "get more data in the same mailing so I'll have it to analyze at another time." Additional, peripherally related questions that add to the length of your questionnaire will decrease your response rate. Remember how important your response rate is to the validity of your study. "Nice to know" data is not worth the expense of a lower return rate. In addition, it is highly unlikely that once you have analyzed the data related to your current study you will go back at some other time to analyze responses to add-on questions.

Response Categories

Response categories can be discrete (nominal), as in Display 8-3, or continuous (ordinal), as in Display 8-4. Discrete categories that contain numbers ordinarily should have equal intervals. The exception to categorization by equal intervals is

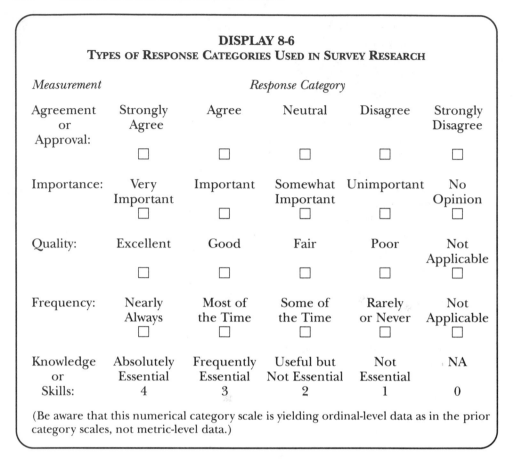

DISPLAY 8-6
TYPES OF RESPONSE CATEGORIES USED IN SURVEY RESEARCH

Measurement   *Response Category*

Agreement or Approval:	Strongly Agree ☐	Agree ☐	Neutral ☐	Disagree ☐	Strongly Disagree ☐
Importance:	Very Important ☐	Important ☐	Somewhat Important ☐	Unimportant ☐	No Opinion ☐
Quality:	Excellent ☐	Good ☐	Fair ☐	Poor ☐	Not Applicable ☐
Frequency:	Nearly Always ☐	Most of the Time ☐	Some of the Time ☐	Rarely or Never ☐	Not Applicable ☐
Knowledge or Skills:	Absolutely Essential 4	Frequently Essential 3	Useful but Not Essential 2	Not Essential 1	NA 0

(Be aware that this numerical category scale is yielding ordinal-level data as in the prior category scales, not metric-level data.)

the first and last category. For example, categories for the question, "How many years have you been in your present job setting?" might be "less than 2 years; 2–4 years; 5–7 years; 8–10 years; and more than 10 years."

Refer to Display 8-6 for examples of various types of ordinal-scale response categories often used in survey research. The American Physical Therapy Association (APTA) monograph *Using and Understanding Surveys,* written by Eugene Michaels, contains a good discussion on the use of nominal and ordinal categories.[10]

Boxes or spaces for answers should be aligned and in a similar location under each question, so that respondents do not have to search for a place for their responses. A vertical arrangement of response categories is usually preferred over a horizontal arrangement because choices are clearly set off from the stem or question. The vertical format also allows for more blank space on the page and thus the question appears easier to complete (see Display 8-3). For a series of questions with the same response categories, such as Strongly Agree, Agree, Neutral, Disagree, Strongly Disagree, arrange the response categories horizontally (see Display 8-4). In addition, be sure to relist each response category (e.g., Strongly Agree) over the response boxes on *every* page of the questionnaire. Also review the questionnaire format to determine how easy or difficult it will be for you to retrieve the data from your questionnaire for computer-entry purposes. Will a different arrangement make it easier for you, as well as for the respondent?

VALIDITY AND RELIABILITY

The most important validity consideration for all questionnaires is *content validity*. Content validity is a way of assessing whether or not the questions you have designed are inclusive of the scope and depth of information you wish to gather. Content validity is most often assessed by a "panel of experts," a group of people who have expert knowledge of the content area being assessed. For example, if you were designing a questionnaire about teaching techniques used by clinical educators, you would have your questionnaire reviewed by a panel of experts who included center coordinators of clinical education, experienced clinical instructors, and perhaps one or more academic coordinators of clinical education. If your questionnaire was designed to measure patient satisfaction in your clinical setting, your panel of experts might include current and former patients and their family members, as well as professional personnel who work in similar clinical units. You would do well to consider including one or more people knowledgeable about questionnaire design on your panel.

The expert panel, usually eight to ten participants, is informed about the purpose of your study, given a copy of your conceptual and operational hypotheses, and asked to fill out your questionnaire. The panel is requested to give you feedback both on substance (e.g., Will the answers to the questions give you sufficient data to accept or reject your operational hypotheses? Do you have too many questions asking essentially the same thing?) and structure (e.g., Are the questions clearly worded? Are the questions stated in an embarrassing or derogatory manner? Do any words have multiple meanings?). If you receive few editorial corrections from this panel, you can make minor revisions and prepare a second draft of the questionnaire ready for pilot testing. However, if you get many substantive suggestions (better now than later!), revise your questionnaire and ask your original panel of experts to review it again. Repeat this process until suggestions are few and nonsubstantive. After your panel of experts has completed its review, you are ready to run your pilot study.

A pilot study is a review of your cover letter and questionnaire by a sample of eight to ten respondents who represent a small subset of the sample you wish to survey. These respondents can give you excellent feedback on the clarity of instructions, the understandability and logical (to them) ordering of questions, the effectiveness of your cover letter, and the approximate length of time it takes to complete your questionnaire. Although pilot testing takes time, it is absolutely essential to the final effective formatting of your questionnaire and cover letter. If you are not willing to do a pilot study, you can *expect* problems with the survey data or response rate.

Clear, well-constructed questions will enhance the reliability of the questionnaire. If the questionnaire will have extensive use, test-retest reliability is generally

TABLE 8-2. Validity of a Questionnaire

Validity:	Were the right questions asked to gain the desired information? Do the questionnaire responses reflect reality, that is, do they really measure a person's knowledge, attitudes, or perceptions?	
Type of Validity	Assessment of Validity	Applicability of Validity Concepts to Questionnaires
Content Validity	Determine if the questionnaire items represent the domain of interest	Use a panel of experts to determine if questionnaire items cover domain of information
Criterion-related Validity (Concurrent and Predictive)	Determine how well "scores" relate to some outside objective information	For self-reported perceptions, opinions, or attitudes, there is no outside criterion
Construct Validity	Determine if a construct, such as burnout, compliance, or job satisfaction, is related to a specific observable/measurable phenomenon, e.g., burnout might be related to absenteeism, depression, and eating disorders	Most questions in survey research are related to demographics, knowledge, and opinions—not to constructs However, construct validity would be relevant if assessing attitudes toward something

(Adapted from Mayerberg, C., *How to Develop a Survey Questionnaire,* 1987 [Didactics, 13 Hartford Rd., Medford, NJ].)

performed. See Moncur's research study "Perceptions of Physical Therapy Competencies in Rheumatology" for an example of the use of a panel of experts, as well as for a presample test of reliability.[11]

Further information on the use of validity and reliability procedures in survey research is presented in Tables 8-2 and 8-3.

DATA ANALYSES

Before you finalize your questions and response categories, set up mock data tables with the data you expect to get. Descriptive data tables or figures are commonly used in survey research to display descriptive aspects of the raw data. Tables might depict, for example, the percentage of subjects who responded to each category under a question (see Table 8-4). Histograms might be used to display data that appear different according to sample subgroup response, for example, different age, educational level, ethnic background, or year (see Figure 8-1).

TABLE 8-3. Reliability of a Questionnaire

Reliability	Is the information derived from a questionnaire dependable or stable over time? Is the respondent motivated to respond accurately? Are the results attributable to characteristics of the respondents or measurement error?

Type of Reliability	Assessment of Reliability	Applicability of Reliability Concepts to Questionnaires
Test–Retest	Determine stability over time	Impractical to do on entire sample Do on subsample during pilot testing phase
Internal Consistency	Determine homogeneity of similar content items (use alpha)	Relevant if using a response scale for related items Do a reliability check on item responses that represent the same idea, i.e., should correlate
Interrater Reliability	Determine level of agreement (Kappa) between two raters who are coding raw data from open-ended questions	Necessary if coding responses from open-ended questions

(Adapted from Mayerberg, C., *How to Develop a Survey Questionnaire,* 1987 [Didactics, 13 Hartford Rd., Medford, NJ].)

TABLE 8-4. Example of a Table Generated from Survey Data

Sources of Pain Management and Pain Theory Information	
Source	Most Useful Source[a]
Continuing education	60 (50.5)
Professional colleagues	26 (21.9)
Reading current literature	16 (13.3)
Salespersons/other	9 (7.6)
Staff inservice training	5 (3.8)
Graduate-level education	3 (2.9)

[a]Percentage of total in parentheses.

(From Wolff, M., Michel, T., Krebs, D., and Watts, N. Chronic pain-assessment of orthopedic physical therapists' knowledge and attitudes, *Physical Therapy* 71:207–214, 1991. Reprinted from *Physical Therapy* with the permission of the American Physical Therapy Association.)

APPLICATIONS TO PHYSICAL THERAPIST PROGRAMS 1980-1990

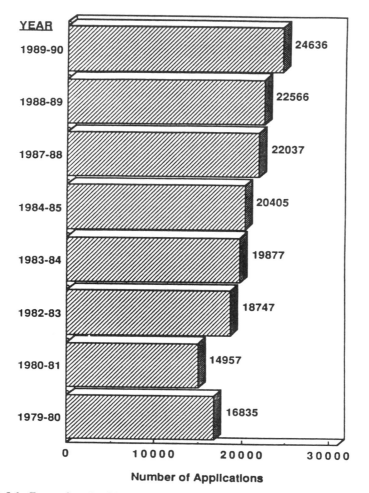

FIGURE 8-1. Example of a histogram generated from survey data. (From Department of Education, American Physical Therapy Association, Alexandria, VA, September 1990.)

Because the data generated by survey research is often massive, there are literally dozens of ways to manipulate it. Hence you must be very clear what analytical statistics you will use *before* you collect the data. Your a priori operational hypotheses will give you explicit guidance on which questionnaire response data to subject to statistical analysis. The most common analytical statistics in survey research are used to determine measures of correlation, association, or difference. You must have at least ordinal-level data to perform a statistical correlation. An association between two variables can be determined for nominal-level data. The chi square is the statistic most often used for determining association between nominal- and ordinal-level data. The differences between responses given by two or more subsamples can be determined by use of parametric or nonparametric statistics. Two or more subsamples are usually differentiated by demographic variables, such as age, gender, job title, primary diagnosis, or functional ability. If the data are nominal or ordinal, nonparametric statistics such as chi square or eta may be used. If the data is metric, parametric statistics such as t-test or analysis of variance (ANOVA) may be used.

After the researcher reviews the descriptive data received and performs analytical statistics to accept or reject each operational hypothesis, additional cross-data analyses may be performed. However, simply to put data in the computer and run all possible combinations is, as a colleague of mine states, "fishing expeditions, not research." Researchers who do not carefully review their raw data and do not use judgment with regard to what combinations of variables are feasible to investigate will end up with nonsensical outcomes as a result of random number crunching.

In addition, remember that the computer does not distinguish among nominal-, ordinal-, and metric-level data. Thus you can ask for, and get, data analyses that have no meaning whatsoever. For example, you can ask the computer to correlate gender (nominal data) with attitudes toward independent practice (ordinal data). The computer will generate for you a correlation value as well as a significance level. However, as you can see, the value that would be generated would make no sense.

QUESTIONNAIRE PRESENTATION

We live in a busy world. Many of us do not have time to complete everything we would like to during the day, much less to participate in someone else's quest that has little payoff for us. Therefore, your questionnaire should intrigue and be pleasurable for the respondent to answer.

Make sure headings, instructions, and questions are easy to read. Bold lettering or press-on letters help set off different portions of the questionnaire. Questions should not be crowded in an attempt to make the questionnaire seem smaller. The questionnaire does not appear smaller; it simply appears crowded and complex, and is more difficult to read.

Keep the total number of pages to a minimum so that the questionnaire appears short and not overly time-consuming. Use the front and back of each page. If you are not mailing to a sample for whom you can predict a high return rate, try to keep your questionnaire to two pages, using both front and back sides. Use of two (or more) large sheets folded in the middle to give you a booklet-like appearance decreases the chance that respondents will forget to turn a page over and complete the other side.

Lightly colored paper that forms an easily readable background is a nice touch and helps your questionnaire stand out on someone's cluttered desk. If you are requesting responses from several different subgroups (e.g., physical therapists, nurses, and physicians), you might want to use different colored paper for ease in sorting. You might also consider the use of a few small, eye-catching graphics at the beginning and end of the questionnaire. Sketches or cartoons capture the interest of our child ego state. The respondent is lured into a questionnaire in much the same way we curiously skim through the pictures in a book we are about to read. For the same reason, brightly colored stamps attract attention and thus should be used instead of an automatic stamp machine.

COVER LETTER

A short, convincing cover letter is vital to ensuring a good response rate. Write the cover letter on the letterhead stationery of the organization in which you are employed or of the school you are attending. Use each respondent's name—spelled correctly—in the salutation. Think about how annoyed you are to receive a letter that begins with "Dear Sir" (especially if you are a woman), "Dear Clinical Director," or even "Dear Respondent." In the first paragraph of the cover letter introduce yourself and state the purpose and value of your study. The other important information in the cover letter should identify why the respondent was selected to participate in the study and to convince the respondent how important his or her participation is.

Each respondent asks and is interested in answers to the following questions: Is this questionnaire of any interest to me? Am I, an individual, important in this mass mailing? Will it really matter if I take time to respond? How much time will this take out of my busy schedule? Will I get anything back for the effort I put in? Is my response confidential? Human Subjects Committees, established to safeguard human rights in research, are also interested in your responses to many of these same questions. Therefore, weave responses to all these potential respondent questions into your cover letter. If you put a code number on envelopes to assist in your follow-up (see follow-up strategies, below), be sure to tell your respondent the purpose of the code number and how it will be used. The letter should contain original signatures of the major investigators. Graduate students may want to consider having the major research advisor also sign the letter to enhance the importance of the request. See Display 8-7 for an example of an initial cover letter.

Respondents are dissuaded from responding if the cover letter sounds demanding or if you appear insensitive to the effort the respondent is asked to put forth in your behalf. Do not say, for example, "Due to my pending graduation this June, it is very important that you return your questionnaire within five days!" Respondents are also less likely to respond when questionnaires are depersonalized and when the follow-up is too soon (pushy) or too late (negligent).

In addition, it is not desirable to give a *specific* return date. If the mail delivery is slow or the respondent is out of town for a few days, she or he will be irritated at being given such short notice. If the respondent does not get to your questionnaire until after a specific date is passed, she or he will likely discard it. Instead, ask your respondent if she or he could please return the response "within the next two weeks."

Follow-up letters requesting responses from those respondents who have not yet returned your questionnaire should carry the same positive and grateful tone as the initial cover letter. Never forget that you are asking a favor. Be humble and appreciative of the time and effort someone puts forth in your behalf.

DISPLAY 8-7
EXAMPLE OF A COVER LETTER USED IN SURVEY RESEARCH

BRANDYWINE UNIVERSITY
COLLEGE OF HEALTH PROFESSIONS
DEPARTMENT OF PHYSICAL THERAPY
55 MAYFAIR COURT
CHESTERTON, PA 55123

Dear Mr. Johansson,

We are physical therapy graduate students at Brandywine University conducting research on physical therapy administrators' views regarding the issue of direct patient access. You have been selected from a list of members either of the Administration Section or the Private Practice Section, APTA.

We understand that you have a very busy schedule and would be very grateful if you could find approximately ten minutes to participate in this study.

Please complete the enclosed questionnaire and return it to us in the stamped addressed return envelope within the next two weeks. Your answers will be anonymous. The return envelope is numbered so that, if necessary, we may send you a reminder. As the questionnaires are returned, the numbers are checked off a master list and the envelopes discarded to ensure anonymity of the respondents.

As our sample size is relatively small, you are vitally important to our study. We appreciate your taking a few minutes of your time to respond to our questions so that we all may gain information about current changes in our profession.

If you would like an abstract of our results, please put your name and address on the enclosed postcard. We expect to complete the study in May 1992.

Thank you for your time and the courtesy of your assistance.

Sincerely,

Amy Feigenbaum, MPT Student   Juan Alverez, MPT Student

Ann Newton, Ph.D., P.T., Faculty Advisor

INDUCEMENTS

Some researchers include inducements to attract the attention of respondents and encourage a high return rate by relying on the inducement to cause a sense of obligation. That is, if people receive a dollar bill or a quarter or a free pencil or a free stamp along with the questionnaire, they will be more likely to feel they have an *obligation* to respond.

If the survey sample consists of your own professional colleagues, the most common inducement is a promise to send a copy of the abstract of the results. To identify those respondents who would like a copy of your abstract, you might enclose a postcard for them to return indicating their desire for the abstract and stating their name and address. An alternative is to have respondents put their names and addresses on the backs of the return envelopes that contain the questionnaires. The return envelopes are separated from the questionnaires and, at the end of the study, abstracts are sent to all the names in the envelope pile. Remember, if your questionnaire is anonymous, you cannot ask the respondents to put their name and address on the questionnaire itself.

It is vital to the reputation of the researcher and the institution she or he represents to fulfill any promises made regarding sharing an abstract of the results with the respondents. One word of caution: *Never* mail a copy of your entire results section to anyone before you have first publicly presented your results under your name(s), either in oral or written fashion.

MAILING THE QUESTIONNAIRE

Costs

Before you finalize your questionnaire, consider carefully the financial costs. Your initial costs will include paper, reproduction services, graphics, and envelopes. Even more expensive are mailing costs. Along with each questionnaire sent out, you must include a self-addressed stamped envelope in which the respondent can return the questionnaire. The weight of the return envelope plus the questionnaire, plus your introductory cover letter, and, perhaps, a postcard for the respondent to use in requesting a copy of your abstract can translate into hundreds of dollars in mailing costs.

Unfortunately, it is difficult to find resources to help defray the expense of printing, reproducing, and mailing. Public or private research foundations that are agreeable to purchasing equipment for experimental research are reluctant to spend money on costs incurred in survey research. These costs, such as mailing or telephoning, are commonly associated with the business of everyday living. Thus mail and telephone costs are difficult for those who make grant decisions to understand and legitimize as "research" costs.

Follow-up Strategies

Before mailing the questionnaires, set up a coding system to identify respondents who return their questionnaires. The purpose of this coding system is to identify which respondents have completed your questionnaire and which will need a follow-up mailing to ensure a satisfactory return rate. At the same time, the respondents' confidentiality must be safeguarded. A common way to do this is to assign each respondent a three-digit (or more, depending upon the sample size) code number. This respondent code number is put on the upper left-hand corner of the return envelope. Be sure to explain the presence of this code number in your cover letter. Keep a list of the names and addresses of your respondents and their assigned code numbers. When the questionnaire is returned, the envelope number is checked against the respondent name and code number list. The questionnaire is then removed from the envelope and put aside for subsequent data analysis. The envelope is destroyed.

In the cover letter you will have requested that the respondent return the questionnaire within a specified period of time, usually about two weeks. All survey research that involves mail questionnaires should have at least two follow-up mailings. One common follow-up pattern is to send a reminder postcard shortly after the return deadline, followed by a second full follow-up mailing a week later. The follow-up full mailing should include a positive cover letter stating how much the respondent's questionnaire is needed and an enclosed second questionnaire in case the respondent misplaced the first one. Cohen and Manion[12] report that a typical response rate pattern to three follow-ups is as follows: Original mailing = 40% return; first follow-up = 20% return; second follow-up = 10% return; and third follow-up = 5% return (p. 88). Obviously, follow-up returns adhere to the law of diminishing returns.

Another survey distribution strategy to consider is to first telephone all respondents, asking them if they would be willing to participate in your study. This is done when the respondents comprise a small, discrete sample, some or many of whom may be known to you, such as patients who have been discharged from your clinical setting within the last year, members of the APTA Section on Neurology, or center coordinators of clinical education in the northeastern United States. The purpose of the phone call is to gain a commitment from the sample, thus ensuring a high response rate and curtailing both initial and follow-up mailing costs.

Time of Year to Distribute

The time of year you distribute questionnaires is also an important consideration. Because filling out a questionnaire looks like (and is) work, do not distribute during summer months. The Christmas and New Year holiday period and the mid- to late-February doldrums are also poor times to distribute questionnaires if you want an enthusiastic response. The best months are September, October, and early November, or late March, April, and May.

QUESTIONNAIRES FOR A CAPTIVE AUDIENCE

The best way to guarantee a high return rate from a select sample is to distribute to and collect your questionnaire from a captive audience. Collecting data from a captive audience also provides you with the opportunity to answer any questions the respondents may have regarding the directions or questions asked in your questionnaire. An audience might be "captured" during an education program, a business meeting, or a special-interest, patient-support group. It is important that the chairperson who introduces you to the group has a clear understanding of what information you want, why you want it, and why you want it from the group that is gathered. (This may best be explained over a lunch that you buy for the chairperson.)

Equally important to your receiving information (data) from a captive audience is what the group might receive in return for its efforts on your behalf. For example, you might offer to give a short presentation on ambulatory aids or general conditioning exercises for a group of people participating in a local Arthritis Club. For practicing clinicians, you might agree to present an inservice program on how to get started on clinical research. Other enticements may include small sums of money donated to the group's special interests ($50 to $100), food (cookies and punch, pizza), or an hour of free consultation.

One serious error made by survey researchers in working with captive audiences is to ask the group to "fill out and return the questionnaire at your leisure" (often by mail). Remember, the primary reason you have located and capitalized on the presence of a captive audience is to secure a high return rate. You ensure that return rate by having members of the audience who agree to participate in the study complete and return the questionnaires to you immediately. The face-to-face contact at the time questionnaires are returned also gives you an opportunity to thank each individual personally for their assistance with your study.

INCREASING THE RETURN RATE

Strategies for increasing the return rate of questionnaires have been of great interest to many social scientists. After all, without a high return rate (70% or above), a study is subject to major problems with sampling error. Can you really draw valid conclusions from a study that does not yield a representative sample return?

Many studies have been carried out in an attempt to define those factors that will increase a response rate. However, the results from these studies are not particularly useful because not all possible response variables have been studied at the same time. Therefore, there are no comprehensive studies on the interactive nature of the many possible variables involved in increasing the return rate. The best strategy for a high response rate is to keep in mind a number of conditions that appear to most strongly influence response: (1) whom you are asking to respond (likely respondents are those with more education and professionals; less likely to respond are physicians, who have a notoriously low response rate); (2) questionnaire construction (few, interesting, closed-ended questions are best); (3) questionnaire appearance (good-quality paper, clear and uncrowded printing, sections well defined, color and graphics help); (4) cover letter (informative, courteous, grateful); (5) time of year sent (fall and spring are good); and (6) how diligently you pursue follow-up procedures (at least two follow-up contacts for the tardy or delinquent). Remember, a few people will refuse to fill out your hard-wrought questionnaire just because they simply will not respond to *any* questionnaires! For an excellent discussion of problems and suggestions on how to deal with bias that may be present because of a low response rate, see Brogan's article "Nonresponse in Sample Surveys."[13]

THE DELPHI TECHNIQUE: CONSENSUAL DATA GATHERING BY QUESTIONNAIRE

The Delphi technique is a method of gathering consensus information about a certain topic from a group of experts.[14] Although this technique was developed in the late 1940s by the Rand Corporation to forecast technological developments, social scientists have since adopted and modified it to gather and collate expert opinions about many different phenomena.

The Delphi technique usually consists of three rounds of questionnaires completed by the same group of experts. The experts are identified and asked to participate in the study before dissemination of the first round. Round 1 of the Delphi consists of open-ended questions. The researcher compiles and consolidates all responses from Round 1 and puts the results into a second questionnaire for Round 2. During Round 2, the respondents have an opportunity to see how other experts responded to the open-ended questions, to validate that their own responses are included in an accurately identified category, and to suggest additional responses that appear to be missing. The researcher then compiles and consolidates all responses from Round 2 and develops a third questionnaire for Round 3. In Round 3, the respondents are asked to order the importance of the information, usually by a Likert-type scale (e.g. Most Important, Important, Least Important, Unimportant). Respondents are sometimes asked to do this ranking in Round 2 and then to note their agreement or disagreement with the collective ranking in Round 3.

An example of the Delphi technique helps to illustrate it. Dr. Jane Walter performed a Delphi survey to determine what physical therapy researchers thought would be the optimal characteristics of a clinical research center in physical therapy.[15] Respondents were asked to list the pertinent characteristics under various components and elements of a research center, such as the organizational environment, the nature of researcher collaboration, and measures of success of the center. See Table 8-5 for an example of how one question from Walter's research was carried through three rounds of the Delphi.

Advantages of the Delphi Technique

The Delphi technique is an inexpensive way to get information about important issues from a group of experts. Because the experts do not meet face to face to discuss the issues, the use of the Delphi prevents the potential problems that often occur in small, consensus-driven groups. These problems include domination by one or several members of the group and "groupthink," which may hinder creative ideas from surfacing. Because the respondents do not interact during a Delphi survey, each participant has the same opportunity to express her or his own views. Further, each response is given equal importance by the researcher, who simply collates and distributes the information for the second and third rounds of data collection.[16]

Although the Delphi technique has been used primarily in the social sciences

TABLE 8-5. Example of three rounds of a Delphi survey used by Jane Walter

---

CLINICAL RESEARCH CENTERS IN PHYSICAL THERAPY
NATIONAL DELPHI SURVEY

Round One

"Clinical research centers in physical therapy have the potential to represent a myriad of designs. The focus of this Delphi survey is to find out from you, the physical therapist researcher, the optimal characteristics of a center. . . . In this first round of the Delphi, you are asked to consider each of the system components and brainstorm the characteristics which you believe identify that component in relation to clinical research centers in physical therapy. . . ."

1. Environment. The setting in which the clinical research center will exist (i.e., independent, within academic medical center, within university, etc.)

Round Two

"The purpose of this round (two) is for you to review the collated responses of the Delphi participants and to add any other responses that you wish to in each section. . . ."

1. Environment
    University affiliated hospital (academic medical center)
    Nonuniversity affiliated hospital
    PT education department in university or college
    PT department in medical school
    Free-standing US government-backed
    Etc.

Round Three

"The purpose of this round (three) is for you to review the collated responses of the Delphi participants and rate the items indicating their degree of appropriateness or importance within specific categories. . . ."

1. Environment	Most Appropriate	Appropriate	Least Appropriate	Inappropriate
University affiliated hospital or rehabilitation center				
Nonuniversity affiliated hospital or rehabilitation center				
PT education department in college or university				
Etc.				

(From Soderberg, G. and Walter, J., Modeling physical therapy clinical research centers, *Physical Therapy* 71:734–745, 1991.)

---

and business, in the past ten years it has become increasingly utilized in the health professions.[17,18] Recent Delphi studies in the field of physical therapy have been performed by Miles-Tapping et al. (priorities for clinical research in Canada),[19] Reed (problems related to teaching electrotherapy in the UK),[20] and Walter (defining the characteristics of a clinical research center).[15]

CONCLUSION

This chapter has included an overview of the process of constructing and using questionnaires to conduct survey research. It is hoped that the ideas presented here will encourage the researcher to develop sound questionnaires in order to gather important information and to use effective techniques to encourage acceptable return rates. As Michaels[10] states, "If done properly, the use of surveys in research is neither quick nor easy, and can be as meritorious and important as the use of any other method in research" (p. 2). Additional resources that may be helpful to the reader in constructing and using questionnaires are included in this chapter's annotated bibliography.

REFERENCES

1. Bork, C. and Francis, J. Developing effective questionnaires. *Physical Therapy* 65: 907–911, 1985.

2. Kemp, N., Scholz, C., Sanford, T., and Shepard, K. Salary and status differences between male and female therapists. *Physical Therapy* 59:1095–1101, 1979.

3. Stelmach, M., Postma, J., Goldstein, S., and Shepard, K. Selected factors influencing job satisfaction of attendants of physically disabled adults. *Rehabilitation Literature* 42: 130–137, 1981.

4. Ballin, A., Breslin, W., Wierenga, K., and Shepard, K. Research in physical therapy: Philosophy, barriers to involvement, and use among California physical therapists. *Physical Therapy* 60:888–895, 1980.

5. Stapleton, K., Tomlinson, C., Shepard, K., and Coon, V. High school coaches' perceptions of their responsibilities in managing their athletes' injuries. *Journal of Orthopedic and Sports Physical Therapy* 5:253–260, 1984.

6. Conoley, J. and Kramer, J. *The mental measurements yearbook*, 10th ed. The Buros Institute of Mental Measurements. Lincoln: University of Nebraska Press, 1989.

7. Uili, R., Shepard, K., and Savinar, E. Physician knowledge and utilization of physical therapy procedures. *Physical Therapy* 64:1523–1530, 1984.

8. Redman, B. *The process of patient education*, 6th ed. St. Louis: C.V. Mosby, 1988, p. 161.

9. Haley, S. and Osberg, J. Kappa coefficient calculation using multiple ratings per subject: A special communication. *Physical Therapy* 69:970–974, 1989.

10. Michaels, E. *Using and understanding surveys: An introductory manual.* Alexandria, VA: American Physical Therapy Association, October 1985.

11. Moncur, C. Perceptions of physical therapy competencies in rheumatology. *Physical Therapy* 67:331–339, 1987.

12. Cohen, L. and Manion, L. *Research methods in education.* London: Croom Helm, 1980.

13. Brogan, D. Nonresponse in sample surveys: The problem and some solutions. *Physical Therapy* 60:1026–1032, 1980.

14. Linstone, H. and Turoff, M., eds. *The Delphi method: Techniques and applications.* Reading, MA: Addison Wesley, 1975.

15. Soderberg, G. and Walter, J. Modeling physical therapy clinical research centers. *Physical Therapy* 71:734–745, 1991.

16. Couper, M. The Delphi technique: Characteristics and sequence model. *Advances in Nursing Science* 7:72–77, 1984.

17. Chaney, H. Needs assessment: A Delphi approach. *Journal of Nursing Staff Development* 3:48–53, Spring 1987.

18. Levine, A. A model for health projections using knowledgeable informants. *World Health Statistics Quarterly* 37:306–317, 1984.

19. Miles-Tapping, C., Dyck, A., Brunham, S., Simpson, E., and Barber, L. Canadian therapists: Priorities for clinical research: A Delphi study. *Physical Therapy* 70:448–454, 1990.

20. Reed, A. An investigation into the problems involved in teaching electrotherapy and their possible solutions: A Delphi technique. *Physiotherapy Theory and Practice* 6:9–16, 1990.

SELECTED BIBLIOGRAPHY

Dillman, D. *Mail and telephone surveys: The total design method.* New York: Wiley-Interscience, 1985.
    Identifies many useful questionnaire preparation and mailing techniques that will help increase questionnaire response rate.

Mayerberg, C. How to develop a survey questionnaire. Didactics, 13 Hartford Road, Medford, New Jersey, 1987.
    An excellent workbook on all facets of questionnaire design. Used in conjunction with a day-long seminar the author presents on this subject.

Michaels, E. *Using and understanding surveys: An introductory manual.* Alexandria, VA: American Physical Therapy Association, 1985.
    Practical guide to questionnaire construction. Contains a good section on how to summarize and analyze questionnaire results.

Payne, S. *The art of asking questions.* Princeton: Princeton University Press, 1951.
    A clear, concise classic work on how to ask questions. As relevant today as when first published.

Rossi, P., Wright, J., Anderson, A., et al. *Handbook of survey research.* San Diego: Academic Press, 1983.
    An advanced work for advanced researchers from very quantitative authors.

Standards for educational and psychological testing. Washington, DC: American Psychological Association, 1985.
    Touchstone document on standards for test construction and evaluation. A must for the serious survey researcher.

Sudman, S. and Bradburn, N. *Asking questions: A practical guide to questionnaire design.* San Francisco: Jossey-Bass, 1983.
    Easy-to-read, comprehensive text on all facets of questionnaire construction. Includes an excellent glossary and a 70-page appendix of questionnaire format examples.

PART III

DATA
ANALYSIS

9

POPULATIONS, SAMPLES, AND STATISTICAL SIGNIFICANCE

Christopher E. Bork

This chapter is the foundation for understanding chapters 10, 11, and 12, which describe statistical tests commonly used in clinical research. I interweave the concepts of population, normality, and chance to introduce fundamental concepts that are the bases for descriptive and inferential statistics. We examine the populations, samples, and methods for describing samples, specifically, measures of central tendency. Normal distribution, its properties, and its relationship to measures of central tendency will also be discussed. Finally, the concepts of normal distribution and chance are related to the concept of statistical significance. My intention is to help the reader understand the underlying logic without the aid of mathematical proofs.

While this approach may appear unorthodox to those who learned statistics in the usual manner, I believe it helps to demystify statistics and research design without distorting the fundamental concepts. For readers who subsequently wish to learn more about and enjoy the mathematical foundations of statistics, abundant texts are available.

POPULATIONS AND SAMPLES

Of the many questions a patient asks a physical therapist, "What is the chance that I'll be normal again?" is the most difficult to answer. The question is difficult because we have only limited understanding of what comprises "normal" function and little knowledge of whether the premorbid function of a given patient is typical of all persons or not. Wouldn't it be wonderful if, as practitioners, we had an idea or were able to estimate the likelihood of success for a patient with a given condition? For example, it would be helpful to know what the passive range of motion (ROM) is for shoulder motion in women in their 50s. With that information, we could ascertain if a particular woman's shoulder ROM was typical or atypical. The information would be even more useful if a physical therapist were rehabilitating movement dysfunction and wished to know how much ROM to strive for. Unfortunately, the information about the people we treat is, at best, incomplete. Nonetheless, there are ways that help us make educated guesses about groups of people or sets of data. First, however, we need to understand some concepts concerning populations and samples.

Populations

A population can be loosely defined to mean an entire group of individuals, an entire collection, or a complete set of measurements. In short, *a population is the entire universe of a given set*. The key in identifying a population is understanding how the set is defined. For example, the population of the United States is the set of individuals who reside within the geographic borders of the land area called the United States. Another population could consist of all the jellybeans in ten kilograms of jellybeans.

It is cumbersome and generally impossible to describe the characteristics of every member of a population. For these reasons, investigators usually describe the most common member of the population: the "average" subject.* Central tendencies, or typical characteristics, of an entire population are used as a shorthand in describing the population and are referred to as *parameters*. For example, the "typical" jellybean may weigh 12.2 grams; this weight is a parameter. This does not mean that every jellybean weighs 12.2 grams but, rather, that if one were to select a typical jellybean, it might weigh very nearly 12.2 grams.

Samples

Because of the effort, time, and expense involved, data from an entire population are rarely gathered in a study. One investigation that gathers data from a population is the census; but even in a relatively wealthy country such as the United States, a census occurs infrequently, perhaps only every decade. For the most part, populations are not studied. Instead, segments of populations, termed *samples*, are examined in order to make inferences about the entire population. A characteristic of a sample is a *statistic*. Statistics are to the sample what parameters are to the population. Both parameters and statistics are a notation, or shorthand, for describing members of a population and sample, respectively.

In clinical research it is virtually impossible to study every member of a set or population that meets the characteristics of a given disease or dysfunction. Instead, the investigator chooses to study a sample and attempts to make inferences (or to generalize from the findings) about the population from which it was drawn. The method of sampling is the choice of the investigator and is chosen on the basis of the study, the availability of subjects, and the strengths and limitations of the sampling method itself.

SAMPLING METHODS

Ideally, a sample contains members of the population in a proportion that resembles, in every way, the population from which it was drawn. In other words, the sample is representative of the population. Although an investigator would like each sample to be representative, there is, however, no way to ensure that a fully representative sample has been drawn. Therefore the investigator makes decisions about how best to represent the population under study when drawing a sample.

Random Sampling

In a random sample, two criteria must be met. First, every member of the population should have an equal probability of being included in the sample. Second, the choice of one member of the sample in no way should affect the choice of another member in the sample; each member of the sample is drawn independently of every other member.[1] The logic of a random sample is that

---

*I have placed "average" in quotes because the word is imprecise and can actually be interpreted in several ways. Later in this chapter, we focus on descriptions of the average, along with their uses.

characteristics within a population have an equal chance of occurring in the sample. Considering all the variations possible in a human population, a researcher can never be absolutely certain that the distribution of attributes in the sample resembles that in the population at large. The researcher must rely upon chance. By ensuring that every member has an equal opportunity to become a member of the sample, the researcher does not introduce a bias. In a random sample, no particular attribute has any more chance of being represented than any other attribute. An example of random sampling is using a computer to select respondents for a survey by generating telephone numbers randomly; each telephone number has exactly the same chance of being selected as any other.

Stratified Sampling

In a stratified sample, the sample resembles the population on one or more critical characteristics. Suppose a researcher knows that a given population with a particular disease is comprised of 40% men and 60% women. The investigator wants to ensure that the proportion of males and females in the sample represents the same proportion as exists in the population at large. Therefore the researcher establishes 40% of the sample as male and 60% of the sample as female. Thus the investigator's stratified sample resembles the population in terms of the proportion of females to males. The researcher could then select the male and female subjects in a random manner.

Cluster Sampling

A cluster sample is obtained when all the members of a particular geographic area or a particular type are studied. Suppose the investigator wanted to look at the effect of a particular exercise program on sixth-grade children. The investigator could obtain a cluster sample by choosing a particular region at random and using all the students in the sixth grade of a particular school or schools as a sample.

Systematic Sampling

Another form of sampling consists of *systematically* selecting every subject for the sample from a particular population. For example, suppose one wanted to investigate physical therapists' attitudes toward direct access to physical therapy. The population consists of all licensed physical therapists in the United States. The investigator in this case could choose to survey every twenty-second physical therapist on a list of all licensed physical therapists in the United States. The investigator thus would have systematically chosen a sample of physical therapists. The "system" is that every twenty-second member of the population is selected for the study.

The Sample of Convenience

Many times in a clinical research study, the investigator does not have access to the entire population or even to a large segment of the population he or she wishes to study. For example, the investigator may be limited to the individuals who come to a particular facility or clinic. In this case, the subjects of the investigation can be termed a *sample of convenience*. The investigator should be cognizant that there may be several biases operating in the selection of the subjects in this situation. For example, the subjects may be only those individuals who have the financial or economic resources to seek health care or, perhaps, only those whose insurance covers physical therapy. Therefore the selection or the sample is biased toward individuals of economic means. Of the methods of sampling discussed, the sample of convenience is the least desirable because (1) it may introduce bias into the study; and (2) it may not represent the population.

Matching

Matching is a method wherein subjects who are considered equal to one another on a number of specified characteristics are assigned to different groups. The purpose is to attempt to eliminate biases by assuring equal representation of certain traits in each group. Matching attempts to achieve a fundamental concept—*random assignment,* the notion that variation within a population will be similarly represented in groups assigned randomly.

Random Assignment

Because a researcher chooses only a segment of a particular population (a sample) to study, there is no way to ascertain if the variations within the population are similarly distributed in the sample. When the researcher will further subdivide the subjects in the sample by assigning them to groups, the concern with bias increases. Yet even if an investigator uses a sample of convenience, there are methods to help minimize biases. One of those methods is random assignment. Random assignment means that the method for placing a subject in a group may be random, for example, a subject may be assigned according to a table of random numbers. In this case, subjects may be assigned to the treatment group because they receive an odd number, while subjects who receive an even number chosen at random may be assigned to the control group.

Random assignment implies not that the groups will be equal in terms of their attributes but that variability or different characteristics will be distributed among the groups in a relatively balanced manner, so that there will be little likelihood of one group being biased toward a certain attribute and thereby affecting results. Suppose one were examining how long it took to learn a specific motor skill using one of three different approaches. If the subjects were assigned randomly to each group, theoretically none of the groups should have a preponderance of highly coordinated individuals.* Rather than implying that the sample groups in this example are equal in coordination, random assignment attempts to preclude imbalances in the distribution of coordination that may affect the internal validity of the study.

*This example assumes that each member of the population had an opportunity to be chosen *and* that the sample group sizes were sufficiently large enough to be representative of the population.

DESCRIBING THE GROUP:
MEASURES OF CENTRAL TENDENCY

Statistics are a shorthand for summarizing or describing the attributes of a sample. Statistics can be subdivided into two broad classifications. The first classification is *descriptive statistics,* which, as the name implies, describe the sample. The second classification is *inferential statistics,* which consist of tests that allow for predictions or inferences about the population based upon the observations of the sample. Inferential statistics are used in hypothesis testing and are discussed in detail in subsequent chapters in this textbook.

Descriptive Statistics

Descriptive statistics are useful to both the investigator and the consumer of research. They give us an appreciation of what the sample looked like for a given set of characteristics. For example, one can know the number of men and women in a particular sample, the sample size, and the average age or the typical age of the individuals in the sample. By knowing what the group under investigation looked like, the reader can compare and contrast the results with her or his experience in dealing with a similar group. The reader is also able to assess whether subjects in different studies are comparable. The ability to make comparisons between studies is important when critically reviewing the literature on a topic.

Descriptive statistics answer relevant questions about the subjects who were studied in an investigation. Depending on the nature and content of the investigation, many characteristics of the sample group(s) may be of interest. Descriptive statistics also enable the reader to make decisions about the generalizability of the results, that is, to what groups or individuals the results may apply. The following statements illustrate some questions that can be addressed with descriptive statistics.

Did the subjects have a certain amount of experience?

Did they come from a particular geographic region?

When initially evaluated, did they have a typical impairment in movement?

Was there a typical loss of strength?

There are several ways to describe a sample. These measures are termed *measures of central tendency.*

The Range

First let us look at how to frame the sample. One way to describe the sample is to describe its boundaries or limits. The descriptive statistic that focuses on the boundaries is the *range*. The range is the difference between the highest and the lowest scores or measurements for a given sample. For example, the range in age from 14 to 64 years of age is 50 years. Note in this case that both the extent of the distribution of age and the highest and lowest ages are of interest.

Central Tendency

The *central tendency* refers to the typical, or middle, subject in the sample. This is commonly described by the *average*. There are three commonly used kinds of "averages," or indices of central tendency—the mode, the mean, and the median.

The Mode

The *mode* is the most commonly occurring value in a distribution. It is most useful when describing discrete variables that are measured with nominal or ordinal levels of measurement. The mode would be the appropriate "average" if, for instance, a physical therapist wished to typify the manual muscle test strength of the quadriceps femoris muscle group for a sample of ten individuals who demonstrated symptoms consistent with post-poliomyelitis syndrome. The manual muscle test is an ordinal-level measurement, so the mode is the best measure of central tendency.

The Mean

When most people speak of the average they are actually referring to the *mean*. The mean consists of the sum of all values that are given in a sample, divided by the number of individuals in that sample. The formula can be represented:

$$\bar{X} = \frac{\Sigma X}{n}$$

wherein,

X = a subject's score or measurement

n = the number of subjects in the sample

Σ (sigma) = the sum of

$\bar{X}$ = sample mean.

The mean is affected by inordinately large scores, becoming inflated. Therefore, if the distribution of scores in a sample includes several very large scores or measurements, the mean is inappropriate to describe the central or average score.

The Median

Sometimes when measuring a continuous variable, several measurements are very large or very small. A distribution of scores that contains an unusual number of high or low scores is called a *skewed distribution*. If the unusual scores are predominantly low, the distribution is skewed to the left; if high, the distribution is skewed to the right. The best measurement of the "average" of the skewed distribution is the value that falls exactly in the middle of the sample when the scores or measurements are arranged from the lowest to the highest. This value, which occurs at the half-way point, is termed the *median*.

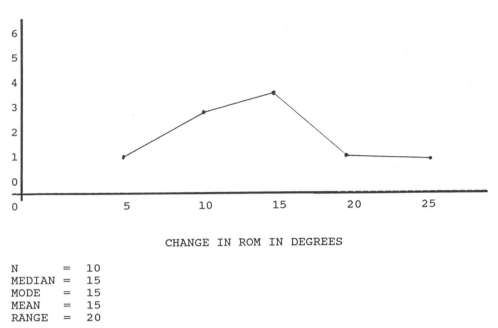

CHANGE IN ROM IN DEGREES

```
N         =    10
MEDIAN  =    15
MODE     =    15
MEAN     =    15
RANGE   =    20
```

FIGURE 9-1. Results in changes in range of motion for a sample of 10 subjects.

For example, if one is looking at the salary for a physical therapist in a given clinical situation, the typical or average salary may be influenced by one or two very large salaries. To present a score that is representative of the typical individual in the sample, the median should be used.

Limitations of the Average: A Practical Example

Suppose an investigator is interested in how much a new exercise program increases the heart rate of the subjects exposed to the exercise. One way of looking at it would be to look at the range of increase of heart rate, that is, the lowest and highest increases in heart rate. That does not, however, reveal much about the sample being investigated. The investigator also could look at the median gain in heart rate or at the mode of gain in heart rate, but because heart rate tends to be a continuous variable and is a ratio-level variable, chances are that there would not be two or more identical gains. Thus the chances of a definite mode occurring are relatively slim. Therefore the researcher may choose to use the mean increase in heart rate to describe the most typical gain in the group.

To illustrate some of the shortcomings of the range, mean, median, and mode distributions, two samples of ten subjects who tried a new exercise machine are compared for gain in range of motion (ROM) in Figures 9-1 and 9-2. As the reader can see, the mean, median, mode, and range are identical. However, the line graphs that depict the distributions of the group are quite dissimilar.

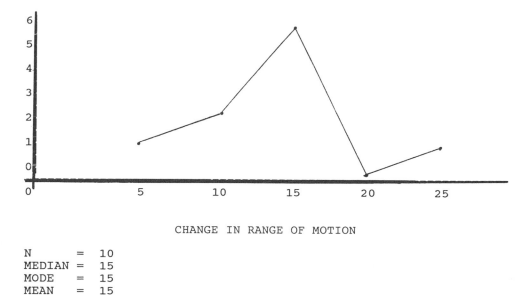

CHANGE IN RANGE OF MOTION

```
N       =   10
MEDIAN  =   15
MODE    =   15
MEAN    =   15
RANGE   =   20
```

FIGURE 9-2. Results in changes in range of motion for a second sample of 10 subjects. Note that all descriptive statistics are identical to those in Figure 9-1.

Variance and Standard Deviation

Clearly, what we need is a statistic that gives the average dispersion about some convenient point of reference on the distribution of scores. If we were to use the mean as the reference point for the dispersion of scores, we would intuitively want a number that expresses the average dispersion about the mean. The most obvious way would be to subtract the mean from each individual increase in range of motion, add up those values, and divide by the number of individuals in the sample. However, the result of this is always zero. This is because the mean represents what can be thought of as a balance point in this example. Zero occurs because the magnitude of the negative scores balances the magnitude of the positive scores, the gains above the mean. What is needed is some way to convert the negative scores and somehow to count the dispersion toward the negative side.* The negative numbers can be easily converted by squaring the scores. When one squares the difference of each score from the mean, adds all the squares together, and divides by the number of subjects, one comes up with the *variance*, more accurately termed the *mean squared deviation*, or dispersion from the mean, a convoluted term that is not used.

While the variance is useful as a concept and, as will be seen in later chapters, very useful in inferential statistics, it is not of much explanatory use to practitioners; for example, consider the usefulness of squared degrees of range of motion or squared gain in heart rate. The obvious way to alleviate the problem of squared

---

*The negative scores are any scores that are lower than the mean. These scores always fall to the left of the mean on a distribution of scores, just as scores greater than the mean fall to the right of the mean on the distribution.

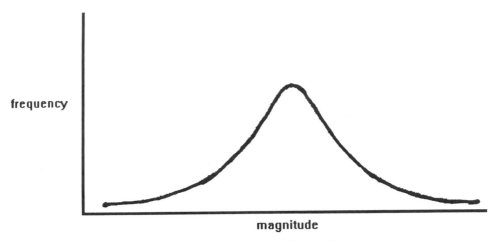

frequency

magnitude

FIGURE 9-3. The normal distribution.

heart rate or squared degrees of ROM is to obtain the square root of the variance. The square root of the variance is termed the *standard deviation*. The formulas are as follows:

for variance (s^2)

$$s^2 = \frac{\Sigma(X - \overline{X})^2}{n}$$

and for standard deviation (s)

$$s = \sqrt{\frac{\Sigma(X - \overline{X})^2}{n}}$$

In other words, the standard deviation is the average dispersion of scores about the mean. A small standard deviation indicates that the scores may be tightly clustered about the mean. A large standard deviation implies that the scores are spread out from the mean. As we will see, the standard deviation is a useful statistic in understanding health populations and samples.

The Normal Distribution

Figure 9-3 depicts the distribution of any characteristic that is randomly distributed within a population. The vertical axis represents the frequency of occurrence; the horizontal axis represents the magnitude of the particular characteristic. There are several universal qualities of the normal distribution. The reader will note that the normal distribution is bell-shaped, symmetrical, and the ends never touch the horizontal axis. Of special note, the mean, median, and mode are identical and are found at the highest point of the bell-shaped curve of the normal distribution.

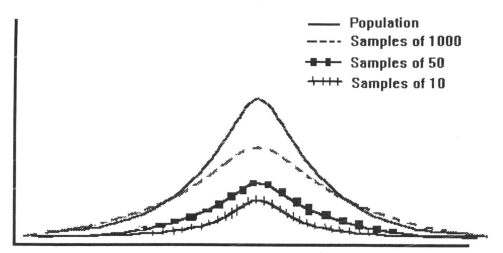

FIGURE 9-4. The effect of sample size on normal distribution.

One of the qualities of the normal distribution that is of particular interest to researchers and statisticians is that if a characteristic is randomly distributed within a sample, it is also described by a bell-shaped, normal curve. The height of the bell-shaped curve is related to the size of the sample. As the sample size becomes larger, the curve of the sample distribution becomes more pronounced and more closely resembles the normal distribution for a population. This phenomenon is referred to as *sampling variation.* Figure 9-4 compares distributions of means for a characteristic from samples of 10, 50, and 1,000 individuals with a normal distribution for a population. The samples for the distribution are drawn at random from the population. The bell-shaped curve on the sample distributions represents a plot of the mean values for sample groups of 10, 50, and 1,000, respectively.

The reader should immediately notice that the mean is identical for each of the normal distributions. The curve, however, is much flatter in the sampling distribution where groups of 10 are used to compute data points than in the groups of 50 or 1,000 or, in fact, than in the population distribution. The figure allows the reader to infer that the standard deviation of the small samples is greater than the standard deviation for the population. In other words, the formula for computing the standard deviation tends to underestimate the standard deviation of the sample, so that a correction factor is needed in the denominator of the formula. The correction factor is the $n - 1$ term, where n equals the number of subjects in the sample.
Standard deviation for samples:

$$s = \sqrt{\frac{\Sigma(X - \overline{X})^2}{n - 1}}$$

With large numbers in the sample, the $n - 1$ correction becomes negligible compared to n. In small samples, where the standard deviation of the population tends to be underestimated, the correction factor acts to correct for the underestimation.

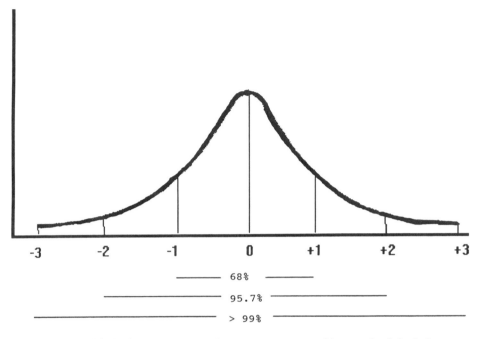

FIGURE 9-5. The percentage of scores encompassed by standard deviations.

The normal distribution is of particular interest in determining the likelihood of the occurrence of a particular score for a given magnitude of a particular characteristic. For a normal distribution, 68% of the scores are described within −1 to +1 standard deviation of the mean. No matter what value the standard deviation is, one standard deviation to −1 standard deviation encompasses 68% of the scores. As seen in Figure 9-5, slightly over 95% of the scores are encompassed within −2 to +2 standard deviations, and over 99% of the scores are contained within −3 to +3 deviations. The distribution, once again, is random, so it is strictly due to chance; there is no bias operating.

The Z Score

The percentage of scores that are contained within certain boundaries of standard deviations can be of substantial use to the investigator and to the physical therapist. Suppose a physical therapist has information on the ROM of a particular joint for a particular group of individuals. This would allow a physical therapist to determine how typical a particular patient's ROM is. The investigator can calculate the number of standard deviations that a given score is from the mean by using a Z score transformation. The value of Z can then be used to compute at what percentile a given score lies on a normal distribution. The formula for Z is:

$$Z = \frac{(X - \overline{X})}{s}$$

For example, suppose after treating 100 patients, a physical therapist plotted a distribution of the increase in ROM for a given joint following the application of a heat treatment. The physical therapist could then measure the patient's response, that is, the increase in ROM after a heat treatment, and would have an idea of how well that particular patient responded to the treatment. In this hypothetical example, let us assign the value of an increase of 50 degrees as the mean and the standard deviation of 10 degrees, that is, ±10 degrees. Consider that a given patient has a response of 35 degrees following a heat treatment. Using the Z score transformation, we note that the Z score is a −1.5 Z. Extrapolating from the Z table, we conclude that the patient's score lies at the 7th percentile. In other words, 93% of the patients who received heat would have a response greater than the 35-degree gain of our hypothetical patient.

The reader will note that in using the table of area under the curve for a normal distribution (Table 9-1), the percentile obtained through the Z score transformation is added to 0.50 (50%). In the example, the value was −0.433. So 0.50 + (−0.43) = 0.07 or 7%. We add to 50% because 50% represents the mean, or the 50th percentile. The reader will recall that the mean, median, and mode are identical in the normal curve. In this example, the physical therapist who examined the given patient can conclude that the response to heat demonstrated by the patient occurs quite rarely; only 7% of the scores are lower than the patient's. This is a rather uncommon response to heat. This knowledge is of use as we will see.

Statistical Significance

In the example above, the physical therapist and patient were able to determine that the patient's response was not the usual one. The usefulness of the normal distribution lies in ascertaining whether a score occurs reasonably often or rarely, strictly due to chance. We can rationally conclude that, if strictly due to chance, a score occurs reasonably often if it falls in the middle of the normal distribution. If a particular characteristic falls at the ends, or tails, of the bell-shaped curve, it can be thought to occur quite rarely. The latter determination is a concept known as statistical significance, and is very useful in research and investigations.

Let us consider a topic of interest to most physical therapists, namely, whether one treatment works better than another. If there is essentially no difference in the response to either of two treatments, comparisons should show that the mean differences between the responses of patient groups exposed to one treatment and those of patient groups exposed to the other treatment occur relatively commonly. In other words, the mean differences will show up on the hump of the bell-shaped curve and be due to chance alone. However, if the obtained mean difference between the two treatments occurs rarely, one would expect it to show up at one end or the other of the curve. Such a difference does not occur strictly due to chance very often. Therefore, perhaps, something other than chance is influencing the results.

In other words, the event is thought to be due not strictly to chance but to something else that is acting upon it. In the latter example just given, because

TABLE 9-1. Areas of the Standard Normal Distribution

					Second decimal place in z					
z	0.00	0.01	0.02	0.03	0.04	0.05	0.06	0.07	0.08	0.09
0.0	0.0000	0.0040	0.0080	0.0120	0.0160	0.0199	0.0239	0.0279	0.0319	0.0359
0.1	0.0398	0.0438	0.0478	0.0517	0.0557	0.0596	0.0636	0.0675	0.0714	0.0753
0.2	0.0793	0.0832	0.0871	0.0910	0.0948	0.0987	0.1026	0.1064	0.1103	0.1141
0.3	0.1179	0.1217	0.1255	0.1293	0.1331	0.1368	0.1406	0.1443	0.1480	0.1517
0.4	0.1554	0.1591	0.1628	0.1664	0.1700	0.1736	0.1772	0.1808	0.1844	0.1879
0.5	0.1915	0.1950	0.1985	0.2019	0.2054	0.2088	0.2123	0.2157	0.2190	0.2224
0.6	0.2257	0.2291	0.2324	0.2357	0.2389	0.2442	0.2454	0.2486	0.2517	0.2549
0.7	0.2580	0.2611	0.2642	0.2673	0.2704	0.2734	0.2764	0.2794	0.2823	0.2852
0.8	0.2281	0.2910	0.2939	0.2967	0.2995	0.3023	0.3051	0.3078	0.3106	0.3113
0.9	0.3159	0.3186	0.3212	0.3238	0.3264	0.3289	0.3315	0.3340	0.3365	0.3389
1.0	0.3413	0.3438	0.3861	0.3485	0.3508	0.3531	0.3554	0.3577	0.3599	0.3621
1.1	0.3643	0.3665	0.3686	0.3708	0.3729	0.3749	0.3770	0.3790	0.3810	0.3830
1.2	0.3849	0.3869	0.3888	0.3907	0.3925	0.3944	0.3962	0.3980	0.3997	0.4015
1.3	0.4032	0.4049	0.4066	0.4082	0.4099	0.4115	0.4131	0.4147	0.4162	0.4177
1.4	0.4192	0.4206	0.4222	0.4236	0.4251	0.4265	0.4279	0.4292	0.4306	0.4319
1.5	0.4332	0.4345	0.4357	0.4370	0.4382	0.4394	0.4406	0.4418	0.4429	0.4441
1.6	0.4452	0.4463	0.4474	0.4484	0.4495	0.4505	0.4515	0.4535	0.4535	0.4545
1.7	0.4554	0.4564	0.4573	0.4582	0.4591	0.4599	0.4608	0.4616	0.4625	0.4633
1.8	0.4641	0.4649	0.4656	0.4664	0.4671	0.4678	0.4686	0.4693	0.4699	0.4706
1.9	0.4713	0.4719	0.4726	0.4732	0.4738	0.4744	0.4750	0.4756	0.4761	0.4767
2.0	0.4772	0.4778	0.4783	0.4788	0.4793	0.4798	0.4803	0.4808	0.4812	0.4817
2.1	0.4821	0.4826	0.4830	0.3834	0.3838	0.4842	0.4846	0.4850	0.4854	0.4857
2.2	0.4861	0.4864	0.4868	0.4871	0.4875	0.4878	0.4881	0.4884	0.4887	0.4890
2.3	0.4893	0.4896	0.4898	0.4901	0.4904	0.4906	0.4909	0.4911	0.4913	0.4916
2.4	0.4918	0.4920	0.4922	0.4925	0.4927	0.4929	0.4931	0.4932	0.4934	0.4936
2.5	0.4938	0.4940	0.4941	0.4943	0.4945	0.4946	0.4948	0.4949	0.4951	0.4952
2.6	0.4953	0.4955	0.4956	0.5947	0.4959	0.4960	0.4961	0.4962	0.4963	0.4964
2.7	0.4965	0.4966	0.4967	0.4968	0.4969	0.4970	0.4971	0.4972	0.4973	0.4974
2.8	0.4974	0.4975	0.4976	0.4977	0.4977	0.4978	0.4979	0.4979	0.4980	0.4981
2.9	0.4981	0.4982	0.4982	0.4983	0.4984	0.4984	0.4985	0.4985	0.4986	0.4986
3.0	0.4987	0.4987	0.4987	0.4988	0.4988	0.4989	0.4989	0.4989	0.4990	0.4990
3.1	0.4990	0.4991	0.4991	0.4991	0.4992	0.4992	0.4992	0.4992	0.4993	0.4993
3.2	0.4993	0.4993	0.4994	0.4994	0.4994	0.4994	0.4994	0.4995	0.4995	0.4995
3.3	0.4995	0.4995	0.4995	0.4996	0.4996	0.4996	0.4996	0.4996	0.4996	0.4997
3.4	0.4997	0.4997	0.4997	0.4997	0.4997	0.4997	0.4997	0.4997	0.4997	0.4998
3.5	0.4998									
4.0	0.49998									
4.5	0.499997									
5.0	0.4999997									

(From *Standard Mathematical Tables*, 15th ed. Copyright CRC Press, Inc. Boca Raton, FL.)

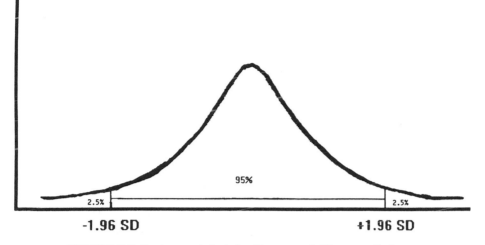

95%

2.5%   2.5%

-1.96 SD   **+1.96 SD**

FIGURE 9-6. Setting statistical significance at 0.05—two-tailed test.

the difference in responses to treatment only occurs very rarely due to chance, the investigator can conclude that a difference is attributable to one or the other forms of treatment. Central to the concept of statistical significance is setting the limit at which one decides the results do not occur strictly due to chance or do not occur commonly. The results are statistically significant if they rarely occur due to chance. That is the key concept. The logic is that if an occurrence is not due to chance, something else (such as the independent variable) may be the cause.

The threshold for determining if there is statistical significance is chosen arbitrarily by the investigator. Most often the 0.05 value is used. In other cases, the 0.01 value is used. These values indicate, respectively, that fewer than 5 times in 100 ($\alpha < 0.05$) or fewer than 1 time in 100 ($\alpha < 0.01$) are the results obtained strictly due to chance. In other words, if fewer than 1 time in 100 the results would be due to chance, the conclusion must be that the results are not due to chance but rather to the differences in treatment.

Finally, if one has read the literature, one sees the low values of p and, every once in a while, the value of α (alpha). Alpha represents the level of statistical significance that is set before the investigation takes place. The investigator sets the level of statistical significance and assigns it to the statistical hypothesis. The p value is the probability of the results occurring strictly due to chance and is obtained from examining the data (results) using a statistical test. When the p (probability) is less than or equal to α (the level for accepting results as statistically significant), the results are statistically significant.

Recall chapter 1, where we noted the three types of statistical hypotheses. Now we have an opportunity for seeing how they relate to statistical significance. For the null hypothesis, the hypothesis is validated if the probability of obtaining the results falls in the hump section of the distribution (Figure 9-6), for the null hypothesis states that the results or differences are due to chance (that is, there will

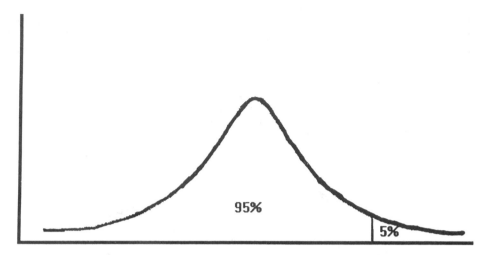

FIGURE 9-7. Statistical significance set at .05—one-tailed test.

be no statistically significant difference). The alternative hypothesis value is validated if the results fall in the "rare" zones, or not very common parts, of the probability distribution; in this case, there will be a statistically significant difference. For the directional hypothesis, only one end of the distribution may be used to achieve statistical significance. Thus, because the directional hypothesis says that there will be a statistically significant difference, if one is using the 0.05 level of statistical significance, then the 95% of the values that will be used to disprove that hypothesis must start from the one end of the normal distribution and proceed until 95% of the scores are included. That is, the entire 5% of scores must be in the direction specified by the hypothesis, as contrasted to the 5% of the scores being distributed equally at either end of the distribution for the alternative and the null hypotheses (Figure 9-7).

In summary, statistical significance has to do with the likelihood of particular results occurring strictly due to chance. If the results occur very rarely strictly due to chance, the investigator may conclude that whatever was manipulated in the investigation may be affecting the outcome. If the scores occur quite commonly because of chance, there may be no difference attributable to the experimental conditions or to manipulation of the independent variable.

I hope that the concept of statistical significance as presented graphically here is understandable and useful. Comprehending the concept of statistical significance permits one to understand what any particular statistical test reveals. Any of the inferential statistical tests indicate how likely one is to obtain similar results due to chance, that is, the probability of obtaining similar results simply because of happenstance.

REFERENCES

1. Shott, S. *Statistics for health professionals.* Philadelphia: W.B. Saunders, 1990.

10

NONPARAMETRIC STATISTICS

Ann F. Van Sant

INTRODUCTION

THE NATURE OF VARIABLES BEING STUDIED AND NONPARAMETRIC STATISTICS
The Nature of Variables and Levels of Measurement

ASSUMPTIONS ON WHICH NONPARAMETRIC TESTS ARE BASED
Parameters and Nonparameters
Distribution-free Tests
Nonparametric Statistics and Research Design

DESCRIPTIVE STATISTICS AND STATISTICAL TESTS
Descriptive Statistics for Attributes and Qualitative Variables

CHI SQUARE
Chi-Square Statistic for a Single Sample
Statement of the Hypothesis
Nature of the Attributes or Variables
Research Design
The Assumptions
The Method
The Two-Sample Chi-Square Test
Statement of the Hypothesis
Nature of the Attributes or Variables
Research Design
The Assumptions
The Method

INTRODUCTION

Nonparametric statistics are a unique set of mathematical procedures used to test research hypotheses. They differ from better known parametric procedures essentially in that they are based on fewer assumptions. Parametric statistical procedures rest on assumptions about parameters or values of a population being studied, such as the population mean or standard deviation from the mean. The assumptions underlying nonparametric procedures are commonly limiting conditions, such as the sample(s) being randomly selected, and elements chosen for study, such as subjects that are independent or not related to one another.

Nonparametric procedures are ideally suited for answering research questions that involve attributes or qualitative variables. As we develop our professional body of knowledge in physical therapy, we must attend to attributes and qualitative variables. Many patient characteristics that are of interest to us have not yet had quantitative measurement scales developed for them. For example, the "quality of a patient's movement," "strength," and "muscle tone" hold important positions in the clinical theories we employ. Each is a qualitative variable.

Basic knowledge of nonparametric statistics is also extremely valuable in studies with small sample sizes, that is, for analyzing results of clinical studies in which relatively small numbers of individuals are studied. Such studies might include patients with a particular disorder or individuals of a specific age group or social background.

An excellent example of this type of situation can be found in our university hospital's physical therapy clinic. Two therapists have been collecting data on hemiplegic patients with shoulder subluxation. The criteria they have used to define the subluxation are relatively restrictive. Despite the large number of hemiplegic patients seen in the clinic, few subjects meet the criteria for entrance into the study. In instances like this, where a small, select group of patients is studied, nonparametric procedures are the most appropriate statistics available to the researcher.

Nonparametric statistics are quite easy to understand. The simple calculations involved in most of the tests can be performed with a hand-held calculator. The logical principles on which the tests are based are easily demonstrated, and they do not require knowledge of calculus or advanced mathematics. A researcher using nonparametric tests often can carry out the statistical tests personally. As a result, the investigator develops a clear understanding of what is done to the data in the statistical analysis. This is not always the case when parametric procedures are used. The models on which parametric procedures are based require knowledge of the calculus for full understanding and often are most practically completed using computers and software packages. Although this technological advance enables rapid analysis of data, the researcher often must expend a large amount of time to understand the technical information that explains how a computer program "handles" or manipulates the data.

In general, for every parametric test there is a similar nonparametric procedure that can be used when the assumptions of the parametric test cannot be met.

Some nonparametric procedures have no parametric counterpart, however, and therefore are the only tests available to the researcher.

To summarize, nonparametric procedures are statistical procedures ideally suited (1) to examine research questions that involve attributes or qualitative variables and (2) for use in studies with small sample sizes. They are easy to understand and apply.

This chapter is a primer for therapists who are acquiring knowledge of the research process and the relationship of statistical procedures to that process. The chapter has two major sections. First, as a start toward understanding some of the most common nonparametric procedures, I discuss elements that are considered when selecting a nonparametric statistical procedure. These include (1) the nature of the variable being studied; (2) the research design or plan used when gathering the data; and (3) the kinds of assumptions that underlie nonparametric tests. Next I introduce examples of commonly employed nonparametric procedures. For each statistical procedure, a statement of the hypothesis being tested is included, the nature of the attributes or variables under study is identified, an appropriate design is reviewed, the assumptions of that specific statistical procedure are explained, and a general review of the methods of the test is presented.

THE NATURE OF VARIABLES BEING STUDIED AND NONPARAMETRIC STATISTICS

The Nature of Variables and Levels of Measurement

As noted, nonparametric procedures are so useful because they help answer questions about many of the variables that interest physical therapists. A significant number of our most interesting clinical variables represent qualities or attributes of people—our patients, their families, and us, as students and therapists. At the present time the majority of these qualities and attributes cannot be measured precisely. These qualities are often described, noted as being present or absent, or classified into one of several categories. If the quality is variable by nature, then instances when the variable occurs are counted, or the property may be judged to be present to a greater or lesser extent.

Attributes and variables represent two different types of characteristics or properties. An *attribute* is a quality that is stable and unchanging. It can be documented on a nominal scale as simply being present or absent. Attributes can also be classified into mutually exclusive subgroups, for example, orthopedic, neurologic, or cardiopulmonary disorders. Both documenting an attribute and assigning it to a subgroup represent the *nominal level of measurement.*

In contrast, a *variable* is a characteristic or property that by its nature varies from one individual or case to another, from one time to another, or from one group of people to another. The ability to discriminate between an unchanging attribute and a variable is quite significant, as the nonparametric statistics used for attributes differ from those used with variables.

Variables may be considered either qualitative or quantitative. *Qualitative variables* are measured using ordered scales, such as mild, moderate, or severe spasticity; or first, second, or third in order of appearance, as might be used to denote a developmental variable or to indicate the order of finishing in a Special Olympics event. Measuring qualitative variables is a process of indicating (1) relatively more or less of the variable, with respect to other cases or individuals, or (2) a relative order in time. Qualitative variables are measured on scales that do not express exactly how much or when in time. The measurement schemes used with these variables are called *ordinal scales*.

Quantitative variables are either measured or counted. In instances where counting is used, the quantitative variable is considered a discrete variable. Discrete quantitative variables are expressed in whole numbers. Example of discrete variables include the number of treatment days, an individual's radial pulse count, or the score on a 100-item, multiple-choice test.

Quantitative variables that could assume an infinite range of values, including fractions of values, are considered *continuous variables*. The concept that a continuous variable could assume an infinite number of values represents a theoretical ideal. No measurement devices exist capable of measuring infinitely small fractions of variables. But the concept of a continuous variable is an important one. How we view the variable determines which statistical test is most appropriate. If a measurement device or counting method exists to help us apply precise values to the variable, we should use it. There are times, however, when this is not the case. For example, if we were to study individuals who took the physical therapy licensing examination, we might not have access to precise scores that measure an individual's knowledge of physical therapy. We might only know the number of individuals who passed and who failed. In this instance, a nominal classification system is the only one available to the researcher. We realize, however, that some individuals "just failed" or "just passed," whereas others hardly missed a correct answer and still others failed royally. If the researcher is interested in the underlying variable "knowledge of physical therapy," then it is important to realize that this is a continuously distributed variable. This is the case despite the fact that a pass/fail classification is being used, which only conveys presence or absence of an attribute. Statistical tests that assume that a continuously distributed variable is studied can be used appropriately even though a nominal classification system is used.

It is important to understand the nature of the attributes and variables that we study as physical therapists. We should be able to discriminate stable attributes from variables. If variables are being studied, we should give thought to whether they possess discrete or continuous properties. Although some statisticians have pronounced that nonparametric tests should be selected on the basis of the specific level of measurement, this is still controversial. In this chapter the view is presented that selection of an appropriate statistical procedure and reasonable interpretation of results of research are dependent on the researchers' understanding of the nature of the variables they are studying, not necessarily the level of measurement of those variables.

As we develop measurement systems in physical therapy, we may discover on close inspection that seemingly stable attributes may be "variable," and that qualitative variables may eventually become measurable by using either discrete or continuous measurement scales. These marks of progress toward a more defined body of knowledge of physical therapy require individuals who are willing to wrestle with the underlying nature of attributes and variables that have clinical relevance. As we struggle with these issues, however, we should not forget that there are nonparametric statistical procedures available to help answer research questions about today's attributes and qualitative variables.

ASSUMPTIONS ON WHICH NONPARAMETRIC TESTS ARE BASED

A set of assumptions underlies every statistical procedure. The most appropriate statistical procedure is selected based on an understanding of the nature of the variables, the design of the research situation, and the assumptions underlying the statistical test. Physical therapists make assumptions about patients and the likelihood that the patients will respond to their interventions. Statisticians make assumptions about the data they manipulate and the likelihood that the data will respond to their mathematical manipulations. Researchers must consider the conditions under which the data were collected. They also must know what statistical procedures are appropriate for a particular research design, just as we understand our patients, the nature of their problems, the conditions under which the problems occur, and the procedures best suited to solve these problems.

Parameters and Nonparameters

The term *parameter* refers to a *value or quantity of a variable within a population.* A parameter is a theoretical idea. This is because a parameter is a value of a *population,* not a precisely known value. It is not usually possible to measure every individual or element in a population to determine the exact value of a parameter. An example of a parameter is the average height of 11-year-old girls. It is not possible to obtain a measure of height for every 11-year-old girl in the world. Because of this impossibility, one must make assumptions about parameters of a population. These assumptions are a distinctive feature of parametric statistics. Nonparametric statistics do not require assumptions about population parameters. This is the reason for the use of the term *nonparametric.*

Because parametric statistical tests rest on a set of assumptions about population values and nonparametric statistics do not, different questions are answered with these different types of statistics. For example, a parametric statistic would answer the question, "*Given the population* of 11-year-old girls, what is the probability that *the average height of these girls is six feet?*" In contrast, a nonparametric statistic would answer the question, "*Given this sample* of 11-year-old girls, what is the probability that *a girl with a height of six feet would be found in my sample?*" The parametric statistic helps answer a question about a population value; the nonparametric statistic assists in answering a question about the sample.

Distribution-free Tests

Nonparametric tests have also been called distribution-free tests. Parametric statistics rest on assumptions about the distribution of values. For example, a statistic may rest on the assumption that the values are normally distributed or form a binomial distribution. The term *distribution-free* refers to statistical tests that do not rest on assumptions about how values are distributed within a population. Very simply, this is because there is no need for the assumption. Distribution-free statistics are concerned with samples, and the form of the sample distribution is known.

To illustrate, consider the situation of measuring the heights in a sample of ten 11-year-old girls. We would admit that if we measured a different sample of ten 11-year-old girls, we would likely obtain a different distribution of heights. However, if ranks were substituted for the girls' heights in the first sample, so that the shortest girl was ranked number 1 and the tallest was ranked number 10, the distribution of ranks would be the same from sample to sample. The distribution of ranks is determined by the number of elements in the sample, in this case, the number of girls. A statistical test that helps answer questions about ranks is distribution-free: it does not depend on an assumption about how the values are distributed.

It has been suggested that the term "assumption free" statistics be used to refer to the statistical tests that do not rest on assumptions about parameters (nonparametrics) or on the form of the distributions of the values within a population (distribution-free tests). Although this term is correct, it does not mean that nonparametric or distribution-free tests are without assumptions. There are theoretical assumptions associated with every statistical procedure. Assumptions on which nonparametric procedures are based relate to the nature of the variable or attribute being studied and processes of sampling and assigning subjects to groups.

Nonparametric Statistics and Research Design

Different research questions and hypotheses require different types of statistics. Not all of these are "test statistics," designed to examine an experimental hypothesis. Researchers are interested in descriptive studies, that is, in describing newly discovered attributes or variables and in describing old variables in new ways. They are also interested in correlational studies, that is, in understanding the interrelationships among various attributes and variables.

In descriptive studies the researcher describes an attribute, characteristic, or variable, or a set of attributes or variables. This may be done at a single point in time or repeatedly, across a series of time intervals. Repeated measures that document the natural course of events during recovery from injury or disease or during the learning or development of some ability also comprise descriptive research.

Correlational studies describe relationships between two or more attributes or variables. Like descriptive studies, correlational studies may be designed to gather one set of measures at a single point in time or may involve repeated measures. Correlational studies can be very helpful in "screening" implausible hypotheses. For example, if one variable or attribute has been hypothesized to cause the other, but in a correlational study no relationship can be demonstrated between the two variables, then the time and effort that would be needed to design and conduct an experimental study of the hypothesis can be saved.

The terms *preexperimental, quasi-experimental,* and *true experimental* have been used to describe three major classes of research design. These research designs all involve applying a treatment, called an *independent variable,* and monitoring its effect on a dependent variable. This system of classification was developed primarily to remind the student of (1) the conclusions that can and cannot be made as a result of each type of design; and (2) the difficulty of conducting a truly controlled experiment in clinical or natural settings, in which we wish to apply our results.

When selecting a statistical test, the most relevant design characteristics are the number of samples studied and the relative independence of the observations of the dependent variable. With these two factors in mind, consider that there are both parametric and nonparametric tests for experimental research involving one, two, and more than two groups. There are also both parametric and nonparametric tests for experimental research involving repeated measures and matched-pairs designs.

DESCRIPTIVE STATISTICS AND STATISTICAL TESTS

Often when thinking of research and statistics, the focus is on computing formulas that are used to test research hypotheses. Statistics is a broader term, however, that includes numbers computed to describe and summarize information.

Descriptive statistics summarize and describe a sample in terms of central tendency and variability. Calculating descriptive statistics is the first step in carrying out any statistical test. When dealing with continuous quantitative variables, the mean or average is the statistic that is the common indicator of central tendency. The standard deviation or variance are the common statistics used to portray variability, or the spread of measured values of continuously distributed variables.

Because statistical tests are designed to examine descriptive statistics that summarize a sample of values, these descriptors are usually calculated first. Consider the fact that statistical tests have the general form of comparing a statistical value that represents central tendency to a statistic that expresses variability of a set (or sets) of observations:

$$\text{test statistic} = \frac{\text{central tendency}}{\text{variability}}$$

This general form of a test statistic is applicable in both parametric and nonparametric tests of research hypotheses. For this reason, before examining nonparametric statistical tests, one needs to understand the descriptive statistics that are appropriately used with qualitative variables and attributes.

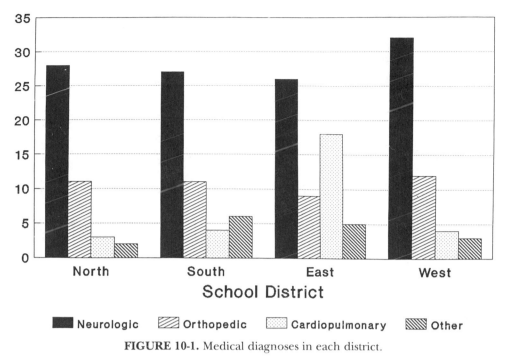

■ Neurologic   ▨ Orthopedic   ▦ Cardiopulmonary   ▩ Other

FIGURE 10-1. Medical diagnoses in each district.

Descriptive Statistics for Attributes and Qualitative Variables

When attributes or discrete qualitative variables are being studied, the statistic that reveals information about central tendency is the mode. *The mode is the most common or frequently occurring class.* To determine the mode, one simply counts the number of observations in each category or class of the attribute studied. The spread or dispersion of the attribute within the sample is expressed by the proportion or percent of cases demonstrating (or not demonstrating) an attribute or the percent of individuals demonstrating each category of the attribute. This simple statistic is determined by counting the frequency with which each class or category appears in the sample and then expressing the frequencies as a proportion or percent of the total number of individuals studied. This information may be expressed in numeric form, as well as in a graphic form called a *frequency histogram* (see Figure 10-1). Graphs are extremely useful when summarizing central tendency and variability of a data set.

The mode is also an appropriate expression of central tendency when discrete quantitative variables are studied. The following example illustrates how important it is to understand the nature of the variable being studied when selecting a statistic.

We all have heard statements such as, "The average American family has 2.1 children." Children do not come in fractions; they are not continuously distributed! Children are a discrete quantitative variable. They can be counted. The central tendency of discrete variables that are counted in whole numbers should be expressed in whole numbers. Therefore, the mode might be used to express central tendency, for example, "Most commonly there are 2 children in an American family," or the proportion of families with no children, one child, two children, and so forth might be presented. Each of these latter statistics is congruent with the underlying nature of the discrete quantitative variable, "children." The strange concept of a fraction of a child is an example of a failure to use a statistic appropriate for the variable when summarizing the data.

The median is the midpoint in a range of values or scores. The median is an appropriate indicator of central tendency when the data represent continuous qualitative variables that are rank-ordered. To determine the median, arrange the values or scores in rank order, from lowest to highest or highest to lowest, according to personal preference or convention. Then count the number of scores. If there is an odd number of scores in the sample, then the middle value in the ordered list is the median. If there is an even number of scores, then the median is the midpoint between the two middle values.

CHI SQUARE

The chi-square statistic has several applications. Each form answers different research questions and is associated with different research designs. Chi square can be used to determine whether two attributes studied in a single sample are related to each other: for example, is there a relationship between the side where hemiplegia occurs and gender within a single group of patients? The chi-square statistic can also be used to determine if attributes among several groups are similar: for example, is the proportion of patients with right hemiplegia the same in one rehabilitation center as in another rehabilitation center? Chi square can also be applied to answer questions about two related samples: for example, do individuals with right hemiplegia remain in the same type of health care facility during the second three-month interval after their stroke (three to six months post-stroke)?

In the following discussion, the chi-square statistic used to examine the attributes of a single sample is presented first, followed by the chi-square test for two independent samples, and, finally, the chi-square test for two related samples.

Chi-Square Statistic for a Single Sample

To appreciate the application of chi square to answer a research question about a single sample, consider the following situation. A therapist working in a large school system is intrigued by the apparent relationship between medical diagnoses of the students and the school district in which they attend school. She believes that the largest number of children with neurologic diagnoses reside in the west district, where large numbers of individuals live below the poverty level. She thinks this group may have a higher incidence of neurologic disorders because of poor prenatal care. She has decided to gather information to determine if her supposition about the distribution of children with neurologic diagnoses is correct.

Statement of the Hypothesis

There is no relationship between medical diagnosis and school district.

Nature of the Attributes or Variables

Here two attributes are being studied: medical diagnosis and school district assignment. These characteristics are not variables. They are considered stable, unchanging traits. The therapist-researcher has decided to study four main classes of diagnosis: neurologic, orthopedic, cardiopulmonary, and "other." The researcher will have to spend time clearly defining each class of diagnosis and deciding what to do if a subject presents with multiple diagnoses. These issues are quite typically encountered when asking questions regarding the classification of individuals' attributes.

Four school districts were mapped out by the school board and staff. Children are not bused between districts. In this study, the therapist is interested in the four school districts (north, south, east, and west).

Research Design

This research is designed as a correlational study and examines the relationship between two attributes. It involves a single sample. This study is an initial step in the attempt to identify an orderly process operating between the two attributes of school district and medical diagnosis. It is not experimental research because nothing will be done to try to change the subjects. The researcher is simply interested in gathering data concerning medical diagnosis and school district at a single point in time.

The Assumptions

The chi-square test of association for a single sample is based on the following assumptions:

1. The subjects are randomly selected from the population being studied. Here the population is all of the children with a medical diagnosis in the school system. Each child in the school system with a medical diagnosis should have an equal opportunity to be included in this sample.
2. The attributes of each subject are independent of the attributes of every other subject. That is, the medical diagnosis of each subject is not related to or determined by the medical diagnosis of any other subject. This should also be true for the school district assignments. The school district of each child is not related to or determined by the school district of any other child. Children have not been purposely assigned to the same school district or purposely separated.

The Method

Prior to carrying out the statistical test, a table is constructed to tabulate the number of subjects in each school district that demonstrate each medical diagno-

DISPLAY 10-1
EXAMPLES OF A CONTINGENCY TABLE FOR A SINGLE-SAMPLE CHI SQUARE

SCHOOL DISTRICT	MEDICAL DIAGNOSIS			
	Neurologic	Orthopedic	Cardiopulmonary	Other
North				
South				
East				
West				

SCHOOL DISTRICT	MEDICAL DIAGNOSIS			
	Neurologic	Orthopedic	Cardiopulmonary	Other
North	28	11	3	2
South	27	11	4	6
East	26	9	18	5
West	32	12	4	3

The two tables above illustrate how a contingency table would be set up for the example in the text of a single-sample chi-square analysis. The top table is ready to receive data; the therapist would keep a tally of both the medical diagnosis and the school district of each child in the sample. A summary of fictitious data is presented in the bottom table.

sis. Each subject on which data were collected is assigned to the appropriate cell or box of the table. This table is termed a *contingency table*. Display 10-1 provides an example of a contingency table that would be used in a study such as this.

The chi-square single-sample test compares the observed frequencies of medical diagnoses in each district to the frequencies expected if diagnoses were randomly distributed across the four school districts. The greater the difference between the observed frequencies and the expected frequencies, the larger the chi-square statistic and the less probable it is that the result occurred by chance alone. Explanations of computational procedures, worked-out examples, and tables of chi-square values can be found in most statistics books, be they parametric or nonparametric texts. The chi-square test is probably the most widely known and applied of the nonparametric tests.

The numeric result of the test does not indicate which diagnoses are related or associated with which school district assignment, and the researcher must look at the distribution of the data among the various categories to make sense of any significant finding.

The Two-Sample Chi-Square Test

In the above example, the therapist who conducted the one-sample chi-square test found that there was a relationship between school district assignment and medical diagnosis. The therapist had originally thought that the neurologic cases would be more predominant in the west district, where there was a greater number of families of lower socioeconomic circumstances. She discovered, however, that this was not the case. Neurologic cases were relatively equally distributed across all districts. There were, however, a large number of children with cardiopulmonary disorders in the east district. After careful analysis and discussions among the therapists she worked with, they decided that this result was likely associated with the location of the Lung Association's after-school swim program for children. They felt the swim program might attract families with children with pulmonary disorders.

There was a similar Lung Association swim program in a city approximately 100 miles away. The therapist had a colleague there who was director of therapy services for the public schools. He was quite interested in the results of the study but did not believe the situation to be similar in his city. He had never noticed the relationship between pulmonary disorders and the swim program, and he believed it existed only by chance in his friend's city. The two therapists decided to collaborate in a study that examined the proportion of children with pulmonary disorders in their two cities who lived and attended school in each city in the district with the Lung Association's swim program.

Statement of the Hypothesis

There is no difference between the two cities in the incidence of children with pulmonary disorders who attend school in districts with and without Lung Association swim programs.

Nature of the Attributes or Variables

One attribute is being studied: types of school districts (those with and without Lung Association swim programs). Children with pulmonary disorders are the subjects of the study. The two cities represent the two independent samples.

Research Design

This is a study of two independent samples. One sample comes from the children in one city. The other sample is drawn from children in the other city.

The Assumptions

1. Individuals in the two samples are independent of one another. Attributes of children in one sample are not determined by the attributes of children in the other sample.
2. Individuals in each sample are independent of one another. Attributes of children in one sample are not determined by the attributes of other children in that sample.
3. Sufficient numbers of cases are studied in each sample to produce an expected frequency of five cases in each classification of the attribute within each sample.

This last assumption is a requirement for use of the chi-square probability tables. If any attribute has fewer than five expected cases within a sample, the *Irwin Fisher exact test* is the most appropriate nonparametric statistic. The Irwin Fisher test addresses the same research question and rests on similar assumptions and design, that is, two independent samples, with each element of the two samples classified into one of the mutually exclusive classes of the attributes. In the Irwin Fisher test, the exact probability of a result is determined. The Irwin Fisher test should always be used if either of the two samples is comprised of fewer than ten observations or cases.

The Method

The procedure for the two independent sample chi-square test is the same as for the single-sample test. It begins with the construction of a contingency table. In this case, the table is a 2×2 configuration, as illustrated in Display 10-2. Again, the observed frequencies are compared to those expected if there were an equal distribution of children in districts with and without swim programs in both cities.

The Chi-Square Test for Two Related Samples (The McNemar Test)

The chi-square test for related samples is the least known version of chi-square. Because it is the only test suited to examining change or stability of "attributes," or unordered qualitative properties, however, it is included here. This test has a basic role to play in the primary identification of variables (as properties or characteristics that have the capacity to vary). The test also is fundamental to examining reliability of unordered classification systems. When used in the latter manner, the statistic is used to answer the question, Are repeated measures of the same attribute stable? This reliability test is termed a *Kappa statistic.*

To understand the application of the McNemar test, consider the following example. Typical work settings for therapists appear to be changing. There appears to be a trend for therapists to leave hospitals and seek work in other types of practice settings. The executive director of a state chapter of the American Physical Therapy Association has been asked by the chapter's board of directors to gather

---

DISPLAY 10-2
EXAMPLE OF A CONTINGENCY TABLE OF TWO-SAMPLE CHI SQUARE

NUMBER OF CHILDREN WITH PULMONARY DISORDERS	CITY	
	A	*B*
In the district with the program		
In another district		

In this table the two independent samples occupy separate columns. The children in each city who are selected for study will be tallied in either the top or bottom row, depending on whether they live in the school district with the swim program or in some other school district in that city.

---

information to determine whether this apparent trend can be verified. The executive director will immediately collect data about who is and is not employed in hospitals and then will repeat the data collection next year, using the same therapists as subjects.

Statement of the Hypothesis

Physical therapists in the chapter are just as likely to change their work settings from hospital to nonhospital settings as they are to change from nonhospital to hospital settings.

Nature of the Attributes or Variables

The work setting is being studied. Work setting is an unordered qualitative variable.

Research Design

This is a repeated-measures design, but in this instance the study is purely descriptive. Like a developmental study, it documents the status of the subjects at two successive points in time. Often-repeated measures are associated with preexperimental or experimental designs. This repeated-measures chi square could be used for preexperimental (pretest, posttest) study of a specific variable that might be thought to cause the apparent change in practice settings. But the study outlined above is not designed to determine the cause of therapists' changing practice settings. Indeed, it is entirely possible that this study might fail to verify change.

The Assumptions

There are three assumptions for this test:

1. The factor being studied is a dichotomous qualitative variable.
2. The subjects in the study were randomly selected from the chapter membership. Here the population being studied is chapter members. Because all therapists in the state do not have an opportunity to be included in the sample, the study results cannot be generalized and no conclusions can be made about all therapists in the state. Conclusions can only be made about chapter members.
3. The work setting of each subject is independent of the work setting of every other subject. This is an assumption that might in reality be violated, for some therapists may choose to work at separate facilities or at the same facility (for a variety of reasons). The extent to which such choices affect the numbers of individuals changing from hospital to nonhospital settings would probably be quite small, and the researcher could reasonably make this assumption.

The Method

As with the other types of chi-square tests, setting up a contingency table is the first step. Display 10-3 illustrates a contingency table that could be used for the study of changing trends in work settings. Paired observations of the same therapist in year 1 and year 2 would be tallied in the contingency table. If there were no changes at all in work setting, everyone in a hospital setting in year 1 would also be in a hospital setting in year 2, and those in nonhospital settings in year 1 would remain in nonhospital settings in year 2. All entries in the table in such a situation would be in the top left-hand box or the bottom right-hand box.

There are procedures like the McNemar test that can be used to examine larger symmetrical contingency tables of repeated or related measures (3×3 tables, 4×4 tables, and so forth). One such statistical procedure is called Bower's test. Explanations of Bower's test can be found in nonparametric textbooks.

MANN-WHITNEY U TEST

The Mann-Whitney U test is a widely used nonparametric test, analogous to the parametric two-sample t-test. It can be used without having to make assumptions regarding the spread of scores about the center of the distributions of the two samples.

Consider this situation: therapists treating patients who have been complaining of dizziness believe that if their patients were more motivated, they would more

---

DISPLAY 10-3
EXAMPLE OF A CONTINGENCY TABLE FOR REPEATED-MEASURES CHI SQUARE

WORK SETTING YEAR 1	WORK SETTING YEAR 2	
	Hospital	*Nonhospital*
Hospital		
Nonhospital		

After the second year of the study, each therapist will be assigned to the appropriate cell. Based on their initial job setting, they will be tallied in either row 1 or row 2. Data from year 2 will be used to decide to which column they will be assigned. Thus a therapist who was working in a hospital at the beginning of the study but switched to a nonhospital setting by the time of data collection in year 2 would be tallied in the upper right-hand cell.

---

quickly learn to overcome their disability. The therapists designed a study in which patients who came into the physical therapy clinic with complaints of dizziness were randomly assigned to either a control or experimental group. Those in the control group received training to enable them to adapt to the dizziness; those in the experimental group received the same training plus a videotape to show how several patients with dizziness were able to overcome their disability and resume functional lifestyles. After two weeks of training, both groups were asked to fill out a questionnaire that contained six items and had been designed to assess the degree of disability. Each question was answered by choosing responses ranging from "strongly disagree" to "strongly agree." These responses were transposed to a five-point scale and summed to produce an indicator of the degree of disability for each subject. High scores were an indicator of a lesser degree of disability.

Research Hypothesis

The hypothesis tested by this statistic is that the difference in the median indicator scores for the two samples (one control and one experimental) is zero. The statistical test is more precisely designed to determine if the two samples have been drawn from the same population. It does this by examining the central tendency of the scores of the groups on the questionnaire. The statistic of central tendency used with ordered qualitative variables is the median.

If the two samples are from the same population, then any difference between the groups can be attributed to the independent variable. One attempts to assure that the two samples were drawn from the same population by random assignment to the control and experimental groups.

Nature of the Attributes or Variables

The test is designed for ordered qualitative variables.

Research Design

The example above is an experimental design with two groups—an experimental and a control group—with both groups receiving only a posttest.

It would be possible to design a similar study involving a pretest, random assignment to either the control or the experimental group, followed by the different forms of management of the patients, and then a posttest. In this case, the scores of the pretest could be subtracted from the scores of the posttest to obtain a *difference score*. The Mann-Whitney U test would then determine if the difference scores arose from the same population by examining the median value of the difference scores. If the videotape made no difference at all, then one would expect the median difference score to be close to zero.

The Assumptions

The following assumptions underlie the Mann-Whitney U test.

1. The underlying variable, "degree of disability," is assumed to be continuously distributed. The questionnaire assigns a rank value to this variable.
2. There is independence among the observations within each sample. Individuals in the control group do not affect one another's scores. The same should be true for the experimental group.
3. There is independence of the observations between the two samples. Scores of the individuals in the experimental group are not affected by the scores of the other group.

The Method

In this test, the scores of the smaller group are compared to the scores of the larger group in the following way. The scores of each group are arranged in rank order and entered on a matrix table. (A fictitious data set and a matrix table for the data are illustrated in Display 10-4.) The matrix table is constructed with the scores of the smaller group listed in rank order along the left side and the scores of the larger group arranged in rank order along the top. The table is filled in by subtracting the scores along the side from the scores across the top. The number of negative values in the matrix is counted. This represents the number of inversions, or instances when the smaller group's scores exceed the larger group's scores. The number of inversions is called U.

DISPLAY 10-4
MANN-WHITNEY U TEST TABLE OF SCORES
FOR THE EXPERIMENTAL AND CONTROL GROUP

Experimental Group	Control Group
13	11
17	14
20	15
21	16
23	18
28	

MATRIX OF ORDERED DIFFERENCES
BETWEEN SCORES OF THE CONTROL AND EXPERIMENTAL GROUPS

Experimental Group		13	17	20	21	23	28
Control Group	11	2	6	9	10	12	17
	14	−1	3	6	7	9	14
	15	−2	2	5	6	8	13
	16	−3	1	4	5	7	12
	18	−5	−1	2	3	5	10

Differences between experimental and control groups.

If there were no difference between the two groups, one would expect the number of inversions to occur approximately half the time, or in one-half of the paired comparisons. This means that it would be just as likely for the smaller group's scores to be larger than the larger group's as it would be for them to be smaller. In contrast, if there is a difference between the groups, the number of inversions should be an extreme value, close to either 0 or the total number of paired comparisons. This would indicate that one group's scores were consistently lower or higher than the other's. The number of inversions is used to compute directly the *p value*, or the probability, of that specific number of inversions, given samples of that size. The formula for that computation is simply

$$p = \frac{U}{n_{\text{(small group)}} \times n_{\text{(large group)}}}$$

where n is the number of individuals in that subgroup. For this example there were five inversions (U), five individuals in the small group, and six in the large group.

$$p = \frac{5}{5 \times 6} = 0.17$$

Thus, this result could be expected 17 times out of 100. If we had decided prior to collecting the data that a significant result would be one that was expected only 5 times or 10 times in 100, then in this study we would have to conclude that these two groups did not arise from different populations, that is, the videotape did not cause a significant difference in the experimental group.

SIGN TEST

The sign test was named because plus and minus signs are counted in computing the statistic. It is an extremely easy test to apply. The sign test may be used to examine the difference between repeated measures of the same subject or the difference between measures of matched pairs. Consider the following example. Preadolescent boys and girls are being screened in a posture awareness program for signs of scoliosis. The physical therapist would like to know if the students learn anything about scoliosis as a result of this program. The hypothesis is that the students are more knowledgeable about scoliosis as a result of being exposed to the postural-screening program. Fourteen fifth graders are given a 20-question quiz about scoliosis. The scoliosis-screening clinic is held, and these same students are then given the same 20-question test again.

Statement of the Hypothesis

The hypothesis tested is that the incidence of improved scores on the posttest is greater than the incidence of lower scores.

Nature of the Attributes or Variables

The characteristic under study is a continuously distributed qualitative variable, in this example, knowledge of scoliosis.

Research Design

Two designs may be appropriately analyzed using the sign test. The first is a preexperimental design in which a single group receives a pretest, a treatment condition or independent variable is applied (the scoliosis-screening session), and the group is then given a posttest.

The other design is a matched-pairs design in which one of each pair receives treatment and then the two groups are compared on the variable of interest. For example, the fifth graders at one school might be matched with fifth graders at another school on the basis of gender and grades in health class. One school undergoes scoliosis screening; the other does not. After screening, the pairs are given the scoliosis-knowledge test and their scores are compared.

The Assumptions

1. The test assumes a binomial distribution, that is, it assumes that the probability of an improved score is equal to the probability of a lower score if the treatment causes no effect.
2. For the preexperimental design involving a single sample with a pretest and posttest, the only additional assumption is that the variable being studied is continuously distributed.
3. For the matched-pairs design, an additional assumption is applied that requires that the pairs be equivalent on the relevant variables used to match them.

The Method

To carry out the test, pretest/posttest scores are compared and a difference score is determined or the differences between the scores of a matched pair are computed. If there is a positive difference—if scores improve on the posttest or are higher for the group who received treatment—a positive sign is substituted for the computed difference. If, however, posttest scores are lower than pretest scores or those who were screened for scoliosis score lower when compared to those who were not screened, a negative sign is substituted. One simply counts the number of minus (-) or plus (+) signs and refers to a table of probabilities that lists the likelihood of such a distribution of minus and plus signs. This table can be found in nonparametric statistics textbooks.

WILCOXON MATCHED-PAIRS SIGNED-RANK TEST

The Wilcoxon test examines the difference between the scores of two groups matched on some attribute or variable, after applying a treatment. Consider the following: Family units attending an infant program were matched into pairs on the basis of attendance at program sessions. A primary caretaker of an infant from each pair of families was then randomly selected and invited to attend a supplemental program on positioning. The other infant-family unit continued with the routine infant program. After eight weeks and a total of four possible sessions given by the physical therapist, each primary caretaker was asked to indicate his or her level of confidence in handling the infant, on a ten-point scale that ranged from "not very confident" to "very confident."

Statement of the Hypothesis

The hypothesis being tested here is that the supplemental program produces greater confidence in handling the infant than the infant program alone.

Nature of the Attributes or Variables

The dependent characteristic under study is "confidence in handling the infant," a continuous qualitative variable that is ranked on a ten-point scale.

Research Design

The study used here as an example is an experimental posttest-only design. There are two randomly selected groups that are matched on the basis of attendance at the infant program. The internal validity of the study rests on the effectiveness of the matching procedure in producing like pairs of infant-family units.

The Assumptions

The assumptions on which this test is based are as follows:

1. The population of differences between the scores of a matched pair is distributed continuously.
2. Sampling from the population is carried out randomly, and therefore each pair is independent of every other pair.
3. The two groups (those receiving the supplemental program and those who do not receive the program) are derived from the same parent population, and thus the difference values are distributed identically and symmetrically about the same central value. This assumption is necessary to restrict the test to one examining central tendency. If the assumption were not adopted, the statistic might be interpreted as detecting differences in the shape of the distributions rather than as detecting differences in location of the central value.

The Method

The data for this study might resemble that in Table 10-1. The pairs of families are tabulated side-by-side with the ratings from the families that received the supplemental program in one column and those that did not in the adjacent column. The difference between each pair's ratings of confidence in handling their infants (d) is computed. These difference scores are ranked, and the sign of the difference is preserved (see the column labeled "Rank of d"). A sum of the positive ranks and a sum of the negative ranks are taken, and the smaller of the two sums is considered a T statistic. Here the negative ranks sum to a smaller number than the positive ranks, so the T value is 6. This value is then compared to a table of predicted sums of ranks to determine if a significant result has been found. In this example, the sum of 6 is significant at the 0.05 level of probability. The hypothesis that the supplemental program improved the caretakers' confidence in handling

TABLE 10-1. Signed-Rank Test Table

Pairs: Family units matched by attendance	Regular program	Supplemental and regular program	d	Rank of d	Rank with – sign
1	3	5	+ 2	3	
2	6	6	0	1	
3	2	6	+ 4	5.5	
4	9	8	– 1	– 2	2
5	5	10	+ 5	7	
6	1	8	+ 7	9	
7	2	8	+ 6	8	
8	3	7	+ 4	5.5	
9	6	3	– 3	– 4	4
				SUM	6

their infants is accepted. Tables of T values to be used in determining significance of the results of the Wilcoxon signed-rank test can be found in nonparametric statistics textbooks.

THE KRUSKAL-WALLIS ANOVA

The Kruskal-Wallis test is the nonparametric test analogous to a parametric one-way analysis of variance (ANOVA). This test enables comparison among more than two samples. It tests the sum of the ranks of each of the samples to determine if the samples come from different populations. That is, it tests to determine if the characteristics of the samples are so different that we would think that their parent populations differed on the characteristic being studied.

As an example of the use of this statistic, an academic coordinator of clinical education (ACCE) at an entry-level physical therapy program wanted to determine if different types of practice settings have an influence on students' attitudes regarding family involvement in therapy. She identified four main practice settings that might affect the students' attitudes in different ways: acute-care hospitals, rehabilitation centers, private practices, and home-health agencies. During the two weeks immediately preceding a full-time, eight-week internship, the students were given a learning module that emphasized the need to involve family in therapy activities, including evaluation, goal setting, and treatment. The 30 senior students then went on to their clinical training and after eight weeks returned to school. When they returned, the ACCE gave the students a test that assessed attitudes toward family involvement in therapy. High scores indicated a positive attitude toward family involvement; low scores indicated a negative attitude toward family involvement.

Statement of the Hypothesis

There is no difference in scores of students trained at acute-care hospitals, rehabilitation centers, private practices, and home-health agencies on a test of attitudes toward family involvement in physical therapy.

Nature of the Attributes or Variables

The dependent variable "attitudes toward family involvement" is a continuously distributed qualitative variable.

Research Design

The study can be classified as a quasi-experimental design. The subjects were not randomly assigned to their clinical sites. Instead, the students and ACCE worked together to select a site for each student that would best serve that student's educational needs.

The Assumptions

Three assumptions underlie the use of the Kruskal-Wallis test.

1. The dependent variable is continuously distributed.
2. The scores of students in one practice setting are independent of the scores of students in all other practice settings.
3. The students' scores within each type of practice setting are not influenced by any other student's scores in that practice setting.

The Method

As a first step, the scores of the 30 students (Table 10-2) are arranged in rank order, preserving the information regarding their training site (Table 10-3). Ranks then replace the actual scores the students achieved. Table 10-4 presents the ranked data separated back into the original four groups. The ranks are summed for each group, and the *H statistic* is calculated and then compared to the values *H* would assume in extreme cases (when the groups are likely from different populations), signifying significant findings. The student needing to apply the Kruskal-Wallis test to examine data should consult a nonparametric statistics text for the formula for computing the *H* statistic, examples illustrating its use, and tables containing lists of significant values of *H* for different numbers of groups.

TABLE 10-2. Score on Test of Attitude Toward Family Involvement in Therapy for Students Assigned to Four Types of Training Sites

Acute Care	Rehabilitation	Private Practice	Home Health
46	51	18	72
32	97	22	104
61	100	39	143
14	86	41	123
38	99	13	141
90	107	44	89
	111	29	120
	121	17	
		49	

TABLE 10-3. Ranking of Scores for Kruskal-Wallis Test

Score	Setting*	Rank	Score	Setting	Rank
13	PP	1	72	HH	16
14	AC	2	86	R	17
17	PP	3	89	HH	18
18	PP	4	90	AC	19
22	PP	5	97	R	20
29	PP	6	99	R	21
32	AC	7	100	R	22
38	AC	8	104	HH	23
39	PP	9	107	R	24
41	PP	10	111	R	25
44	PP	11	120	HH	26
46	AC	12	121	R	27
49	PP	13	123	HH	28
51	R	14	141	HH	29
61	AC	15	143	HH	30

*PP = private practice, AC = acute care, R = rehabilitation center, HH = home health agency.

TABLE 10-4. Summing of Ranks for Kruskal-Wallis Test

Acute Care	Rehabilitation	Private Practice	Home Health
2	14	1	16
7	17	3	18
8	20	4	23
12	21	5	26
15	22	6	28
19	24	9	29
	25	10	30
	27	11	
		13	
Sum 63	170	62	170

THE FRIEDMAN TEST:
A TWO-WAY ANOVA

The Friedman test is the nonparametric equivalent of a two-way ANOVA. Like the Kruskal-Wallis test, the Friedman test examines ranks. However, in the case of the Friedman test, more than two measures are obtained from each subject. Note that if only two observations were obtained from each subject, a difference score might be computed and used to examine the differences between groups.

The following example will illustrate an application of the Friedman test:

In the study of the effect of training site on the attitude toward family involvement in therapy, the students who were assigned to home-health settings were given equivalent forms of the attitude test five weeks after returning from the clinic and then again ten weeks after their return. Thus their attitudes were assessed three times.

Statement of the Hypothesis

The hypothesis being tested is that there is no systematic change among the home-health students in their attitudes toward family involvement in therapy after their return to the academic setting.

Nature of the Attributes or Variables

As in the example used to illustrate the Kruskal-Wallis test, the dependent variable, "value of family involvement," is considered a continuously distributed qualitative variable.

Research Design

This is a repeated-measures design, with subjects serving as their own control. It would also be possible with this statistic to compare groups of students at several

TABLE 10-5. Students' Attitude Scores Across a 10-Week Period
Following a Home-Health Clinical Internship

Student	Immediately after return from home-health clinical site	5 weeks post	10 weeks post
1	72	69	70
2	89	90	80
3	104	100	99
4	107	88	110
5	120	123	124
6	123	121	116
7	141	130	111
8	143	150	119

different times. For example, the median score of the subjects assigned to each type of clinical site might be compared repeatedly across the same time intervals outlined above.

The Assumptions

Two assumptions underlie the use of this test:

1. The dependent variable is continuously distributed.
2. The observations of one subject (or block of subjects) are independent of the observations of other subjects.

The Method

The scores of each subject on each of the different test occasions are ranked as is illustrated in Table 10-5. The ranks are summed for all subjects at each time of testing to determine if systematic change in the students' attitudes occurs across time (see Table 10-6). The test statistic is calculated and compared to a table of chi-square values. As with the parametric ANOVA, the finding of a significant result would have to be followed with a post hoc analysis to determine where any significant difference might lie. Nonparametric statistic texts should be consulted for complete descriptions of procedures for the Friedman test and associated post hoc comparisons.

It is also possible, when blocks of subjects are compared, to examine the data for interaction. Interactions could occur in this instance when the attitudes of a

TABLE 10-6. Ranks of Students' Attitude Scores Across a 10-Week Period
Following a Home-Health Clinical Internship

Student	*Immediately after return from home-health clinical site*	*5 weeks post*	*10 weeks post*
1	1	3	2
2	2	1	3
3	1	2	3
4	2	3	1
5	3	2	1
6	1	2	3
7	1	2	3
8	2	3	1
Sum	13	18	17

group of students who experienced one type of clinical setting changed in a different way than the attitudes of students who experienced other clinical settings. Examining interactions under the Friedman model is a long and tedious mathematical process. The beginning researcher should realize, however, that it can be done.

BIBLIOGRAPHY

Bradley, J.V. Nonparametric statistics. In Kirk, R.E., ed., *Statistical issues: A reader for the behavioral sciences.* Belmont, CA: Wadsworth, 1972, 329–338.

Campbell, D.T. and Stanley, J.C. Experimental and quasi-experimental designs for research. In Gage, N.L., ed., *Handbook of research on teaching.* Chicago: Rand McNally, 1963, 171–246.

Clarke, D.H. and Clarke, H.H. *Research process in physical education,* 2nd ed. Englewood Cliffs, NJ: Prentice Hall, 1984, 149–244.

Hays, W.L. *Statistics,* 3rd ed. Philadelphia: Holt, Rinehart and Winston, 1981.

Marascuilo, L.A. and McSweeney, M. *Nonparametric and distribution-free methods for the social sciences.* Monterey, CA: Brooks/Cole, 1977.

Rothstein, J.M. Measurement and clinical practice: Theory and application. In Rothstein, J.M., ed., *Measurement in physical therapy.* New York: Churchill Livingstone, 1985, 1–46.

Seigel, S. *Nonparametric statistics for the behavioral sciences.* New York: McGraw-Hill, 1956.

Winer, B.J. *Statistical principles in experimental design,* 2nd ed. New York: McGraw-Hill, 1971.

11

COMPARISON OF MEANS:
ONE SAMPLE,
TWO INDEPENDENT SAMPLES,
PAIRED OBSERVATIONS

Wanda C. Wilkes

INTRODUCTION

SAMPLING DISTRIBUTION OF MEANS

TWO SAMPLES: COMPARISON OF MEANS

TWO INDEPENDENT SAMPLES

COMPARISON OF MEANS OF NONINDEPENDENT PAIRED SAMPLES

INTRODUCTION

Statistics can be divided into two major categories: descriptive statistics and inferential statistics. Following the collection of data, we must resort to techniques that enable us to extract meaningful information from that data. Merely inspecting and comparing individual measurements or observations is useless and inefficient. To be useful, data must be organized and summarized with one or two meaningful values. The same data can also be condensed and presented in tabular or graphic form. The techniques associated with organizing, summarizing, and presenting data are the basis of *descriptive statistics*. Annual hospital reports utilize the techniques of descriptive statistics in summarizing patient data collected over a one-year period to yield such relevant, descriptive measures as the average daily census, occupancy rate, average length of stay, death rates, nosocomial infection rates, and consultation rates. Tabular and graphic displays can convey information about the frequency and distribution of age groups, patients' gender, and sources of payment.

Inferential statistics is that branch which allows us to draw conclusions about an entire population on the basis of sample results. Various opinion polls utilize the results obtained from a carefully selected sample of people to draw conclusions about the preferences of an entire population from which the sample was drawn. Similarly, in a clinical trial designed to study the efficacy of an antihypertensive drug, the results obtained from a random and representative sample of subjects with hypertension can be used by the drug manufacturer to draw conclusions about the effectiveness of the drug in treating all people with hypertension. This process of drawing inferences from sample to population is especially relevant to clinical medicine and allied health disciplines, where study of an entire population is neither feasible nor cost-effective, necessitating the use of carefully selected samples.

SAMPLING DISTRIBUTION OF MEANS

If one collected measurements on a population of subjects and examined the distribution of measurements, the result would be a *population distribution*. Because researchers typically deal with samples, the distribution of measurements obtained from random samples taken from a defined population would represent a *sampling distribution*. The sampling distribution of means is one example of such a distribution.

The random sampling distribution of means is generated by a process that involves taking a random sample of a fixed size (n) from a defined population. The mean of this sample is calculated, and the n items or subjects are returned to the population. A newly selected sample of the same size is chosen randomly, its mean is calculated, and the n items are again replaced in the population. This process is repeated indefinitely until we have gathered a large collection of samples of the same size n from which the mean of each has been computed. The result is a large series of sample means that can be grouped, ordered in a frequency distribution, and plotted to generate a sampling distribution of means of size n. Thus we can identify a large population of male athletes, ages 21 to 35 years; select repeated random samples of 25 from this universe; measure serum cholesterol levels; and compute the mean cholesterol for each sample of 25 men. The array of means can then be plotted to produce a random sampling distribution of mean cholesterol values of samples of 25 male athletes, age 21 to 35 years. Obviously, in practice, it would be foolish for researchers to compute a vast number of mean cholesterol values of male athletes from repeated samples of the same size simply to generate a sampling distribution of mean cholesterol values. However, the sampling distribution of means possesses unique characteristics that allow us to use this distribution to make inferences about a defined population, such as the cholesterol values of all male athletes, based on the results of a single random sample of male athletes of a given size, such as 25.

Properties of the Sampling Distribution of Means

From the collection of sample means obtained from repeated sampling of the population, one can compute the overall mean value. This value would be the same as the value of the population mean (μ). Examining the same collection of sample means would reveal variability among the values. We would intuitively expect that the extent of this variability would depend not only on the variability of the values in the population but also on the size of the samples selected from the universe. Repeated samples of 100 would show less variability among the mean values than samples of 10 selected from the same population, since a greater proportion of the population in which we are interested is included in the larger sample. Thus we can expect that the variability among means of repeated samples will decrease with increases in sample size.

Having considered the central tendency and dispersion of the sampling distribution of means, we must finally examine the shape of the distribution. While the shape of the parent population distribution may be asymmetrical, it is rather astonishing to note that the sampling distribution of means will be symmetrical and bell-shaped if the sample size is large enough. Of course, if the underlying population distribution were normal, it would not be as surprising to note that the sampling distribution of means would also be Gaussian (normal).

Hence the properties of the sampling distribution of means can be enumerated as follows:

1. The mean of the sampling distribution of means will be equal to the population mean, μ.
2. The variability of the distribution can be determined from the standard deviation (SD) of the mean values. With any sampling distribution, the SD is given a special name—the standard error (SE) of that distribution. Thus the SD of the sampling distribution of means is termed the *standard error of the mean* and is denoted by $SE_{\bar{x}}$ or $\sigma_{\bar{x}}$. We have learned that the variability among means will be dependent both on the variability of the population values as determined

by the population SD (σ_x) and on the sample size (n). Therefore $SE_{\bar{x}}$ may be computed as follows:

$$SE_{\bar{x}} = \sigma_{\bar{x}} = \frac{\sigma_x}{\sqrt{n}}$$

The denominator of this term utilizes sample size, which can be manipulated by the investigator, while the numerator requires use of the population SD, whose value is beyond control of the investigator. Further, because the denominator involves the square root of the sample size, it should be apparent that an inverse relationship exists between the size of $SE_{\bar{x}}$ and sample size n. Therefore, if the sample size is quadrupled, the $SE_{\bar{x}}$ will be reduced by half. This provides a formal expression of our earlier, intuitive impression that increases in sample size would result in less variability among sample means.

3. The shape of the sampling distribution of means will be approximately normal regardless of the shape of the parent population and provided that the sample size is large enough. The basis for this property is a significant statistical principle called the *central limit theorem*. The importance of this theorem is that it allows us to make inferences about population means on the basis of a single sample mean, even when the measurements in the population are not normally distributed.

The proviso that the sample size be sufficiently large before the sampling distribution adheres to normality raises the question of how large a sample must be drawn. If the parent population is itself normally distributed, any sample size will be sufficient, as the sampling distribution will likewise be Gaussian. However, in cases where the underlying distribution is not normal, the degree of departure from normality will dictate the sample size required to ensure approximate normality of the sampling distribution of means. It has been shown that, with underlying distributions that are rectangular (uniform), bimodal, or skewed in either direction, repeated samples of sizes three to five are sufficient to produce a sampling distribution that is approximately Gaussian (Figure 11-1). These three qualities are collectively referred to as the *central limit theorem*.

Use of the Sampling Distribution of Means

Provided that sample size is sufficient, the central limit theorem assures us that the sampling distribution of means will be approximately normal. Therefore we can conveniently convert the normal distribution of sample means to the standardized normal curve by use of the Z transformation. Because the values of the sampling distribution are means and since the mean and SD of the distribution have already been enumerated, the equation for Z becomes:

$$Z = \frac{\bar{x} - \mu}{\sigma_x / \sqrt{n}}$$

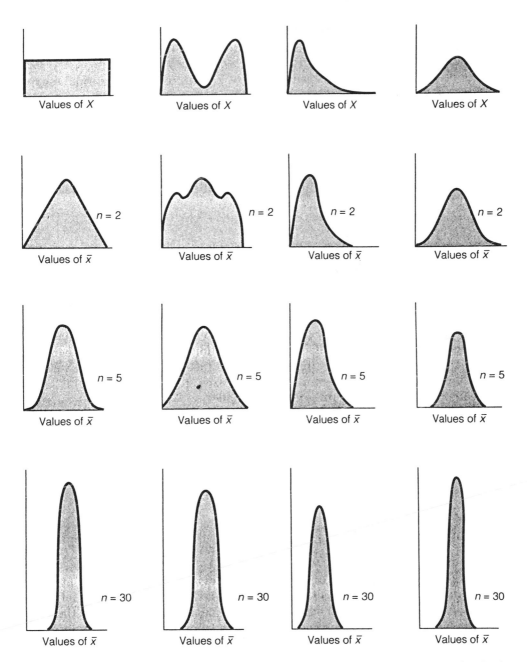

FIGURE 11-1. The effect of shape of population distribution and sample size on the distribution of means of random samples. (From Kuzma, J.W., *Basic Statistics for the Health Sciences,* 2nd ed., Mayfield Publishing Co., 1992.)

From the computed Z value we can determine either the area under the curve or the relative position of a sample mean in the distribution of means. Thus we have a process that allows us to test hypotheses about sample means and to draw inferences about an entire population on the basis of a single sample mean.

Suppose we wish to determine whether the mean HDL-cholesterol (HDL-C) level of a defined group of men who participate in a prescribed exercise program is higher than that of a comparably matched population of sedentary men who exercise minimally. Further, assume that the latter population has been well investigated and is known to have a mean HDL-C of 50 mg/dl, with a standard deviation of 12 mg/dl. If we now select a random and representative sample of 64 male subjects from the exercise program, measure their HDL-C, and compute a mean of 54.5 mg/dl, we would have sufficient data to determine whether the mean HDL-C level is higher for men who exercise. We hypothesize that the mean HDL-C level of men who exercise is no different from that of the population of sedentary men (50 mg/dl). The sampling distribution of means would represent the means of all possible samples of size 64 (the single sample size), with an overall mean equal to 50 mg/dl (the population mean) and $SE_{\bar{x}}$ equal to 1.5 mg/dl ($SE_{\bar{x}} = \dfrac{\sigma_x}{\sqrt{n}} = \dfrac{12}{\sqrt{64}}$). The equation for Z is:

$$Z = \frac{54.5 - 50}{1.5}$$

$$Z = \frac{4.5}{1.5}$$

$$Z = 3.0$$

From the computed Z value, we can determine that the chance of obtaining a mean HDL-C of 54.5 mg/dl or larger is 0.1%. This gives us sufficient reason to reject the null hypothesis and to conclude that mean HDL-C levels are significantly higher in men who participate in a prescribed exercise program.

Student's T Distribution

In most studies it seldom happens that the value of the population standard deviation (σ_x) is known. Therefore we usually must use our best estimate of σ_x, namely, the sample standard deviation s_x. Under these conditions, when one uses the sampling distribution of means for an analysis, the $SE_{\bar{x}}$ would be calculated in the same fashion, except that s_x would replace σ_x. Thus $SE_{\bar{x}} = s_x/\sqrt{n}$, when σ_x is unknown. Will the substitution of s_x for σ_x in the $SE_{\bar{x}}$ term affect the analysis of means? The analysis will be similar, but it will require use of a new distribution called *Student's t distribution*.

Student's t distribution was discovered over 80 years ago by William S. Gossett. Gossett was a junior employee of the Guinness Brewery in Dublin, Ireland. His employer, thinking that the brewery might profit from the application of statistical methods to its industrial processes, selected Gossett to go to London to study statistical principles under Karl Pearson, a noted mathematical scholar and a famous contributor to the field of statistics. Gossett proved to be an exceptionally talented student of theoretical and applied statistics. On his return to the brewery, he implemented statistical procedures that were of immediate commercial benefit.

What Gossett had discovered was a family of distributions that accommodated the limitations imposed by the use of small samples. This allowed his employer to use small samples to project the readiness of his product for market. Not only did this reduce labor costs but it also minimized delays in shipping the product to taverns. Gossett's further theoretical applications were of no benefit to his employer, and he wanted to share those findings with other mathematical scholars through publications. His employer, however, feared that any published report by his employee would alert other brewers that statistics could be profitably applied in their industry. Unwilling to reveal this secret to his competitors, the brewer forbade Gossett from publishing his findings.

Gossett was fiercely determined to make his theoretical findings public. Consequently, he protected his identity as an employee of the Guinness Brewery by adopting the pseudonym "Student," and he published his work under this name in the journal *Biometrika*. So though the study of statistics is reputed to have driven many students to drink, from this historical anecdote the reader can see that drink drove "Student" to study statistics!

The *t* distribution resembles the normal distribution in that it is bell-shaped and symmetrical and extends from negative to positive infinity. It differs from the normal in terms of dispersion, being more spread out with small sample sizes and approaching the dispersion of the standardized normal curve as *n* increases. Consequently, the *t* distribution will assume different shapes depending upon a quantity called *degrees of freedom (df)*.

The Concept of Degrees of Freedom

The substitution of the sample standard deviation for the population value in the $SE_{\bar{x}}$ term invokes the use of the *t* distribution for making inferences about means. Degrees of freedom refer to the quantity $n - 1$, in which n represents the sample size on which the calculation of a *sample variance* (s^2) and, hence, a sample standard deviation is based. Thus

$$df = n - 1$$

Recall that $n - 1$ is the denominator in the formula for obtaining an unbiased estimate of population variance:

$$s^2 = \frac{\sum (x - \bar{x})^2}{n - 1}$$

and

$$s = \sqrt{\frac{\sum (x - \bar{x})^2}{n - 1}}$$

The numerator of these formulas represents a sum of squared deviations from the sample mean. The sum of the deviations around the mean is always equal to zero:

$$\Sigma \, (x - \bar{x}) = 0$$

Thus if we have a sample of three ($n = 3$) and were to determine the values of the three deviations from the mean, we could freely assign any value to the first two deviations (D). For example, we might choose the following:

$$D_1 = -4$$

$$D_2 = 8$$

Having selected these two deviation values at will, we cannot freely select the third value, because it will be fixed and determined for us. Thus

$$x - \bar{x} = D$$

and

$$\Sigma \, D = 0$$

When $n = 3$ and D_1 and D_2 are -4 and 8,

$$(-4 + 8 + D_3) = 0$$

$$D_3 = -4$$

The third deviation value can only be -4. Because we were free to choose any two deviation values, the degrees of freedom for any sample size of three must be $n - 1$, or 2.

We can generalize this concept by considering the values of deviations from the mean for any sample size. It should be apparent that $n - 1$ of these deviations are "free" to be any numbers of our choosing but that the final deviation will then be automatically fixed. Therefore we say that we have $n - 1$ degrees of freedom, and this is identical to the value of the denominator ($n - 1$) in the formulas for determining sample variance and sample standard deviation. Because degrees of freedom are used in these estimates of population variance and standard deviation, they indicate the reliability of our sample estimate. When n increases, the reliability of s_x as an estimator of σ_x increases as well. This explains why the spread of the t distribution decreases as df (and the reliability of s_x as an estimator of σ_x) increases, to the point where, with infinite degrees of freedom, the t and normal distributions are identical.

Although the spread of the t distribution varies with changes in df, the area under the transformed curve is still equal to 1.0. The transformation is similar to that of a normal curve representing the distribution of means, except for the substitution of s_x for σ_x in the $SE_{\bar{x}}$ term:

$$t = \frac{\bar{x} - \mu}{s_x / \sqrt{n}}$$

Conventional tables for the t distribution (see Table 11-1) are presented differently from tables of areas of the normal curve, because there is a different t distribution for every df. The volume of pages that would be required to present t values for all possible tail areas with every possible df up to infinity would be prohibitively large. Consequently, we usually use an abridged table, which lists df consecutively up to 30 with a few selected df beyond 30 and selected tail areas corresponding to those commonly used in tests of significance. The body of the table contains the t values corresponding to the df and selected tail area.

Like a Z value, t indicates the relative distance above or below the mean that a particular value falls and excludes a specified tail area of the distribution. From the table, note that for any specified tail area, the t values decrease with increasing df. Since the t values represent relative distance above or below the mean, this observation supports the fact that the spread of the t distribution is greatest with small df (large t) and decreases with increasing df (progressively smaller t values).

If one compares Z and t values for specific tail areas excluded in the corresponding distribution, one finds that t approaches Z with increases in df. For example, to exclude a tail area of 0.025 in the standard normal distribution, the Z value would be 1.96. If one examines the column from the t-distribution table that specifies the same tail area exclusion of 0.025, with $df = 1$ ($n = 2$), the t value is 12.706. However, for the same area, as df increase, the t value becomes progressively smaller until, with infinite df, t is identical to Z (1.960). This means that with increasing df, the t distribution approaches the normal distribution until, with infinite df, the t and normal distributions are identical. Comparison of t and Z values for any specified tail area shows close agreement between the two when df exceed 30. Therefore for most practical purposes, because the normal and t distributions are reasonably close when df exceed 30, one can use the normal distribution instead of t when sample sizes exceed 30.

Examples of Significance Tests on a Sample Mean

Example 1

A large population of healthy adults who do not exercise is known to have a mean serum lactate level of 5.0 mg/dl ($\mu = 5.0$). To determine whether the mean serum lactate is higher in adults who regularly run 50 km per week, an investigator selects a random sample of 25 adults who regularly run 50 km, measures their serum lactate, and computes a mean and standard deviation of 5.6 and 1.5 mg/dl respectively. The investigator seeks to ascertain whether the data support a claim that the serum lactate for runners is higher at a 1% level of significance ($p < 0.01$).

TABLE 11-1. Distribution of t Probability

df	Level of Significance for One-Tailed Test					
	.10	.05	.025	.01	.005	.0005
	Level of Significance for Two-Tailed Test					
	.20	.10	.05	.02	.01	.001
1	3·078	6·314	12·706	31·821	63·657	636·619
2	1·886	2·920	4·303	6·965	9·925	31·598
3	1·638	2·353	3·182	4·541	5·841	12·941
4	1·533	2·132	2·776	3·747	4·604	8·610
5	1·476	2·015	2·571	3·365	4·032	6·859
6	1·440	1·943	2·447	3·143	3·707	5·959
7	1·415	1·895	2·365	2·998	3·449	5·405
8	1·397	1·860	2·306	2·896	3·355	5·041
9	1·383	1·833	2·262	2·821	3·250	4·781
10	1·372	1·812	2·228	2·764	3·169	4·587
11	1·363	1·796	2·201	2·718	3·106	4·437
12	1·356	1·782	2·179	2·681	3·055	4·318
13	1·350	1·771	2·160	2·650	3·012	4·221
14	1·345	1·761	2·145	2·624	2·977	4·140
15	1·341	1·753	2·131	2·602	2·947	4·073
16	1·337	1·746	2·120	2·583	2·921	4·015
17	1·333	1·740	2·110	2·567	2·898	3·965
18	1·330	1·734	2·101	2·552	2·878	3·922
19	1·328	1·729	2·093	2·539	2·861	3·883
20	1·325	1·725	2·086	2·528	2·845	3·850
21	1·323	1·721	2·080	2·518	2·831	3·819
22	1·321	1·717	2·074	2·508	2·819	3·792
23	1·319	1·714	2·069	2·500	2·807	3·767
24	1·318	1·711	2·064	2·492	2·797	3·745
25	1·316	1·708	2·060	2·485	2·787	3·725
26	1·315	1·706	2·056	2·479	2·779	3·707
27	1·314	1·703	2·052	2·473	2·771	3·690
28	1·313	1·701	2·048	2·467	2·763	3·674
29	1·311	1·699	2·045	2·462	2·756	3·659
30	1·310	1·697	2·042	2·457	2·750	3·646
40	1·303	1·684	2·021	2·423	2·704	3·551
60	1·296	1·671	2·000	2·390	2·660	3·460
120	1·289	1·658	1·980	2·358	2·617	3·373
∞	1·282	1·645	1·960	2·326	2·576	3·291

The data are summarized below:

μ lactate, nonexercising, healthy adults = 5.0 mg/dl
n = 25 adults who regularly run 50 km per week
$\bar{x}$ = 5.6 mg/dl
s_x = 1.5 mg/dl

We hypothesize that the mean lactate of the runners is higher than that of non-exercising, healthy adults and proceed to the analysis of means.

Because the population standard deviation (σ_x) is unknown, we must use our sample value (s_x) as its best estimate, and we calculate the $SE_{\bar{x}}$ accordingly:

$$SE_{\bar{x}} = \frac{s_x}{\sqrt{n}} \qquad \frac{1.5}{\sqrt{25}} = 0.3$$

Since we have substituted s_x for σ_x, we must consider use of the t distribution and its transform for the analysis. Because $n < 30$, we select the t transform and complete the analysis as follows:

$$t = \frac{\bar{x} - \mu}{s_x/\sqrt{n}}$$

$$= \frac{5.6 - 5.0}{0.3}$$

$$= 2.00$$

The tabular t value would be identified from the entry corresponding to 24 df ($n - 1$) and an excluded upper-tail area of 0.01. The tabular t value is listed as 2.492. Because the relative position of the sample mean is below that indicated by the tabular value for the upper-tail area exclusion, we do not have sufficient reason to reject the hypothesis or to claim that mean lactate levels are higher for adults who run 50 km per week.

Example 2

The range of motion (ROM) of the wrist extension of a population of healthy women is known to have a mean of 70 degrees. An investigator suspects that wrist extension is decreased in women diagnosed as having carpal tunnel syndrome. A random sample of 64 women with carpal tunnel syndrome is examined, and the ROM for wrist extension of the involved extremity is measured. The mean ROM for wrist extension in the sample is 62°, with a standard deviation of 5.3°. The data are summarized below:

Population: μ wrist extension ROM for healthy women = 70°
Sample: n = 64 women with carpal tunnel syndrome
              $\bar{x}$ = 62° of wrist extension ROM
              s_x = 5.3°

The investigator posits the following directional hypothesis: the women who have been diagnosed as having carpal tunnel syndrome will have a statistically significant decrease in ROM for wrist extension. The level chosen for statistical significance is set at the 1% or 0.01 level. The $SE_{\bar{x}}$ term, computed from the sample estimate of σ_x, becomes:

$$SE_{\bar{x}} = \frac{s_x}{\sqrt{n}} = \frac{5.3}{\sqrt{64}} = 0.66$$

The substitution of s_x for σ_x should alert us that we are dealing with Student's t distribution. However, because the sample size is reasonably large, greater than 30, the t and Z values are close enough to permit the use of the Z transform.

$$Z = \frac{\bar{x} - \mu}{SE_{\bar{x}}}$$

$$Z = \frac{62 - 70}{0.66}$$

$$Z = -12.1$$

The Z value for all but the lowest 1% on the standard normal curve is -2.33. From the computed Z value of -12.1, it is apparent that the sample mean lies well beyond the cutoff point; in fact, the probability of obtaining a sample mean this low or lower is less than 0.001. Therefore the investigator can accept the hypothesis that women diagnosed as having carpal tunnel syndrome do have less ROM in wrist extension.

Summary of One-Sample Cases Involving Inferences About Means

We have introduced and discussed the random sampling distribution of means, whose unique properties allow us to use the normal distribution and its transform to make inferences about population means on the basis of a single sample. When the sample standard deviation is used in place of the population value to compute $SE_{\bar{x}}$, the distribution of means is no longer Gaussian but becomes a Student's t distribution, which assumes different shapes and spread depending on degrees of freedom. When the sample size exceeds 30, the t and normal distributions become reasonably proximate, as do the t and Z values. Thus when sample sizes exceed 30 and s_x is used in place of σ_x in calculating $SE_{\bar{x}}$, the normal distribution of means can be used instead of Student's t distribution. Table 11-2 summarizes the tests of significance used to draw inferences about population means from a single sample.

TABLE 11-2. One-Sample Case: Tests of Significance on Means

Indication for Use	Type of Distribution	Transform Equation for Test of Significance
Population SD known	Normal	$Z = \dfrac{\bar{x} - \mu}{\sigma_x / \sqrt{n}}$
Population SD unknown; substitute sample s_x $(n < 30)$	Student's t	$t = \dfrac{\bar{x} - \mu}{s_x / \sqrt{n}}$
Population SD unknown; substitute sample s_x $(n > 30)$	Student's t, which will be reasonably close to normal	$Z = \dfrac{\bar{x} - \mu}{s_x / \sqrt{n}}$

TWO SAMPLES: COMPARISON OF MEANS

It is more common for investigators to compare the means of samples drawn from two parent populations, to determine whether a significant difference exists between the two values, than to compare the mean of one sample to some hypothesized value, as in the one-sample case. Hence investigators may wish to compare mean HDL-cholesterol levels in exercising and nonexercising women or mean oxygen consumption during ambulation for two comparably matched groups of patients with total hip replacements, each group having received a different type of prosthesis. In both examples, the objective would be to determine whether a significant difference exists between the means of two samples. We may learn, for example, that mean HDL levels are higher in nonexercising women or that the type of hip prosthesis does not affect mean oxygen consumption while ambulating.

Application of a test of significance to these data requires use of a sampling distribution with unique characteristics. The sampling distribution is generated by selecting a random sample of given size from each of two populations; measuring some characteristic, such as HDL-cholesterol levels or energy expenditure; computing the mean of each sample ($\bar{x}_1$ and $\bar{x}_2$); and, finally, computing the difference between the two means ($\bar{x}_1 - \bar{x}_2$). The subjects are returned to their respective populations, new samples of the same size are again randomly chosen from each population, and the difference between these two sample means is calculated. This process would be repeated indefinitely until an array of differences between two sample means is obtained. This array would consist of sample differences ($\bar{x}_1 - \bar{x}_2$) that are positive values, negative values, or zero. The null hypothesis would assume that the two populations being tested have identical means; hence we would hypothesize that the difference between the means of the two populations is zero ($\mu_1 - \mu_2 = 0$). If we group and plot the distribution of all possible differences between sample means ($\bar{x}_1 - \bar{x}_2$), the result would be the sampling distribution of differences between means. This distribution possesses three unique characteristics:

1. Under the assumption that the population means are identical, the mean of all possible differences between sample means (positive and negative values, as well as zero) is equal to zero—the difference between the two population means ($\mu_1 - \mu_2 = 0$).
2. With sufficient sample size and knowledge of the population standard deviation of the two groups being compared, the distribution of differences between two means will be normal. In the more common case, where the population SDs are unknown and sample values are substituted, the differences between means would follow the t distribution.
3. The array of differences would show variability among the values. To estimate the extent of this variability, we must recognize that the variability in the array of differences between means will be greater than the variability in the separate array of mean values for either of the two groups. When we estimated the variability among means of all possible samples of a given size, we computed a special standard deviation, termed *standard error of the mean*—$\text{SE}_{\bar{x}}$. The square of this standard deviation would represent the variance of the mean values:

$$(\text{SE}_{\bar{x}})^2 = \left(\frac{\sigma_x}{\sqrt{n}}\right)^2 = \frac{\sigma_x^2}{n}$$

Thus the variance of the mean values obtained by selecting samples of a fixed size from one of the two populations being compared would be

$$\frac{\sigma_{x_1}^2}{n_1}$$

The variance of the mean values obtained from the second population would likewise be

$$\frac{\sigma_{x_2}^2}{n_2}$$

We have stated that we expect the variability in the differences between two sample means to exceed that of either of the two listings of mean values. From fundamental laws of probability that govern the sums or *differences* of independent random variables, we would find that the variance of the differences between two groups is the *sum* of the two separate group variances. Thus the variance of the *difference* between two sample means would be equal to the *sum* of the variances of the means of each group:

$$(\text{SE}_{\bar{x}_1 - \bar{x}_2})^2 = (\text{SE}_{\bar{x}_1})^2 + (\text{SE}_{\bar{x}_2})^2$$

and

$$(\text{SE}_{\bar{x}_1 - \bar{x}_2})^2 = \frac{\sigma_{x_1}^2}{n_1} + \frac{\sigma_{x_2}^2}{n_2}$$

To convert the variance of the difference between two sample means to a standard deviation value, we would simply extract the square root. Consequently,

$$SE_{\bar{x}_1 - \bar{x}_2} = \sqrt{\frac{\sigma_{x_1}^2}{n_1} + \frac{\sigma_{x_2}^2}{n_2}}$$

This special standard deviation is termed *standard error of the difference between two sample means,* and it estimates the spread of the values that make up the sampling distribution. Thus the third unique characteristic of the sampling distribution of the differences between two sample means is that the variability in these differences can be described by $SE_{\bar{x}_1 - \bar{x}_2}$.

TWO INDEPENDENT SAMPLES

We have introduced a new sampling distribution that will allow us to test the differences between the means of two independent samples to determine statistical significance. This sampling distribution of differences between sample means will have a mean equal to 0 ($\mu_1 - \mu_2 = 0$), a standard deviation termed $SE_{\bar{x}_1 - \bar{x}_2}$ (described in the previous section), and a shape that will be approximately normal, with sufficient sample size and use of population values in the standard error term. Under these conditions, we can convert the normal distribution of differences to the standardized normal curve by a Z transformation that will give the following:

$$Z = \frac{(\bar{x}_1 - \bar{x}_2) - (\mu_1 - \mu_2)}{SE_{\bar{x}_1 - \bar{x}_2}}$$

and, since

$$\mu_1 - \mu_2 = 0 \text{ and } SE_{\bar{x}_1 - \bar{x}_2} = \sqrt{\frac{\sigma_{x_1}^2}{n_1} + \frac{\sigma_{x_2}^2}{n_2}}$$

then

$$Z = \frac{(\bar{x}_1 - \bar{x}_2) - 0}{\sqrt{\frac{\sigma_{x_1}^2}{n_1} + \frac{\sigma_{x_2}^2}{n_2}}}$$

It is unlikely that we would ever know the values of the population SDs, however. Because we would then have to substitute sample values for these parameters, the distribution of differences between two sample means would be that of Student's t and the transform equation would become:

$$t = \frac{(\bar{x}_1 - \bar{x}_2) - 0}{\sqrt{\frac{s_{x_1}^2}{n_1} + \frac{s_{x_2}^2}{n_2}}}$$

To determine degrees of freedom (df) for this case of using two independent samples, consider that the df for the sample drawn from the first population would be $n_1 - 1$. Similarly, the df for the second sample would be $n_2 - 1$. The total df would then be additive:

$$df = (n_1 - 1) + (n_2 - 1)$$

$$= n_1 - 1 + n_2 - 1$$

$$= n_1 + n_2 - 2$$

When conditions prevail that mandate the use of the Student's t, rather than the Gaussian, distribution for comparison of two means, the statistical test is called *t-test for the comparison of two independent means.*

When this *t*-test is invoked, we face additional considerations in the use of the sample SDs in the calculation of $SE_{\bar{x}_1 - \bar{x}_2}$. The *t*-test for comparing independent means assumes that if only differences between two sample means are being judged, these differences should not be affected by differences in the variability of the two groups of measurements being compared. Hence the *t*-test assumes that the two population variances are equal (i.e., $\sigma_{x_1}^2 = \sigma_{x_2}^2$). Such an assumption of equality of variability (homoscedasticity) would ensure that any observed differences between sample means would emanate solely from differences in central tendency, not from differences in dispersion. This assumption is reasonable in many cases where we expect that the observations that distinguish one sample from the other will have an effect on the mean values but will not appreciably affect variability.

For example, when we compare survival times of two groups of women with breast carcinoma where each group has been treated with a different chemotherapeutic mix, it is reasonable to expect that each of the two therapies being evaluated might tend to affect the duration of survival but not the variability in survival values. Therefore, because the *t*-test assumes equality of population variances (homoscedasticity), use of sample estimates must be reevaluated.

Each of the two sample variances ($s_{x_1}^2$ and $s_{x_2}^2$) may be regarded as an independent estimator of the corresponding population variance ($\sigma_{x_1}^2$ and $\sigma_{x_2}^2$). Although the sample variances may appear to differ considerably, under the assumption of homoscedasticity the numerical differences are judged to be due to sampling variations in $s_{x_1}^2$ and $s_{x_2}^2$. If an investigator is doubtful about the equality of variances, it is always possible to test the assumption of homoscedasticity by applying a test of homogeneity of variability. Thus an F test, which compares the ratio of the two sample variances to a tabular value with appropriate degrees of freedom and a specified level of significance, often precedes a *t*-test for comparison of two independent means. A nonsignificant F will support the assumption of equality of population variances and assure us that any subsequent, significant difference in the means of the two groups being compared is solely the result of differences in central tendency of the values.

There may be cases where an investigator is reluctant to assume equality of population variances or where a test of homogeneity suggests that the variances differ considerably. In such cases it may be possible to work with a transformed scale of measurement, such as the logarithmic scale, which may reduce the disparity in the variances without appreciably affecting the differences in means. In other cases the disparity in variances may not be resolved by any valid transformation. Several solutions have been developed to deal with this problem. These approaches are approximate methods that permit us to test the differences between two means while accommodating the inequality of variances. Such methods are beyond the scope of this text.

When the assumption of homoscedasticity is justified, we can turn our attention to obtaining a more reliable estimate of $SE_{\bar{x}_1 - \bar{x}_2}$. Because each sample variance estimates its corresponding population variance and because the two population variances are assumed to be equal, we have two independent estimates of a common variance, σ_x^2. Therefore, it is reasonable to pool both sample variances to obtain a single, more reliable estimate of σ_x^2, which can then be used to compute $SE_{\bar{x}_1 - \bar{x}_2}$. The pooled sample variance (s_p^2) is obtained by computing a weighted average of the two sample values. If the sample sizes of the two groups were the same, s_p^2 would simply be the mean of the two sample variances. However, when the sample sizes differ substantially, weights must be considered in deriving an average of the two variances, greater weight being given to the larger sample. The weights selected for the computation of s_p^2 are the degrees of freedom in each sample variance, and the result is termed *the pooled estimate of common variance:*

$$s_p^2 = \frac{(n_1 - 1)s_{x_1}^2 + (n_2 - 1)s_{x_2}^2}{(n_1 - 1) + (n_2 - 1)}$$

and

$$s_p^2 = \frac{(n_1 - 1)s_{x_1}^2 + (n_2 - 1)s_{x_2}^2}{n_1 + n_2 - 2}$$

This pooled estimate of common variance can also be written in a more convenient computational form by replacing each s_{x_2} with the formula for sample variance (p. 257). Thus

$$s_p^2 = \frac{\Sigma (x - \bar{x}_1)^2 + \Sigma (x - \bar{x}_2)^2}{n_1 + n_2 - 2}$$

Finally, having now obtained a single, reliable estimate of the common variance, we can use this value to compute $SE_{\bar{x}_1 - \bar{x}_2}$ as follows:

$$SE_{\bar{x}_1 - \bar{x}_2} = \sqrt{\frac{s_p^2}{n_1} + \frac{s_p^2}{n_2}}$$

or

$$= \sqrt{s_p^2 \left(\frac{1}{n_1} + \frac{1}{n_2}\right)}$$

The t transform equation would then take the form:

$$t = \frac{(\bar{x}_1 - \bar{x}_2) - 0}{\sqrt{s_p^2 \left(\frac{1}{n_1} + \frac{1}{n_2}\right)}}$$

We now have developed a procedure for comparing the means of two independent samples.

Examples of T-Test for Comparing Two Independent Sample Means

Example 1

Serum cholesterol levels (mg/dl) were measured in a simple random sample of 40 healthy women, who were subsequently subdivided according to activity: those who exercised regularly and those who did not exercise. The investigator wished to determine if, at the 2% level of significance, there was any difference in mean cholesterol levels between the two groups. The data are summarized below:

	Do Not Exercise	Exercise Regularly
n	25	15
$\bar{x}$	230	209
s_x^2	729	1225
s_x	27	35

In this comparison of the means of two independent samples, we would select the t-test for the analysis. The sample sizes differ considerably. Note that, as we might expect, there is more variability in cholesterol values of the smaller sample (women who exercise regularly). We would obtain a pooled estimate of common variance as follows:

$$s_p^2 = \frac{(n_1 - 1)(s_{x_1})^2 + (n_2 - 1)(s_{x_2})^2}{n_1 + n_2 - 2}$$

$$= \frac{(24)(27)^2 + (14)(35)^2}{25 + 15 - 2}$$

$$= \frac{17,496 + 17,150}{38}$$

$$= 911.7368$$

Note that s_p^2 is an average of the two separate sample variances (729 and 1,225), which has been weighted by *df.* Having obtained s_p^2, we can now calculate $SE_{\bar{x}_1 - \bar{x}_2}$:

$$SE_{\bar{x}_1 - \bar{x}_2} = \sqrt{s_p^2\left(\frac{1}{n_1} + \frac{1}{n_2}\right)}$$

$$= \sqrt{911.7368\left(\frac{1}{25} + \frac{1}{15}\right)}$$

$$= 9.86$$

Finally, use of the *t* transform yields the following:

$$t = \frac{\bar{x}_1 - \bar{x}_2}{SE_{\bar{x}_1 - \bar{x}_2}}$$

$$= \frac{(230 - 209)}{9.86}$$

$$= 2.130$$

With $(n_1 + n_2 - 2)$ or 38 *df,* the tabular *t* at the two-tailed level of significance specified by the investigator (2%) is between 2.457 and 2.423. The computed *t* value of 2.130 indicates that the 21 mg/dl difference in mean cholesterol levels in the two groups of women is not sufficiently distant from the mean of the sampling distribution of differences to be judged significant. Hence we do not have reason to claim that the mean cholesterol levels of the two groups of women are different.

Example 2

Aspirin is thought to decrease blood clotting, which might be advantageous in the prevention of certain vascular diseases. Prothrombin times (in seconds) were compared in a selected group of 25 healthy subjects who abstained from aspirin for one week and a group of 25 comparably matched individuals who ingested two aspirin tablets daily for one week. At the 5% level of significance, is the mean prothrombin time longer for the individuals who ingested aspirin? The data are summarized below:

	No Aspirin	Two Aspirin Tablets Daily
n	25	25
$\bar{x}$	20 seconds	26 seconds
s_x^2	6.25 seconds	9.0 seconds
s_x	2.5 seconds	3.0 seconds

Once again, because we are comparing the means of two independent samples, we would analyze the data by the t-test. The pooled variance is computed as follows:

$$s_p^2 = \frac{24(6.25) + 24(9.0)}{25 + 25 - 2}$$

$$= \frac{150 + 216}{48}$$

$$= 7.625$$

Note that because the sample sizes of the two groups are identical, the value of s_p^2 is the same as what we would obtain by calculating the mean of the two variances—$(6.25 + 9.0)/2$. We now compute $SE_{\bar{x}_1 - \bar{x}_2}$ by:

$$SE_{\bar{x}_1 - \bar{x}_2} = \sqrt{7.625 \left(\frac{1}{25} + \frac{1}{25} \right)}$$

$$= 0.78$$

Use of the t (or we can consider using Z in this case) transform gives the following:

$$t \text{ (or } Z) = \frac{26 - 20}{0.78}$$

$$= 7.692$$

It should be apparent that this computed value, whether it be t or Z, reveals that the six-second difference in mean prothrombin times $(26 - 20)$ lies 7.7 standard deviation units above the mean of the sampling distribution of differences! Such a sampling difference would be extremely unlikely to arise from populations with identical means. To be precise, at the specified 5% level of significance, the one-tailed tabular Z value is 1.65, while the corresponding tabular t value (for 48 df) is nearly identical (1.678). Therefore the six-second difference in mean prothrombin times is highly significant and allows us to claim that the mean prothrombin time is significantly longer in individuals who ingest two aspirin daily for one week.

Example 3

An investigator wishes to compare the effects of two treatments for bicipital tendinitis. Thirty males with bicipital tendinitis are randomly assigned to one of two treatment groups. One group receives continuous ultrasound with a placebo ointment, while the other group receives ultrasound phonophoresis of 1% dexamethasone. Their pain-free ROM for shoulder external rotation with the shoulder abducted 90° is measured prior to the first treatment and at the end of nine treatments. The investigator hypothesizes that there will be a significantly greater increase ($p < 0.01$) in pain-free ROM in the group receiving phonophoresis with dexamethasone. The data are summarized below:

	Ultrasound with Placebo	Phonophoresis Dexamethasone
n	14	16
$\bar{x}$	26	40
s_x^2	256	225
s_x	16	15

After selecting the t-test for comparison of two independent sample means, we proceed to calculate s_p^2:

$$s_p^2 = \frac{(13)(256) + (15)(225)}{14 + 16 - 2}$$

$$= \frac{3328 + 3375}{28}$$

$$= 239.3929$$

Substituting s_p^2 in the formula for $SE_{\bar{x}_1 - \bar{x}_2}$,

$$SE_{\bar{x}_1 - \bar{x}_2} = \sqrt{239.3929 \left(\frac{1}{14} + \frac{1}{16} \right)}$$

$$= 5.66$$

Finally, application of the t transform would yield

$$t = \frac{(40 - 26)}{5.66}$$

$$t = 2.473$$

At the specified 1% level of significance, with 28 df, the one-tailed tabular t value would be 2.467. Therefore our observed difference in mean gain in pain-free range of motion just barely lies in the area of exclusion and permits us to conclude that phonophoresis of dexamethasone increases pain-free ROM significantly better than ultrasound alone.

COMPARISON OF MEANS OF
NONINDEPENDENT PAIRED SAMPLES

The previous section discussed the comparison of means computed from two independent samples. There are also situations in which we wish to analyze observations or measurements derived from nonindependent samples. Such an analysis is termed a *paired comparisons test,* in which each observation in one of the samples has a matching observation in the second sample. Often, due to the nature of a study, observed differences between the means of two independent samples may be the result of extraneous factors. In these cases the process of pairing observations will reduce the variability contributed by these extraneous factors by matching the pairs with respect to as many relevant variables as possible. Thus we attempt to identify and eliminate as many outside sources of variation as possible. Although pairing will reduce the amount of variability and yield a smaller standard error, we have lost independence of the two samples. Additionally, even though we have two sets of measurements, the analysis is applied to the number of paired observations. Compared to the analysis applied to two independent means, the analysis of these paired observations leads to a 50% reduction in degrees of freedom.

Paired observations can be made in a variety of ways. Before-and-after experiments use subjects who serve as their own controls. In this self-pairing process, a group of subjects or items is randomly selected for study, and measurements are made before a treatment is applied. Following a prescribed period of treatment, measurements are again made to determine whether any significant change occurred from before the measurement to after. Thus to determine effectiveness of a weight-reduction program, we can select a group of obese subjects, measure their initial weights, subject them to the weight-loss regimen for the specified period of time, and remeasure their weights at the end. The changes in weight from before to after the program would then be analyzed.

Similarly, to evaluate the efficacy of a glucose-lowering drug, we might select a sample of non-insulin-dependent diabetics and measure their blood glucose levels before and after administration of the drug. The mean change in blood glucose would then be analyzed statistically. Likewise, effectiveness of specific exercises designed to increase passive range of motion in patients with limited mobility can be evaluated by measuring ROM in a selected sample of such patients before and after the exercises.

Another way in which paired observations can be made is by applying a treatment to two individuals or items that share a common experience. Thus two animals of the same sex can be selected from a litter, and each litter mate can then be assigned to a particular treatment. Twins or siblings can be paired so that one member receives one treatment while the other member of the pair receives an alternate treatment. Some retrospective studies use medical records of patients with a specific diagnostic code (test group), each of which has been matched with a medical record of a patient without the specified diagnosis (control group) but with the same demographic composition as the test record. Comparison of analytical methods, such as two different methods for measuring serum cholesterol, is often performed by dividing each selected serum sample and measuring the aliquots by each of the two methods. The differences between the pairs are then analyzed.

A final method of pairing is to select a test group that possesses characteristics that might be relevant to the outcome under investigation and to match each member of the test as closely as possible with respect to the identified, relevant characteristics. The latter subjects would comprise the control group. Such artificial pairing is often difficult to achieve because of (1) the need to identify a priori the characteristics that might affect outcome, and (2) the difficulty in finding a matching control who possesses as many similar traits as the test subject.

Regardless of the method of pairing, we have two groups of observations or measurements—before/after, test/control, or some other relevant labels for the pairs. The comparison of the means of the paired observations can be treated as a one-sample case of the analysis of means, which has been discussed previously. The data are reduced to a single-sample set of values by finding the *difference* between the paired observations—before value minus after value; or test value minus control value. When all differences have been computed for each pair, the list of differences may contain values that are positive, negative, or zero. We now have a single list of sample differences (d), and these become the values on which the analysis is based. Both the mean of the sample differences ($\bar{d}$) and the standard deviation of the sample differences (s_d) are calculated. It can be shown that $\bar{d}$ is identical to the difference between the sample means of the two original sets of measurements ($\bar{x}$ before $-\bar{x}$ after). Because we have reduced the two sets of observations to a single list of sample differences, only one variance (s_d^2) is involved; hence, unlike the t-test for comparing two independent means, there is no need to be concerned about equality of variances.

The null hypothesis would assume that the population difference between pairs is zero ($\mu_d = 0$). The sampling distribution of differences would be generated in the same manner as those previously discussed under the one- and two-sample cases. The sampling distribution of differences would possess three characteristics:

1. The mean of all possible mean sample differences is equal to the population difference of 0 ($\mu_d = 0$).
2. The standard deviation of all mean differences of a fixed size is termed the standard error of the difference ($SE_{\bar{d}}$) and, similar to $SE_{\bar{x}}$ in the one-sample case, is equal to $\frac{\sigma_d}{\sqrt{n}}$
3. The distribution of mean differences will be approximately Gaussian with sufficient sample size and knowledge of σ_d. In the common case, where s_d is substituted for σ_d, the distribution of differences follows Student's t distribution with $n-1$ df, where n *refers to the number of pairs. In this case, the test for analyzing the differences of paired observations is known as the paired* t-test.

When σ_d is known, the transform equation takes the following form:

$$Z = \frac{\bar{d} - \mu_d}{\sigma_d/\sqrt{n}}$$

and, since

$$\mu_d = 0,$$

$$Z = \frac{\overline{d}}{\sigma_d/\sqrt{n}}$$

When s_d is substituted for σ_d, the transform equation becomes

$$t = \frac{\overline{d}}{s_d/\sqrt{n}}$$

Both equations resemble those used in the one-sample case of analyzing means. This is to be expected, as we have successfully reduced our paired observations to a single set of differences, which is then treated as a one-sample problem.

Examples of the Paired T-Test

Example 1

One problem of prolonged weightlessness may be the loss of calcium from bones. Serum calcium levels (mg/dl) were measured in a sample of 12 astronauts who were subjected to 20 days of simulated space flight. The study was performed to determine whether calcium levels increased after 20 days in space. The data are summarized below:

	Calcium Levels Prior to Flight	Calcium Levels 20 Days After Simulated Flight	Differences
$\overline{x}$	9.4	10.0	+0.6
s_x	0.72	0.78	0.48
n	12	12	12

At the 2.5% level of significance, have the serum calcium levels of these astronauts increased?

Note that the only values required for the analysis are those representing the *differences* in calcium levels from before to after flight. It can be verified that the computed mean difference of +0.6 mg/dl is identical to the difference between the mean levels before and after flight (10.0 − 9.4). $SE_{\overline{d}}$ is computed using the s_d value:

$$SE_{\overline{d}} = \frac{s_d}{\sqrt{n}}$$

$$= \frac{0.48}{\sqrt{12}}$$

$$= 0.14$$

The test statistic then becomes

$$t = \frac{\overline{d}}{SE_{\overline{d}}}$$

$$= \frac{+0.6}{0.14}$$

$$= 4.29$$

The tabular t value for a one-tailed test of significance at the 2.5% level and 11 df is listed as 2.201. Hence our sample difference of +0.6 is significant and allows us to claim that mean serum calcium levels increase after 20 days of space flight simulation.

Example 2

One benefit of continuous passive motion (CPM) following total knee joint replacement (TKR) is believed to be a decrease in edema. A randomly selected group of 16 patients who underwent a TKR had the circumference of their knees measured before and after four hours of CPM. The results are summarized below:

	Knee Circumference Prior to CPM in Inches	Knee Circumference After 4 Hours of CPM in Inches	Differences
n	16	16	16
$\bar{x}$	17.4	15.8	−1.6
s_d	3.7	4.5	0.8

It is hypothesized that at the 1% ($p < 0.01$) level of significance, there will be a decrease in edema, as measured by circumference after four hours of CPM.

The test selected for the analysis is the paired t-test, because the same subjects have been measured at two different points in time. Again, the only statistics required for the analysis are the values representing differences between the paired measurements. The mean difference of −1.6 inches can be seen to be identical to the difference between the means of the values obtained from the two measurements. $SE_{\overline{d}}$ is computed as follows:

$$SE_{\overline{d}} = \frac{s_d}{\sqrt{n}}$$

$$= \frac{0.8}{\sqrt{16}}$$

$$= 0.2$$

TABLE 11-3.

Indication for Use	Type of Distribution	Transform Equation for Test of Significance

A. INDEPENDENT SAMPLES

Population SDs known	Normal	$Z = \dfrac{(\bar{x}_1 - \bar{x}_2) - 0}{\sqrt{\dfrac{\sigma_{x_1}^2}{n_1} + \dfrac{\sigma_{x_2}^2}{n_2}}}$
Population SDs unknown but assumed to be equal; use of pooled variance (s_p^2)	Student's t with $df = n_1 + n_2 - 2$	$t = \dfrac{(\bar{x}_1 - \bar{x}_2) - 0}{\sqrt{s_p^2 \left(\dfrac{1}{n_1} + \dfrac{1}{n_2} \right)}}$
Population SDs unknown and not equal	Approximate methods available; discussion beyond the scope of this text	

B. PAIRED SAMPLES

Population SD of differences known	normal	$Z = \dfrac{\bar{d} - 0}{\sigma_d / \sqrt{n}}$
Population SD of differences unknown; use sample s_d ($n < 30$)	Student's t with $df = n - 1$ where n = number of pairs	$t = \dfrac{\bar{d} - 0}{s_d / \sqrt{n}}$

Use of the t transform gives

$$t = \frac{-1.6}{0.2}$$

$$= -8.0$$

With 15 df and a one-tailed area of 0.01 the tabular t value is −2.602. Because our sample difference falls 8 standard deviation units below the mean of the sampling distribution, it is well beyond the 2.6 limit of exclusion. Hence the directional hypothesis that edema will decrease after four hours of CPM is validated.

Summary of Two-Sample Cases Involving Inferences About Means

This section has introduced and discussed the t-test for comparison of two independent means and the paired t-test. Table 11-3 summarizes both tests of significance.

12

A GENERAL, MULTIVARIATE APPROACH TO RESEARCH DESIGN AND INFERENTIAL STATISTICAL ANALYSIS

David E. Krebs

INTRODUCTION: THE MULTIVARIATE DATA ANALYSIS "FOREST"

Multivariate data analysis can make clinical researchers feel stranded in an unfamiliar environment, out of the comforting unpredictability of clinical mysteries and into the arcane world of statistical, systematic order. Particularly in drawing inferences about the effects of two or more variables, the rules for statistical analysis may seem to vary without reason for each problem examined and research method used. Too often, researchers lose their way in the data analysis forest because they focus myopically on the trees—the details of the statistical analysis which, of course, vary from problem to problem.

The purposes of this chapter are to present a coherent, general approach to research designs that use inferential statistical analyses and to illustrate this general method with examples of data that physical therapists have (or might have) collected. Because this is not a statistical textbook, however, the presentation is an overview; its goal is to be superficial enough to be a broad-based approach, yet deep enough to permit applied understandings. To accomplish these objectives, the reader should be familiar with the concepts presented in chapters 2, 7, 9 10, and 11, where descriptive methods and inferential statistics have been covered; this chapter assumes you are familiar with those concepts.

Usually, researchers want to do two things with data. First, they want to describe data—by generating means and standard deviations, ranges (high and low values), and, perhaps, percentages and correlations. They also want to draw *inferences* from data—by assigning probability (*p*) values and confidence levels to the observed differences or similarities in the data. Going beyond mere description of data requires inferential statistics; a consistent and coherent approach to inferential analysis requires general, robust research designs and statistics, as are presented below.

Purpose of Inferential Statistics

The purpose of inferential statistics is to help one decide, or infer, whether apparent, or described, differences or similarities in data are likely to be real (significant) or likely to be flukes (insignificant). A *t*-test (see chapter 11) is an example of an inferential statistical test; it tests whether two means differ significantly from chance expectations. Inferential statistics are assigned a probability value, ranging from close to 0—signifying that there is little likelihood the observed differences or similarities are due to chance—to close to 1—signifying that the observations are likely to be "chancy." The usual *p* or probability values accepted as signifying a real, nonchance difference are 0.05, or 1 chance in 20, and 0.01, or 1 chance in 100, that the observed results could have occurred by chance alone.

The purpose of all inferential statistical tests is to determine how well independent variable(s) relate to, or go along with, dependent variable(s). After collecting data, researchers are not usually satisfied with merely describing the results; we usually want to determine if a statistically significant relationship can be found between some presumed cause—the independent variable(s)—and some presumed effect—the dependent variable(s).

For example, suppose we wish to study the relationship between age and the number of falls per year. Such relationships could be described with means (annual number of falls per person for ages 61 to 65, 66 to 70, etc.) and correlations (the correlation between an individual's age and the annual number of stumbles). But such descriptive statistics alone could not tell us whether the observed relationships could be expected to be due to chance alone or whether they are unlikely to occur by chance.

In fact, we almost always wish to draw conclusions about or study some population (all geriatric individuals, for example). It is usually impossible, however, to study the entire population. As a trade-off for not being able to describe the phenomenon of interest in the entire population, we accept some risk of making erroneous conclusions by sampling, or studying, only part of the population. This risk can be mathematically estimated as a probability (*p*) value. The larger the number of subjects studied, the more sample size approaches the population size and, in turn, the less the risk of inferring erroneous conclusions from the data gathered. Conversely, the smaller the sample size, the greater the possibility or risk of inferring that, for example, falling frequency increases with age when it does not. In short, we sample a number of subjects from a population, measure their age and falling frequency, and examine this information to draw inferences about falling in the population of geriatrics. These inferences are usually of the form,

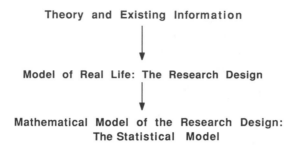

FIGURE 12-1. Schematic relationship between theory, research design, and statistical analysis.

"The frequency of falling increases with age more than one would expect by chance alone."

In other words, we want to conclude that we can explain the variability, or variance, in falling frequency in a sample of subjects by knowing their age, but we also expect some variability to occur even in the absence of a real cause for difference: things in the real world simply are not so precisely constant. These minor, uncaused differences per se are usually not of major importance to us; we say they are caused by chance alone or unexplained factors. Unexplained variability, however, can form the basis of an estimate of chance variability, which together with estimates of the amount of variability explained and of sample size are the fundamental elements of any inferential statistical test. We will return to the concepts of sample size and explained versus unexplained variation many times in this chapter.

Why General, Multivariate Designs?

It should be clear from the other chapters in this book that logic guides the prudent researcher's course of action. Optimally, a research design is logically deduced from existing theory and previously published information; statistical procedures are deduced from or at least interrelated with the research design. In other words, the research design models real-life clinical events, and the statistical paradigm models the research design (Figure 12-1). As more information and better theory become available, studies become more sophisticated and complex, and the statistical demands are commensurately increased.

Advantages of Multivariate Studies

If more than one independent and one dependent variable are manipulated and measured, respectively, an empirical study can be a better paradigm of real life, because most often more than one cause and more than one outcome measure are needed to adequately model reality. By manipulating more than one independent variable (IV) or measuring more than one dependent variable (DV), the researcher's and subjects' time is used more efficiently, because more than one cause can be studied and more than one effect can be measured. Furthermore, interrelationships and interdependencies among the IVs and DVs can be examined—a feat not possible if only one IV and one DV are studied.

Greater statistical efficiency is another happy result of multiple independent variable studies, if only because the degrees of freedom of the statistical test usually increase as more independent variables are added to the study. Perhaps of greater importance, however, is the ability of multivariate statistics to control experiment-wise error rates.

When a univariate statistic is used, the nominal p value of .05 is valid only if one and only one comparison is made in a given experiment. As will be discussed in more detail later, if more than one comparison is made, the experimentwise p value becomes artifactually inflated, distorting the real p value. Multivariate statistics permit multiple comparisons to be made *without* inflating the nominal p value.

Disadvantages of Multivariate Studies

While it is true in general that studies involving more than one IV generate more degrees of freedom and thus enhance statistical power, the same is generally not true when more than one DV is measured. One sense of "multivariate" implies a set of multiple dependent variables, and statistical power is sometimes *reduced* in multivariate studies where sets of dependent variables are analyzed. In essence, the researcher pays a price for not knowing the one best dependent variable to study and thus to which to apply the more powerful univariate statistics. This multivariate penance—loss of statistical power—is extracted to a greater or lesser extent depending upon the relationship, or correlation, between the DVs.

Another disadvantage of multivariate studies is the relative paucity of literature on the subject of multiple dependent variables. The precise nature of multivariate probabilities, chance, and sampling errors, and even the p value distribution characteristics have not been so completely studied as in univariate statistics. Thus while an exact F or t value and its corresponding p value can be established for a univariate comparison of two means of one DV or a single regression line predicting one DV from one IV are well known, the so-called Monte Carlo simulations of multivariate statistics, particularly with complex interactions and mixed models, are still being studied by statisticians.

Lest the researcher be discouraged by the disadvantages cited and the seeming enormity of multivariate applications, we should keep in mind that the goal of all good research is to model real life accurately. Real life is complex and multivariate in nature. If we strive to oversimplify research designs to fit simple statistics, the value of the research is vitiated.

A Brief History of Multivariate Statistics

As recently as the beginning of this century, statistical analyses were accepted only by scholars who were willing to admit that error was a normal and prevalent part of empirical research. Student's *t*-test and Pearson's correlation were the most sophisticated inferential tests available; calculating anything more complex than means and standard deviations was impractical because the arithmetic had to be done by hand. The rudiments of multivariate statistics were developed by the third decade of this century by social scientists studying such complex phenomena as human intelligence, but hand calculations of the required matrix algebra rendered the results error-prone and suspicious. Not until computer power was widely available could one reasonably hope to achieve accurate results from, say, a multivariate analysis of variance, so, until recently, researchers in all fields by and large shunned multivariate techniques.

Until the 1960s, physical therapy research rarely reported any statistic more sophisticated than a *t*-test. Complex interactions and the effects of confounding variables (covariates) such as gender or prior exposure to some treatment, which cannot be manipulated by the experimenter, were simply ignored instead of being accounted for using appropriate statistical techniques. Recently, however, more attention has focused on the appropriateness of our field's inferential analyses, and it has become increasingly rare—although unfortunately not impossible—to find reports of multiple comparisons using only univariate *t*-tests or ignoring covariates in our literature. As our researchers have become more sophisticated, reports of naively simple research designs that violate statistical principles shrink to their rightful ignominy.

Completing this historical tale, development of more powerful computer hardware and statistical software now allows virtually any research design to be analyzed—*controlling* p *values experimentwise*. The importance of this technological development is hard to overstate. Whereas prior to this development we had to memorize and apply the sometimes arcane rules and procedures peculiar to each type of "named" statistical design (such as the *t*-test, ANOVA, and regression), we now have readily accessible a conceptually coherent and general approach to statistical analysis, the general linear model.*

THE GENERAL LINEAR MODEL: THE MULTIVARIATE "TREES"

Perhaps you have shared this experience: when I first took a statistics course, I wished there were some alternative to having to apply a different statistical test to each unique research design. After all, if the one purpose of inferential tests is simply to assign a probability value to observed differences and similarities, why was there more than one statistical approach? Fortunately, the general linear model (GLM) is one such integrated, general approach. Although the GLM cannot be applied to all research and statistical designs, it effectively applies to virtually all situations encountered in physical therapy research.

The general linear model, as its name implies, is a statistical approach whose

---

*No one should conclude that all scientists agree that the General Linear Model approach is the final answer in statistical analysis. Indeed, Bayesian theorists disagree with the very premises of the GLM (and, more generally, the usual methods of testing of null hypotheses). It is fair to say that most statisticians support GLM approaches.

purpose is to create a mathematical, or statistical, model that to the maximum extent possible describes and assigns probability values to all causes and effects under study. The GLM approach assumes that the variability in the dependent variable can be explained by linear and additive relationships among the independent variables. This general approach therefore permits researchers to include all variables manipulated or measured in one, single, overall statistical analysis. After developing the overall model, specific comparisons are made among the independent and dependent variables.

For example, if we wish to study the relationship between flat-footedness and causes of knee pain, we could study the weightbearing and nonweightbearing behavior of the lower limb to determine if arch height (which will decrease during weightbearing) varies directly with tibial torsion and Q-angle. In this example, weightbearing (WB/NWB) would be the main independent variable, and measures of arch height, tibio-fibular torsion (TFT), and Q-angle (QNGL) would be the dependent variables. The subjects' age and gender might be other important IVs. Using a GLM approach prevents the researcher from having to develop separate analyses for each of the dependent variables, perhaps involving some convoluted test of each IV by creating separate *t*-tests of the gender and weightbearing effect on each DV, with separate correlations of age with each DV. Using the GLM approach, however, the researcher would create a single statistical model of all variables thus:

arch height, TFT, QNGL = WB/NWB + sex + age + error

which should be read, "Variance in arch height, tibio-fibular torsion angle, and Q-angle can be explained, or accounted for, by knowing the subjects' WB/NWB status, their gender, and their age." The error term is essentially a trash bin in which to collect variability in the DV(s) for which the IV(s) cannot account. The extent to which the error term is small is the extent to which the GLM model is a good one.

In general, the GLM approach provides the opportunity to reflect the research paradigm in a single statement of the form:

Variance in the Dependent Variables = Variance in the Independent Variables + Error

where, again, the equals sign is interpreted as "is explained by."

Hypotheses are tested within this overall model by indicating which of the independent variables are the main effect(s) (e.g., WB/NWB) and which are covariates (e.g., age and gender). Again, the purpose of inferential analyses is to determine if the observed similarities or differences differ statistically from error or chance expectations, so by specifying the IVs and error terms, particular hypotheses (e.g., of the differences between weightbearing and nonweightbearing while statistically holding constant the effects of age and sex) can be tested on all the DVs as a set or on any particular DV.

Because the GLM deals with variance, the researcher learns (1) whether the IVs are significantly related to the DV(s) or not; and (2) the percent of DV variance "explained" by the IVs. The statistical way the GLM permits this flexibility is by treating variance as information.

Variance as Information

Variance, the variability in data, is the statistical equivalent of verbal information. When data are collected and recorded, the information they contain can be partitioned or analyzed in a variety of statistical ways.

For example, if we wish to describe the average score for a group, perhaps to characterize the group's response by a single number, we could calculate a mean. That single mean, however, would only properly characterize the response of the group when every subject in the group responded identically. In this case the mean would contain all the information we could wish to know; the variance would be zero. Most often, subjects in a group respond somewhat differently and thus do not all achieve the same score. This differential response gives rise to dispersion, or variance in the scores. As long as the variance conforms to statistical rules (e.g., as long as the scores are normally and symmetrically distributed), that variance contains information that can be exploited mathematically as systematic information in inferential analyses.

Partitioning Variance

Variability of dependent variable scores is usually assumed to be caused by one of two factors: (1) a factor controlled by, or at least measured and identified by, the experimenter; or (2) factors independent of the experimenter's intervention and knowledge.

The type of variance presumed to be caused by the experimenter's intervention is sometimes called *explained variance* (or the *effect variance* or *between-groups variance*). This type of data variability is information in the best sense of the word: the distribution of the scores in Figure 12-2 *informs* the researcher that, if he or she performed the other aspects of the research properly, one treatment (that received by group B) is substantially better than another treatment (the treatment given to group A). Thus the dispersion or clumping of the scores—their appearance as two discrete clusters—in Figure 12-2 indicates that group membership (group A vs group B) "explains" why some scores fall into the high cluster and the others fall into the lower (group B's) cluster.

The type of variance that is unaccountable by or unattributable to experimental intervention is called *unexplained* (or *error variance* or *within-groups variance*). This unexplained type of variation in data is generally presumed to be caused by random events, such as naturally occurring differences between human subjects. For example, the variability of the scores *within* group A and group B in Figure 12-2 is most likely due to sampling or chance factors, idiosyncratic to each subject's peculiarities, physique, mood, or other characteristics. This within-groups variance is called *error variance*, and it is used to estimate the variation due to chance alone, that is, occurring in the absence of any treatment intervention. It is error variance

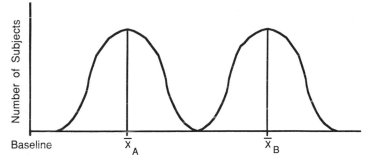

CHANGE IN ROM (PRE-POST TREATMENT)

FIGURE 12-2. Hypothetical scores from applying treatments A and B; note that the scores do not in any way overlap, so it is clear that by simply knowing which treatment a subject received the researcher knows whether change in ROM was relatively small (group A) or large (group B).

not in the sense that it is a mistake but rather in the sense that it is not due to the treatment effect under our control.

Partitioning the total variance into effect, error, and other variances is schematically described by specifying these sources in a regression equation of the form, $Y = B_1 X_1 + B_2 X_2 + \ldots + E$, where Y is the dependent variable (or set of variables); B represents a weighting factor, or regression coefficient; X represents the values of the independent variable; and E represents residual (unexplained) variance. The techniques for actually computing these factors are not germane here, because we are assuming that a computer program will carry out the calculation instructions. The important message is that the researcher instructs the GLM how to assign and partition the variance in the dependent variable(s). This partitioning effectively permits the researcher to determine (1) whether the IVs significantly affect the DVs; and (2) the effect size or degree of relationship (amount of information known or variance explained). Both of these topics are covered in more depth later in this chapter.

Significance Testing

Significance tests require that effect variances and error variances be clearly differentiated. Identification of the effect variance is usually straightforward, because the experimenter manipulates an IV that is intended to "cause," or effect, a change in the DV. Identification of error variance is not always so simple, however. To restate the principle, error variance is variability due to chance alone or to unexplained variance: variance "left over" that cannot be attributed to the treatments or IVs. In the case of the two-groups comparison depicted in Figure 12-2, the best estimate of the error variance in the DV (change in ROM *not* due to group membership) is the variance unaccounted for by knowing the treatment group. This unexplained variance is assumed to be what we *would* have found if no intervention had been made. Because we cannot know what the variance would have been had we not intervened, we use the spread of the scores *within* each group as an estimate of variability due to unexplained factors. Thus in the usual case we take the average variance within each group to estimate error variability, because we assume that the within-groups variance is the result of factors not under our control. Therefore we use the average within-groups variance as our estimate of naturally occurring, or chance, variance. We recognize, of course, that this is something of a polite fabrication, but we have no other estimate of the amount of variability purged of the effects of our intervention.

Conceptually, by randomly assigning subjects to groups and then introducing either treatment A or B to each group, we "caused" the ROM to change. Our treatment effect caused differences in the data greater than the average differences within groups. If the treatment effect exceeds chance, or within-groups variability, we conclude that the treatments are effective, that is, statistically significant.

How do we test whether the difference between the group means (i.e., the average difference induced by the treatment) is statistically significant? Simply compute the ratio of the effect variance to the error variance and multiply it by a function of n (the total number of observations in the study). This "variance test" is applicable to virtually all inferential tests; their precise formulas differ only in detail.

In general, the essence of any parametric inferential test is the variance, or F, ratio:

$$F = \frac{\text{Variance Explained}}{\text{Variance Unexplained}} \times f(n) \qquad \text{(Formula 12.1)}$$

Formula 12.1 applies to any set of variances. If this variance ratio (F ratio) is less than 1.0, meaning that variance unexplained or variance due to chance factors exceeds the variance explained, we conclude that the treatment was "statistically insignificant." If the ratio exceeds 1.0 by a sufficient amount,* then we can conclude that the treatment effect was "significant." In other words, if the variance due to the example treatment (between the groups) sufficiently exceeds the variance due to the natural variations among the subjects (within the groups), we conclude that the treatment is effective for the subjects in this experiment.†

Sample Versus Population Variance

Both treatment and error variance—explained and unexplained variance—are intended to be population variance *estimates*. Most often, we wish to make a

---

Sufficient here means that the ratio's value exceeds chance expectations for that n of comparison (here, the number of subjects); in this example, significance could be determined with a *t*-test whose t ratio would be compared with a theoretical F curve for that n.

†Strictly speaking, we would conclude that there was at most a .05 probability that the same size difference between groups would occur by chance alone. In practice, this amounts to saying that it is unlikely that this difference "just happened" by chance; rather, we might ascribe the difference to the treatment effects.

statement about the effect of the treatment in the general population and not merely limit our conclusions to statements about the effect of the treatment on the sample studied. Because we cannot study the entire population but only a subset (sample) thereof, we must be satisfied with making statements on the basis of the variance observed and measured within our samples, which are only estimates of the population variances. Such estimates would be much more accurate if we could repeatedly sample the population and repeat the experiment on these new samples. Because repeated sampling and estimation are usually impossible, however, the probability or significance levels effectively restrict our inferences so that they can be based on the size of the sample studied. In effect, if the sample size is large, we have more confidence in concluding that small differences are real or significant. These same mathematical rules dictate that if the sample size is small, a large effect size must be observed to permit confidence in its significance. Thus by making certain assumptions we make an intuitive leap from samples to populations and from variance estimates to conclusions about the effect of the IV.

Assigning Variance Estimates to Population Sources: Assumptions of the Variance Test

The mathematical equivalent of verbal information is variance. For information to be believable, certain conditions must be met. First, we assume that the variance estimates fairly represent the population's response; second, we assume that the mathematical requirements of the statistical tests are met. Inferential statistical procedures depend on the mathematical properties of the effect and the error variances to determine the significance of an IV's influence.

Logical Assumptions

The sample's variance estimates must be representative of the population's variance to permit inferences that relate meaningfully to the population. The chief means of satisfying this logical assumption is by *randomly selecting* subjects from the population to participate in the sample being studied. It is also possible to draw characteristic samples by other methods and still meet the assumption of representativeness. Random selection does not guarantee representativeness; nor is random selection a guarantee that the error variances, or within-groups variances, will conform to the mathematical requirements described below. Further, we may not always wish to generalize back to the population. Thus, random selection is neither a necessary nor a sufficient condition for an inferential test to be valid.

A sufficient condition for an inferential test to be valid is *random assignment* of subjects to the various groups or conditions being studied. Here again, it is not necessary to randomly assign the subjects to groups or conditions, but random assignment is usually advisable to avoid compromising the integrity of the inferences being drawn. In other words, some bias might be responsible for both our group assignments and the results of the experiment if an unbiased method such as random assignment is not employed.

For example, if I hypothesize that ultrasound is more effective than hot packs for treating tendinitis and I assign subjects to one or the other treatment, I will likely err toward assigning subjects who will probably get better sooner to the ultrasound group. Despite the fact that I am honest, I am also human and my psychological makeup prevents unbiased or random assignment. As another example, even if an inferential test indicates that gender is responsible for most of the variance in the DV, we should be very careful in making such a conclusion unless the sample fairly represents the population. Because we are unable to assign sex randomly to our sample, it is possible that some other factor, such as strength or size (males generally but not invariably having more of both), is causal. To make sexist or indeed any other conclusions without logical and physiological evidence that fit a theoretical model consistent with the observed results of an experiment is bad science.

Independence of Variance

The fact that we do not analyze the actual (population) error variance demands stringent quality and integrity of the error variance estimate that *is* analyzed. Therefore one assumption in any inferential variance test is that the error variance estimates are independent of any effect of the IVs. That is, we generally assume that the effect variance but not the error variance is altered by the IV. For example, if the scores tend to spread out substantially more or substantially less in one treatment group than in the other, then the inferential test might be invalid, because its within-groups variance component would not be independent of the effect variance and thus would not be a fair estimator of the population's error variance independent of any treatment. Figure 12-3 shows a situation where group variances are not independent. Most often, however, we do not know the characteristics of the population variance and so cannot determine whether the assumption of variance independence is met. Further, the *F* or variance ratio, or test, does not require the assumption to be satisfied; it is neither necessary nor sufficient that group variances be independent in most research situations encountered. Instead, we generally assume variance homogeneity and normality.

Homogeneity

In most cases, it is sufficient to assume or prove that the variances within all comparison groups are equal, or homogeneous. This "homogeneity of variance" is a useful safeguard because if the error variance is affected by the treatment, then the denominator comes to reflect not just the error variance but also the treatment effect.*

Normality

The variance test assumes a normal distribution of the population's scores on the test for the same reason as use of the mean and standard deviation to character-

---

*Practically, the researcher is responsible for assuring that the error variances are homogeneous by examining the distribution of scores within groups. The statistical examination most frequently used is Bartlett's test for variance homogeneity. This test is computed automatically by a number of computer statistical programs; however, see Winer (1971, 208-210) for criticism of tests of homogeneity. Furthermore, as the structural equations approaches, discussed later in this chapter, become the computational algorithms of choice, neither variance homogeneity nor normality will need to be assumed by variance tests.

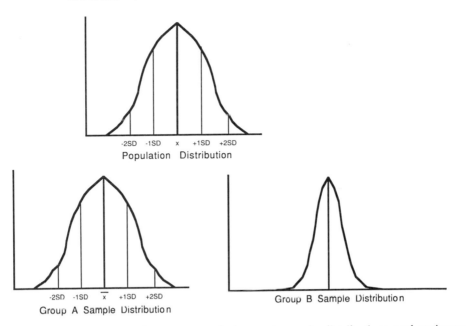

FIGURE 12-3. Relationship between population and sample distributions and variances. The mean ($\bar{x}$) and standard deviations (*SD*, square root of the variance) are listed for the population and the two sample groups. Prior to treatment application, both groups had means and standard deviations equal to that of the population. Note that following the treatment intervention, group A's variance is similar to its parent (population) variance but that group B's variance was apparently affected by the treatment in such a way as to narrow the spread of scores. Therefore to average the variance from A and B would be to misrepresent the population variance: B's smaller variance would cause the average within-group variance to plummet. Analysis of variance tests might therefore mistakenly conclude that the group's means differ when, in fact, their variances differ.

ize a group's scores assumes normal distribution of the scores. The mathematics of the variance test may not work properly unless the population's scores are normally distributed. Further, if the scores are not normally distributed, we can be virtually assured that the error variances do not represent chance variation: chance distributions are normal distributions.*

Caveats

Some authors list several other assumptions of the variance test, including the necessity of equal *n*'s (numbers of observations) in each comparison group. Assumptions other than homogeneity and normality, however, are chiefly imposed by the computational algorithms. Because most readers today will not be calculating their statistical results "by hand" but will be using a computer program, such

---

*Remember that this chapter describes only "parametric" or population inferential tests. It is these assumptions about the distribution of the underlying scores that characterize parametric tests. Distribution-free, or nonparametric, tests are described in chapter 10.

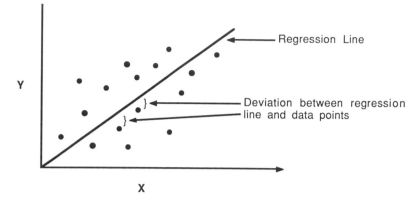

FIGURE 12-4. Scattergram for two variables, including regression line. The regression line is the line of best fit between continuous independent variables and dependent variables. Here, for simplicity, only one IV and DV are represented. Note that the regression line is the single best choice for minimizing the average distance between it and the data points; any other line would not fit as well.

restrictive computational algorithms are rarely an issue (most computer programs allow a "least squares approach" that does not require equal n's).

There is ample evidence that gross violations of the assumptions of homogeneity, normality, and equal n's are important only when all three violations occur simultaneously. For example, if the within-groups variances are unequal (not homogeneous) but the scores are normally distributed and based on equal n's, the result from an F test is sufficiently robust as to be essentially unaffected. Similarly, the F test results are valid even if the assumptions of homogeneity and normality are moderately violated but are based on equal n's.

Statistical Procedures: Overview

The remainder of this chapter will focus on specific applications of the general linear model. Each "named" procedure will be presented separately for clarity, but the reader should bear in mind that many of the computational procedures and assumptions are common to all of these tests.

The two main branches in the GLM family are (1) multiple correlation/regression, typically used to assess the degree of association between two or more continuous variables, and (2) analysis of variance, typically used to assess group mean differences (Figures 12-3 and 12-4). The GLM approach actually computes the F ratio very similarly for all members of this statistical family. The researcher's responsibility is to specify the correct error and effect terms to permit the computer to perform the appropriate comparisons.

Multiple Correlation/Regression

Perhaps the most straightforward use of the general linear model is with correlation and regression. The GLM, as indicated previously, is essentially a mechanism for partitioning variance to determine effect size and statistical significance. Thus the GLM permits researchers to answer such questions as, To what extent are two or more predictor variables related to a DV? and, Can this relationship can be attributed to chance?

Because bivariate correlation is a special case of multiple regression, I will consider here only those aspects of it necessary to understand its generalization to multiple regression.

Relationship of Bivariate Correlation/Regression to Multiple Correlation/Regression

As you will recall from the literature, the Pearson correlation technique permits the researcher to assess the extent to which a linear relationship exists between two variables; regression is similar to correlation in that it assesses the extent to which variables "fit" a straight line, called the *regression line*. The GLM for Pearson's correlation, or univariate regression, would be

Dependent Variable = Independent Variable + Error

or, in similar algebraic terms,

$$Y = bX + a$$

where Y is the dependent variable, a is the intercept, X is the independent variable, and b is the regression weight or slope of the regression line. Generalizing this bivariate regression to multiple regression is conceptually simple: merely add independent variables to the right side of the GLM statement. For example, suppose "treatment group" accounts for 20% of the variance in the GLM; if another factor is added and it independently accounts for an additional 10% of the variance, then we will have decreased our ignorance—or increased our explanatory power   to 30% by using both factors. The computational complexity is unimportant to us, as a computer will perform the calculations. The conceptual issues, however, are important: how does one interpret the calculated results? The primary interpretive tools are effect size and statistical significance.

Effect Size

Just as bivariate correlation and regression permits estimation of the percent variance shared between the two variables (i.e., r^2), so too does multiple correlation. In Pearson's correlation r is used to represent the degree of relationship; in multiple correlation/regression R is used. R^2 represents the percent of dependent variable variance explained by the independent variables. One could, of course, calculate a series of bivariate correlations between sets of predictor, or independent, variables and the dependent variable. The chief contribution of multiple regression, however, is to estimate the relationship between the DV and a *set* of IVs as they *in concert* explain variance in the DV.

Significance Testing

Lastly, just as this chapter assumes that a computer will be used to calculate the r or R values and the t or F ratios, it is also assumed that a computer program will calculate the probability or p values associated therewith. The GLM, and therefore this chapter, assumes that the classical null-hypothesis tests are desired, in which the probability of the sample result is compared to a p value specified prior to collecting data. Given a calculated p value of less than .05 or .01 (the usual a priori p values), we conclude that the sample result is unlikely to have occurred by chance and therefore supports our research hypothesis. In simpler language, if a variable such as patients' age accounts for more variance in the dependent variable than chance alone, we will generate a significant p value and conclude that age has a significant effect. The magnitude of effect, or effect size, is calculated by r^2 or R^2.

Applied Multiple Correlation/Regression

Multiple correlation/regression analysis permits researchers to estimate the degree of relationship between several independent variables and one dependent variable. Strictly speaking, a regression analysis is used to "predict" one or more dependent variables from one or more independent variables; correlation analysis estimates how well the variables relate to one another. Therefore, in practice, correlation and regression analyses are usually conducted simultaneously.

In other words, multiple regression is used to generate an equation relating the IVs and DVs in such a way as to describe a line that is the best fit possible, given the data collected. This regression line is constructed so as to minimize the deviation between the data points and the line, thereby maximizing the correlation between the predictors (IVs) and the predicted variable (DV) (Figure 12-4). The minimal deviation between the data and the regression line is found by squaring each deviation from a trial regression line; the line with the least squared deviation total will therefore best fit the data, so regression analysis is sometimes called a *least squares approach* to data analysis.

The least squares approach is also applied to finding a line that fits one IV to one DV or several IVs to a DV. Imagine the scattergram depicted in Figure 12-4 being extended to include another predictor variable. To do so, imagine the axis for that variable running perpendicular to this book; the scatter of data would then form a three-dimensional cloud. Alternatively, imagine the scattergram of Figure 12-4 projected onto the wall; the y axis would run from floor to ceiling and the x axis would run along the floor, and the data would be projected onto the wall. Now imagine your second predictor variable as having an axis originating at the same corner as the first, but running along the other wall. The data might now appear in the center of the room, in a cloud shaped like a football.*

For example, if we wish to study pulmonary function tests (PFT), such as FEV_1, we would probably determine the age, gender, and height, along with FEV_1, of a large group of subjects. We would use age, gender, and height to predict

---

*Even if you cannot imagine this 3-D scattergram, you at least have an appreciation for why you never see multiple regression scatterplots in textbooks or journal articles!

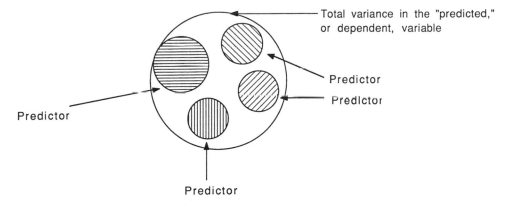

FIGURE 12-5. Venn diagram depicting total variance in the dependent variable (large circle) and the variance explained by the independent variables (small circles). Note that this schematic represents the ideal case, where the predictors (the independent variables) are independent: they do not overlap one another and they explain a large portion of the variance in the dependent variable (hatched area). The area of the large circle represents the pool of variance in the variable to be predicted, so the unhatched areas represent unexplained variance. In GLM terms, the unhatched areas represent error variance, because we cannot account for it with any of our predictor variables.

FEV_1. Regression analysis would thus generate an equation to weight and combine the IVs (age, gender, and height) in such a way as to generate a number that comes very close to the measured DV values (FEV_1). The high correlation—the strong relationship—of the IVs to PFT values makes them essential considerations. Indeed, this regression technique is exactly what is used in modern PFT machines that require the operator to enter subjects' age, gender, and height; these machines then print out a "percent normal" value, after accounting for (controlling for) the variance in FEV_1 attributable to age, gender, and height. In other words, age, gender, and height are assigned a regression *weight*—a value determined by the regression equation to calibrate their relative importance—and these regression weights are used to help explain the variation in FEV_1 measurements.

Multiple regression is most efficient if the individual IVs (the predictors) are highly correlated to the DV but poorly correlated to one another. Therefore the researcher ideally chooses predictor variables that have high correlations to the dependent variable but low intercorrelations among themselves. In less technical terms, the researcher would choose predictors that "go along with" the variable he or she wishes to predict but which tend to be independent of one another (Figures 12-5, 12-6, and 12-7). In the preceding example, you might expect some redundancy, or *multicollinearity*, among the predictors, because men are usually taller than women, so knowing the person's gender overlaps some of the information contributed by height (tall women and short men are exceptions but not nonexistent). You would not, however, enter both height and lung volume, because these measures are almost completely redundant; knowing a person's height tells you almost exactly what the lung volume is. Besides, lung volume is difficult to measure, but height measurements are practical and convenient.

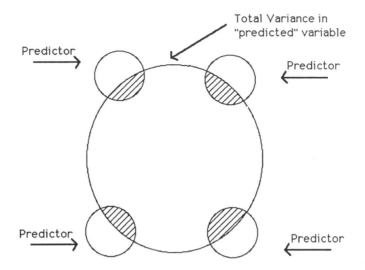

FIGURE 12-6. Example of predictor variables having little relationship to the dependent variable. Note that the total variance in the dependent (predicted) variable is largely unhatched. The independent (predictor) variables' (small circles) small hatched area of overlap with the pool of dependent variance is intended to indicate that even if we possess information about the predictors, we gain relatively little knowledge about the dependent variable.

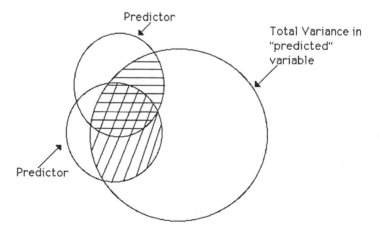

FIGURE 12-7. Example of a situation where the predictor variables are not independent; their overlap, or multicollinearity, is depicted by the doubly hatched area. These two predictor variables explain less than half of the variance in the dependent variable, in part because each one alone contributes only slightly more than the two together. That is, one variable explains almost as much about the dependent variable as two variables together, because the two variables are quite redundant with each another.

Multiple regression uses all the information inherent in the independent variables to produce the largest possible correlation with the dependent variable. The combination of regression weights and independent variables that generate the largest correlation form a prediction equation that looks very similar to the GLM.

The GLM for multiple correlation/regression is

$$\text{dependent variable} = IV_1 + IV_2 + \ldots + \text{error}$$

or, in similar algebraic terms,

$$Y = b_1 X_1 + b_2 X_2 + \ldots + a$$

where Y is the dependent variable, a is the intercept, the Xs are the independent variables, and the bs are the regression weights. Note that the last term in the GLM is *error*, whereas the last term in the algebraic regression equation is the *intercept*. This difference is traceable to the fact that the GLM statement is a theoretical model intended to explain variance in the dependent variable and compare the IVs' effect to error variability, whereas the regression equation is an empirical description of the data you have collected. In the PFT example above, the GLM would be

$$FEV_1 = \text{age} + \text{gender} + \text{height} + \text{error}$$

and the regression equation would be

$$FEV_1 = (b_1 \cdot \text{age}) + (b_2 \cdot \text{gender}) + (b_3 \cdot \text{height}) + \text{intercept}$$

In other words, the GLM can *test* the degree of relationship between the FEV_1 and age, gender, and height by comparing them to one another and to the error estimate to determine if they were useful predictors. The regression equation, by contrast, *describes* the relationship by saying, "If you multiply a person's age by b_1, add that to the gender value (where male is assigned 0 and female a value of 1) multiplied by b_2, add that to height times b_3, and add that to the intercept value, you will come up with a number that is close to that person's measured FEV_1 value." (The bs in the regression equation are the regression weights.)

Consider another example: Suppose we have percent-body-fat data, estimated by two measurement techniques—(1) nuclear magnetic resonance techniques (NMR), and (2) skin calipers at three body sites—on a large number of subjects. We wish to use the skin-fold thickness caliper measurements as a proxy for the cumbersome and costly NMR techniques. To test the relationship between the noninvasive measurements and the NMR's percent-body-fat data, we could measure wrist diameter (WD), elbow diameter (ED), iliac diameter (ID), and skin-fold thicknesses at the ilium (IS) and triceps (TS) in a large group of subjects. Our goal is to find the fewest number of variables that we must measure to be 95%

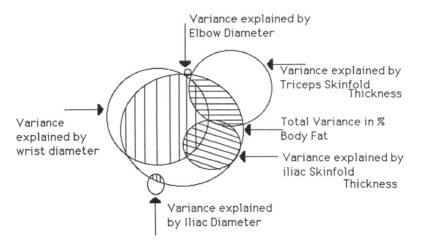

FIGURE 12-8. Schematic representation of the relationship between total variance in percent body fat and its predictors. Note that the elbow and iliac diameter measurements are poor predictors; they explain little of the variance body fat. Note also that some overlap exists among the triceps skin-fold, iliac skin-fold, and wrist diameter predictors, indicating that the predictors are correlated among themselves, so they are not ideal predictors, as are those shown in Figure 12-5.

accurate in predicting percent body fat as measured by NMR. The initial GLM would be

% body fat = WD + ED + ID + IS + TS + error

Suppose we find that IS, TS, and WD combined correlate well with the NMR measurements, so that together they explain 95% of the variance in percent body fat. That relationship would look schematically like Figure 12-8. We would drop ED and ID from our search for predictors, because they do not contribute much to our predictive knowledge, and we would construct a predictive mathematical model* based on the regression (*b*) weights, such as the following:

% body fat = (0.5 · wrist diameter) + (.08 · iliac skin fold) +
(.07 · triceps fold) + 0.0014

where 0.0014 is the constant, or intercept, and .05, .08, and .07 are the regression weights for WD, IS, and TS, respectively.

How are the regression weights determined? We merely ask the computer program to determine the weight values in such a way that the IVs' predictions of

---

*The astute student of body-composition physiology will, I hope, forgive the liberties I have taken with the Sloan, Burt, & Blyth and Wilmore and Behnke approaches to percent-body-fat estimation.

the DV values will be as stable as possible over samples. They essentially choose the weights that minimize the discrepancy between the predicted and measured DV values.

Variance Partitioning Techniques

Multiple regression offers a variety of ways of predicting the dependent variable. At its heart, multiple regression is a kind of statistical tournament, where the various predictors are kept in or eliminated from the tournament based on their performance in predicting the dependent variable. The methods by which the predictors are entered into this statistical tournament—the rules of the game— offer different costs and benefits, depending on the empirical design and the extent to which the researcher is willing to capitalize on chance factors.

The variance partitioning techniques are *natural* and *hierarchical variable entry methods*. Although hierarchical entry is perhaps the most commonly used, natural entry is usually preferable, particularly when the researcher has a causal model in mind.

Natural methods enter all the predictor variables into the statistical tournament simultaneously. The researcher hence uses theory and prior research to decide which variables ought to be entered into the model. In this sense, regression can be used as a real test of the relationship between the dependent variable and predictors; the theoretical model is translated into empirical variables, and the statistical model is tested using a sample of the population. Just as in real life, where all independent variables are typically applied to the subjects simultaneously, in natural regression no one independent variable is treated preferentially by being entered first.

Hierarchical regression allows each variable to be entered into the statistical tournament one at a time; the researcher may or may not elect to control the order of the variables' entry. Leaving this hierarchical control decision to chance or to the sampled data themselves is called *stepwise regression*. If stepwise hierarchical regression is chosen, the variable with the highest bivariate (Pearson) correlation to the dependent variable is retained from the first round of competition. During the ensuing steps, the remaining variables have a shot at currently unexplained variance (Figure 12-9). Various criteria are made available by statistical programs for retaining or eliminating variables, but you should avoid stepwise techniques except for exploratory or descriptive data analysis, where the goal is to generate the equation with the fewest variables that obtains the largest possible R or R^2. The reason for this caution is simple: stepwise techniques capitalize on chance factors unique to the sample of data at hand and therefore tend to produce unrealistically high R^2 values and unreliable regression weights (and therefore unreliable regression equations and predictions).*

---

*Monte Carlo simulations of regression equations on truly random data often generate very high R values for stepwise regression criteria, despite the absence of any true relationship. These simulations generate different regression weights and include/exclude different variables based on chance differences alone, so the predictions thus generated are perforce unreliable. The difficulty for the researcher employing stepwise regression techniques with real data is that it is impossible to know if the stepwise procedure is generating random or real relationships. See Hocking, R.R., Developments in linear regression methodology: 1959–1982, *Technometrics* 25: 219–230, 1983, for a review of these and other multiple regression difficulties.

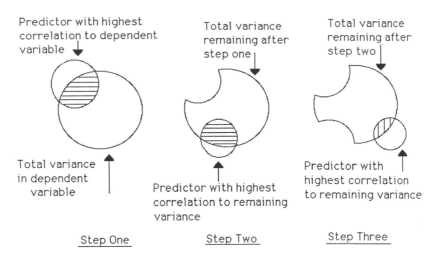

FIGURE 12-9. The workings of hierarchical regression techniques. Each predictor variable is a chance to explain variance in the dependent variable on the first step; the one best predictor is chosen. On the next step, the remaining variables are tested, in the same way, to determine their relationship to the remaining variance. Notice that the variance pool changes after each step; the variance to be explained on that step depends on the explanatory effect of the variables entered previously. The process is repeated until the variables remaining fail to explain variance. Note, however, that if an artificially high relationship between one predictor and the dependent variable occurs (by chance) in your sample data set, the variance remaining steps will be incorrect. Furthermore, the variance remaining after each step depends on the variance accounted for by the preceding variables, which can vary substantially, by chance, from sample to sample. Thus hierarchical techniques can capitalize on chance factors inherent in a given sample.

Covariance and Partial Correlation

Hierarchical techniques are not always evil. Occasionally, theory and the empirical design require a statistical adjustment to the model prior to significance testing. Before entering the independent variables of interest, one can remove, or *partial out*, the variance due to a predictor variable and then run the regression tests on the remaining variance.

For example, suppose that the researcher is interested in how well height and age explain FEV_1, independent of the gender of subjects. A hierarchical technique could be employed to enter the gender variable first, thus purging the dependent variable of gender effects. Figures 12-10 and 12-11 depict the use of gender as a *covariate,* a variable to be statistically controlled before giving the other variables a shot at explaining the remaining variance.

Analysis of covariance (ANCOVA) is similar to hierarchical regression in that both enter a "noise," or a *confounding variable*, on the first step and then enter the remaining variables. Confounding variables are effects that cannot be experimentally controlled but can be measured and statistically controlled as covariates. In ANCOVA, the predictor variables remaining after the covariates are partialed out are usually categorical variables. As will be explained in the discussion of analysis of

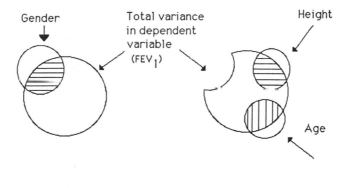

Step One   Step Two

FIGURE 12-10. Schematic depiction of covariate analysis. The variance due to subjects' gender is removed in step one, thus leaving a pool of dependent variable variance purged of variance due to gender. In step two, the height and age predictor variables are entered, and their effect is assessed. By step two, however, the variance pool has been shrunk by removing variance explained by gender, so the same absolute amount of variance explained by height and age becomes relatively greater. Compare to Figure 12-11.

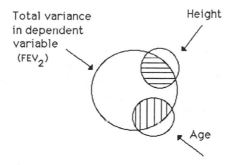

FIGURE 12-11. Effect of the same analysis performed in Figure 12-10 but without first partialing out the variance due to gender. Note that now the error variance (unhatched area) is much larger in Figure 12-10, step 2, and, in turn, the relative amount of variance explained by knowing height and age is diminished.

variance (ANOVA), below, it is simply the use of categorical variables rather than continuous variables that distinguishes ANOVA from regression. This artificial distinction becomes completely blurred in ANCOVA. Typically, the covariate is a continuous variable, such as age, but there is no statistical reason why the covariate cannot be a categorical variable, such as gender or presence or absence of a disease. After removing the variance due to the covariate, all the rules of ANOVA obtain: One can perform classical ANOVA, repeated-measures ANOVA, or even regression analysis on the remaining variance.

For example, you could argue that the gender covariate should *not* be removed on the first step; subjects retain their gender despite most experimental efforts, so it may be most appropriate to leave gender in the model to battle it out with your presumed treatment effects. A strong case can be made, however, in favor of removing the variance due to gender if it is considered a preexisting variable of no interest to the experiment.

Conceptually, the same process is used to create partial correlations. The effect of some confounding variable is partialed out of the model and then correlation coefficients are calculated from the remaining variance. For example, suppose we are interested in the relationship between triceps skin-fold thickness and percent body fat without regard for frame size (as represented by wrist diameter). We would calculate a partial correlation between the triceps skin-fold measures and percent body fat, after removing the variance due to wrist diameter. This partial correlation behaves like Pearson's r: it varies from 0 to ± 1, the partial correlation squared yields the proportion of variance explained, and $1 - r^2$ yields the proportion of variance unexplained by the predictor variable.

Several variables can be partialed out prior to analyzing the remaining variance. For example, a partial correlation can be calculated between two variables after partialing out two or even more variables; several covariates can be employed in an ANCOVA. Clearly, however, the more variables that are partialed out of the model, the more artificial the model because these confounding effects have been statistically removed. It is almost always preferable to control for confounding influences by means of the research design rather than through covariate or partial correlation statistical analysis.

A final word of warning: Using ANCOVA or partial correlation analysis to control confounding covariates requires that the covariables are highly related to the dependent variable. If they are not, covariate or partial correlation analysis decreases statistical power, because valuable degrees of freedom are wasted by controlling for a variable that is unrelated to the model.

A Comment on Measurement Scale Requirements

Multiple regression assumes at least interval-level DV measurement. Both the independent and dependent variables are usually continuous variables. It is, however, possible to use a discrete IV, or predictor, such as gender, in the regression or GLM equation. The use of discrete predictors is easily understood if you simply consider them as sources of information; the variance attributable to gender, for example, is no less a source of information than, say, the variance attributable to continuous variables such as height or age.

When the measurement scale for a predictor variable is dichotomous, as in the case of gender, assign the numbers 0 and 1 to the two levels measured. For example, assign 0 to males and 1 to females. In so doing, you have created a ratio-level measurement from a nominal-level measurement! In other words, if you consider gender to represent "femaleness," then a true zero exists (males have no "femaleness") and there are equal intervals between the levels of measurement, by definition, because the interval between female and not-female is the only interval on the measurement scale.

Even if a nominal variable can take on three or more values, regression can still be used. For example, if you have A, B, and C treatment groups, create two "dummy" variables, D_1 and D_2. Assign 0s and 1s to D_1 and D_2 as follows:

Old Variable	New (Dummy) Variables	
Treatment Group	D_1	D_2
Group A	0	0
Group B	0	1
Group C	1	1

This is the technique computer programs use to include categorical variables in GLM or regression approaches. The general rule is: All the information about an N-level nominal variable can be maintained by assigning 0s and 1s to $N-1$ dummy variables. The computer program then recombines the variance attributable to each of the dummy variables to provide an estimate of the variance explainable by the original categorical variable.

In summary, multiple correlation/regression can be used for many parametric research designs. If only nominal or categorical IV measurements are available, multiple regression can use dummy variables to calculate F and the effect size. Alternatively, a separate procedure, called ANOVA, can be used.

Analysis of Variance

Analysis of variance (ANOVA) is used to assess the effect of one or more categorical independent variables on a continuous dependent variable. As implied by its name, ANOVA partitions variance into explained and unexplained variability, analyzing it according to causes identified by the researcher. For example, if we randomly assign patients with frozen shoulders to mobilization or hot pack treatments, we could determine if the treatments made a significant difference in shoulder ROM by using ANOVA.*

Analysis of variance is classically employed for experiments with nominal-level independent variables. For example, if one independent variable such as body type had three levels or categories, such as thin, normal, and fat, a one-way (one independent variable or factor) ANOVA would be the inferential statistical test of choice. One could argue that three t-tests would also be sufficient, comparing thin vs normal, thin vs fat, and normal vs fat, but such an approach would violate the nominal alpha or p value†. As another example, if our frozen shoulder patients are

---

*The astute reader might point out that these data could be examined using a t-test and, further, that the above definition of ANOVA sounds suspiciously like that used to define multiple regression/correlation. In fact, the t-test is a special case of ANOVA, and ANOVA, in turn, is a special case of multiple regression/correlation. Interested readers should consult any mathematical statistics book for formal proof of this assertion. Informal proof of the relationship between t and F can be established by comparing a table of t to a table of F values. At $F_{1,n}$ and t_n you will find that $t^2 = F$! Indeed, at $n = \infty$ both t and F follow a normal, or Z, distribution.

†With three t-tests, the actual p-value would be .143 ($1-.95^3$), rather than nominal or a priori .05 level.

assigned to no treatment, joint mobilization, or hot pack treatment and the groups are balanced according to gender, then we have two independent variables (treatment type and gender) that may help explain ROM. This two-way ANOVA is called a 3 × 2 factorial analysis of variance. In two-way or higher ANOVA, applying multiple t-tests loses its appeal altogether; the sheer number of t-tests required to perform all the possible mean comparisons would virtually guarantee that at least one would be significant.*

Perhaps the most compelling reason for using classical ANOVA calculations rather than multiple regression/correlation is history. Historically, ANOVA approaches determine *sums of squares (SS)* and *mean squares (MS)*, or variance estimates, assignable to independent variables, and then determine if the effect of the independent variables and their interactions significantly explain variance in the dependent variable. Sums of squares, in turn, were used because they are easily calculated with an adding machine. Mean squares are sums of squares divided by degrees of freedom (*df*). Degrees of freedom are defined as in chapter 11. Some professional journals require that any ANOVA results reported must include not only the *F* ratios (variance ratios) of interest but also the *SS*, *MS*, and *df*.

Many modern computer statistical packages *display* ANOVA summary tables that include these sums of squares, but they typically *calculate* the requisite *F* ratios based on a GLM or regression analysis! You should be aware, however, that classical ANOVA calculation approaches assume equal numbers of observations within each category or level of a main effect and across each interaction cell; regression approaches impose no such requirement. Therefore you should investigate whether or not your computer's statistical program uses the more modern GLM approach; if not, you may have to interpret the results more carefully.

Significance Testing

Significance testing proceeds generally by investigating each effect and then performing post hoc pairwise comparisons among the means or levels of any overall effect that is found significant.

Tests for Overall Significance of an Effect

The significance of a given factor in ANOVA is determined by comparing the variance attributable to the treatment or the effect to variance not due to treatments or error. In general, the mean square (*MS*) of interest (main or interaction effect) is divided by the error mean square:

$$F = \frac{MS_{\text{effect}}}{MS_{\text{error}}} \qquad \text{(Formula 12.2)}$$

As you might expect, Formulas 12.1 and 12.2 are algebraically equivalent. The *variance explained*, in GLM or regression jargon, is the *effect variance* in ANOVA

---

*Furthermore, as we shall see later, t-tests could not test interaction effects.

terminology; regression's *variance unexplained* is ANOVA's *error* term. The F ratio thus determined is assigned a p value, just as in regression, using the same techniques of determining degrees of freedom and thus the critical p value.

You should be aware, however, that a significant F ratio here merely indicates that a probable non-zero difference exists among the means of the groups being compared. Therefore if three treatment groups are being compared, a significant F ratio implies only that at least one of the means differs significantly—by greater than the difference expected by chance alone—from the other means. In other words, it is possible that all three treatments differ from one another, or that only two of the three differ. To determine which means are significantly different, post hoc tests are used.

Post Hoc Tests

Post hoc tests are used to compare specified pairs of means to determine which are responsible for generating the overall significance. These pairwise tests are essentially t-tests that are corrected to compensate for the fact that multiple comparisons are being performed. Useful post hoc tests include—from most to least conservative—Tukey's Honestly Significant Difference, Sheffé's post hoc test, and Bonferroni's test. Some of these post hoc tests require equal n's in each group; others make strenuous requirements concerning equality of variance.

Bonferroni's post hoc test is general, simple to calculate, and reasonably powerful. You (or the computer) simply perform a t-test for each mean comparison of interest and divide the calculated p value by the number of comparisons being made. The result is the new, corrected p value. For example, if you compare three means, using a nominal $p = .05$ critical value, then any of the three t-tests will have to reach $.05/3$ or $p = .0167$ to be called significantly different.

In summary, the most important aspect of ANOVA significance testing is to identify the correct main effects, interaction effects, and error terms. If an effect is found to be significant, a post hoc analysis is performed to compare the means within each main effect.

Main Effects

Main effects in an ANOVA are the independent variables identified in the research design. The variance attributable to or caused by the independent variables in an ANOVA model is also called *main effects*. Main effects are typically the results of interest in the research design. Essentially, in ANOVA jargon, the main effect of a treatment is presumed to be a difference between group *means*. That is, we assume that the dependent variable's mean score for each category of a main effect best represents the group's response to a main effect (see Figures 12-2 and 12-3). For example, in a 2×3 (e.g., gender by treatment group) ANOVA, the two levels of gender would be one main effect and the three levels of group would be the other main effect. The mean DV score of male versus female and the means among the three treatment groups are the statistical manifestations of the main effects.

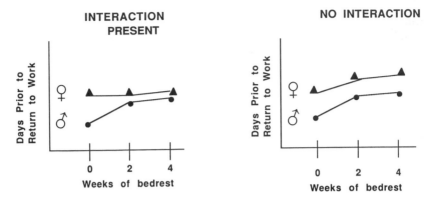

FIGURE 12-12. Interaction effect. Note that in the graph at the left, the relationship between the treatment—weeks of bedrest randomly assigned following back pain onset—and the dependent variable—days prior to return to work—interacts with or depends on patient gender; that is, males (▲) seem to respond differently to treatment than females (●). In the graph at the right, males and females respond symmetrically to the treatment; there is no interaction between treatment and gender. Thus we can say that females tend to return to work later than males, irrespective of treatment, and that early mobilization is best, irrespective of patient gender.

Interaction Effects

An interaction effect is the result of the combination of two or more main effects. In GLM terms, an interaction occurs when the *joint* effect of two or more main effects accounts for variance in the dependent variable beyond the additive composite variance explained by the main effects *separately*. In research design terminology, if the relationship between a dependent variable and one independent variable depends on another independent variable, an interaction is present (Figure 12-12).

One of the main advantages of ANOVA using more than one main effect, or factor, is the ability to study not only the main effects, as could be done in separate experiments, but also the interactions or interrelationships among the main effects. If an interaction is present between the main effects, then one cannot normally draw conclusions about one main effect independent of the other main effects. In other words, the key point about interactions is to determine if conclusions about the main effects can stand alone or if the conclusions need to be qualified by saying, "The effect of 'this' IV depends on 'that' IV."

For example, suppose we wish to study how soon male and female patients return to work following no bedrest, two weeks of bedrest, or four weeks of bedrest. The variability in the dependent variable, days before return to work, would be examined with a 2 × 3 ANOVA, or gender by treatment ANOVA. The GLM would be

Days prior to return to work = gender + treatment +
gender × treatment + error

which is read, variance in days before returning to work is accounted for by knowing the subjects' gender, the treatment group, and the joint effect or interaction of gender by treatment. If the ANOVA results indicate the interaction effect is insignificant, then you can generally conclude that the slopes of the lines connecting the treatment effect means are parallel (Figure 12-12). If the interaction effect is statistically significant and large, then you cannot draw conclusions about the efficacy of the treatment or the effect of gender without saying, "The effect of gender and treatment on days prior to return to work are interdependent," or making some such qualifying statement.

The same logic applies to interpreting higher-order interaction effects and IVs. In an A × B × C (e.g., 2 × 3 × 4) three-way ANOVA, there would be three main effects, A, B, and C; three two-way interactions, A by B, A by C, and B by C; and one three-way interaction, A by B by C. The two-way interactions are interpreted as described above. For example, if the A by B interaction is significant, then you should not try to make inferences about the effect of A or B alone; the effect of A or B would depend on the other. A significant three-way interaction would indicate that each two-way interaction depends on the others. Four-way and higher-order ANOVAs can compel even more complex interpretation, but most often interactions higher than two-way interactions are pooled into the error term.* This pooling has subtly become routine in the now-common practice of statistical computer programs to enter main effects and then ascending orders of interactions into the regression model.

Note that interaction effects are not limited to categorical IVs; one or both of the IVs being examined for interaction can be continuous. Therefore one should examine the interrelationship of age and treatment effect not by artificially throwing away precious degrees of freedom and information by categorizing age into "young and old" or "young, medium, and old" but rather by entering the subjects' actual ages into the model.

Effect Size

An important gauge of an effect's (factor's) influence is *effect size*. Effect size is the mathematical estimate of the magnitude, or importance, of a main effect. Effect size estimates are used for both main effects and interaction effects. Effect size can be estimated directly from the means or from variance units.

For example, suppose the effect of a treatment is to generate a mean of 37, compared to a mean of 33 in the control group. The effect size would be 37 − 33, or 4. Unfortunately, this direct method of calculation does not take into account variability within groups: Is a mean difference of 4 large or small compared to the error variance? Effect size is therefore usually based on effect variance components.

---

*More interactions examined yield a greater chance for finding significance where none exists and yields fewer degrees of freedom for the error mean square. A five-way ANOVA that entails five main effects comparisons and 26 interaction comparisons would consume most of the limited degrees of freedom available in many clinical research studies. Because the higher-order interactions generally possess little explanatory power, I join most statisticians in recommending their variance and *df* be pooled into the error term.

When effect size is estimated from variance components, it provides some perspective, or relative scale, of the magnitude of the effect. The usual method of estimating effect size is eta^2. Eta^2 is the ratio of the main effect variance to the total variance, or

$$eta^2 = \frac{SS_{effect}}{SS_{total}}$$

where SS stand for *sums of squares.* Just as r^2 or R^2 represent the variance estimate or effect size in regression, eta^2 is sometimes called a *correlation coefficient.* Indeed, multiple R^2 is identical to eta^2; they are given different names in some texts and computer packages simply to distinguish the regression approach (R^2) from the *classical,* or *fixed-effects,* ANOVA approach (eta^2). Note that the effect SSs sum to the total SSs in any ANOVA, so eta^2 can estimate the percent variance explained for any effect, including the error or unexplained variance. Note that $1 - eta^2_{total}$ is the residual or error variance, just as $1 - r^2$ in regression analysis is the error variance.

Fixed Versus Correlated Effects

Most texts on ANOVA consider chiefly the *fixed-effects model,* in which equal numbers of observations appear in each level of a given factor and the experimenter is assumed to control the independent variables. The essential premise is that these IVs are the only ones of interest; they do not represent a sample of a larger domain of categories of the IV, and the experimental factors (main effects) are independent of one another. Indeed, a necessary and sufficient condition of fixed effects ANOVA calculations is that the main effects are uncorrelated with, or orthogonal to, one another. *Random effect* is sometimes used to refer to an IV whose levels are selected at random from a population; for example, the "subjects" term in repeated-measures studies may be called a random effect. Gender is a good example of a possible fixed effect because the levels studied, male and female, are the only genders of interest. However, unequal numbers of males and females may prevent a fixed-effects approach.

When a fixed-effects model is used with balanced data—that is, an equal number of observations in all cells—some texts and computer programs use a computational formula that increases power. This extra statistical power may trifle with the etiquette of proper data analysis, depending on the underlying conceptual model, because the fixed-effects computation technique assumes that the independent variables are independent of, or uncorrelated with, one another. Thus if you randomly assign equal numbers of post-fracture subjects to hot packs or ultrasound, each of which is followed by either active exercise or massage, both of the IVs of this 2 × 2 ANOVA would be independent of each other (Display 12-1). That is, by assigning equal numbers of subjects at random to one of the four different treatment cells, you have forced the independence of the treatment effects. If the number of subjects is not identical across cells, however, or if the variance attributable to one main effect is not independent of the other main effect(s), then a correlation will exist among the cells so that their resulting within-cell variances will

DISPLAY 12-1
TREATMENTS TO BE EXAMINED

Treatment 1 (Type of Heat)   *Treatment 2 (Type of Exercise)*

Hot Packs   Active Exercise

Ultrasound   Massage

RESEARCH DESIGN

Treatment 2

	Active Exercise	Massage
Treatment 1 Hot Packs	A	C
Treatment 1 Ultrasound	B	D

Schematic appearance of 2 × 2 ANOVA (two-by-two) with the orthogonal (uncorrelated) independent variables. To provide balanced comparisons of all effects, four cells must be used. Subjects should be randomly assigned to one of the four cells, A, B, C, or D.

not be independent of one another. If the within-cell variances are not independent of one another, then the error term is invalid and the calculation techniques used for a fixed-effect ANOVA will err; therefore a least-squares or regression approach should be used.

You may see reports that describe *mixed models*. This unfortunate term is intended to convey the fact that correlated effects are included in the model. Happily, the GLM makes no such distinction and thus does not burden the user with this unnecessary jargon. The GLM typically does not assume that the IVs are independent and can use fixed-effects, classical regression, or hierarchical regression approaches to partition the variance.

Typically, computer programs denote the calculation method by differentiating between the *sums of squares types*. They are said to be different types of sums of squares (*SS*s) because *SS*s are estimates of variance; different methods of determining variance are called *different types of SS*s. Many programs automatically print both the fixed-effects type of *SS*s and the regression *SS*s. It is interesting to note how frequently the fixed-effects *SS*-type algorithms generate artifactual significance because they make the blind, a priori assumption that the ANOVA cells are independent.

The classical regression approach determines the incremental amount of variance attributable to a given IV accounting for all other effects simultaneously.

The error term is calculated from the residual variance unaccounted by any other source. Hierarchical regression approaches require that the researcher specify which term should be entered first, assuming there is a causal order to the statistical problem; the error term for a given effect is the residual variance unexplained at that step. For example, if the two IVs are gender and treatment type, it may be reasonable to use a hierarchical model, entering gender first. The gender effect would thus be tested against all the remaining variance, including any variance due to the treatment.

In summary, the important question to ask of your research design is whether the variance accounted for by the IVs should be partitioned as if the IVs are independent of (uncorrelated with) one another, as in the fixed-effects approach, or whether the IVs are not independent of one another, necessitating a regression approach, as when an unequal number of subjects appears in each treatment effect or when the factors, or effects, are correlated with one another.

Covariates

Although analysis of covariance (ANCOVA) was described previously, it is reasonable, if you are familiar with classical discussions of statistics, to expect that it would also put in an appearance in the ANOVA section of this chapter. Further, covariates may have a special responsibility in ANOVA approaches to data analysis. As described previously, a covariate is an independent variable that statistically adjusts for inequities that could not be controlled in the research design.

For example, to compare DeLorme and isokinetic quadriceps exercise programs, subjects could be randomly assigned to six weeks training with one or the other regimen. If muscle power were measured following the interventions, a significant difference might result simply because more powerful subjects were by chance assigned to one group. A pretest measure of quadriceps power could be used to adjust posttreatment differences, and the variance remaining could be analyzed for the effect of treatment differences.

In this simple case, it would be equivalent and equally correct to subtract the pretest from the posttest value and then to analyze the resulting change score. However, if the pretest measurement were of a different *metric* (scale) than the posttest, ANCOVA would be most appropriate. In other words, if no pretest measure of quadriceps power were available, you could use the subjects' weight, knowing that weight correlates well with muscle power. Because they are of a different metric, you could not subtract one from the other; you must therefore use ANCOVA.

In general, a hierarchical or classical regression approach is used to calculate ANCOVA. The covariate(s) are partialed out of the model first, then the main effects and ascending orders of interactions are entered. Thus, in the example above, the variance in posttreatment muscle power due to pretreatment differences would be removed on the first step of the analysis; then analysis of variance proceeds for determining the influence of group membership on the remaining variance.

Repeated-Measures Designs

Repeated-measures ANOVA is perhaps the most common design in physical therapy. Because of their complexity, however, space permits only a rather brief survey of repeated measures. Repeated-measures designs are often called *within-subjects* or *within-groups designs*, to distinguish them from the classical *between-groups experimental design*.

Advantages

In general, within-subjects designs are more powerful than between-subjects designs because the effect of a set of treatments applied to a subject repeatedly can be compared to an error term that is considerably smaller than that of a between-subjects design. This difference of the error term size results from the fact that subjects differ more when compared to one another than when compared to themselves. In short, within-subjects designs are more powerful and efficient. They are better able to detect treatment effects with fewer subjects.

Disadvantages

The basic repeated-measures design involves exposing a subject to two or more treatment conditions and analyzing the different responses to each condition. The chief conceptual problem with this approach occurs if there is carryover from one treatment to another. For example, if learning occurs in the first trial, performance in the second trial will probably be better, regardless of which treatment is used in the first vs the second trials.

Statistical restrictions can also be problematic in repeated-measures designs. The typical method of analyzing repeated measures with ANOVA assumes not only homogeneity and normality of variance within cells, but also compound symmetry: the covariances among all cells must be equal. In practice, these restrictive assumptions are rarely satisfied. As you may have guessed by this point in the chapter, the GLM not only can handle repeated measures, it can relax the compound symmetry assumption, by using a multivariate, least-squares calculation approach.*

Example

For example, imagine you want to investigate the patellar tendon pressures in two different types of below-knee prosthetic sockets during walking. You could take two groups of six subjects and randomly assign them to wear one or the other socket, but the more powerful within-subjects research design would have one group of six subjects wear one or the other socket alternately. Of course, you would balance the design so that half of the subjects will wear one socket first and the other three subjects will wear the other socket first, then have each subject cross over and wear the other socket (the one not yet worn). The reason this design is more powerful is that we can attribute part of the variability in subjects' pressure

---

*This multivariate approach unfortunately decreases power slightly. However, you can have more confidence in the repeatability of your findings if you report the results of GLM-generated repeated-measures ANOVA.

data to between-subjects factors which would, in a between-groups design, be buried in the error variance. In other words, in a classical two-group experiment, each subject is exposed to only one treatment, so the variability due to the treatment is inextricably linked to the between-subjects variance. In repeated-measures designs the response to each treatment is measured within each patient, so the between-subjects variance is estimable.

In this example, all the variability in pressure (the variance in the dependent variable) can be attributed to either (1) between-subjects factors, including such possible covariates as gender or which socket was worn first, or (2) within-subjects factors, in this case, variance in pressures due to differences in socket type.

For purposes of this example, all the between-subjects effects (for example, gender and which socket was worn first) are assumed to be noncontributory; that is, we assume that males and females respond similarly to the laws of biomechanics, so there is no need to examine variance due to gender, and we balanced the effect of which socket is worn first through the research design, so that variance should be zero. Therefore, the only variance remaining is due to within-subjects factors, that is, variance due to the socket and residual, or error, variance.

Specifying the Model

The two primary ways of calculating repeated measures ANOVAs are (1) univariate ANOVA or (2) multivariate ANOVA (MANOVA). The univariate ANOVA approach is most frequently used and is sometimes called the *Winer approach* after B. J. Winer, whose book (referenced at the end of this chapter) is considered something of a classic for ANOVA design. The latter, MANOVA, is simply the analysis of more than one dependent variable by using otherwise conventional ANOVA strategies.

The univariate approach treats the repeated measurements on the dependent variable as a single outcome with multiple causes, including the subjects' and the treatments' contribution to variability in the dependent variable. That is, the between-subjects effect becomes one of the independent variables; the differences in the dependent variable attributable to between-subject differences is partialed out, and the treatment effect variance is compared only to the within-subjects variance (Figure 12-13). The GLM statement for the univariate approach to the example would be:

$$\text{pressure} = \text{subject} + \text{socket} + \text{subject} \times \text{socket}$$

That is, we would generate a two-way ANOVA, even though the only main effect of interest is the socket's influence on pressure. Note there is no error term because there is no residual variance; this is a fully saturated model, where all the variance is accounted for. In other words, variance not attributable to socket type is attributable to idiosyncrasies within each subject. The subject's interaction with the socket becomes the error term. The *MS* for the socket effect is divided by the *MS* for the subject $\times$ socket interaction to form the *F* ratio; the usual degrees of freedom and comparison to tabled *F* values then pertain.

The MANOVA approach is easier to describe than the univariate ANOVA, albeit harder to calculate. We treat both pressure readings from each subject as if

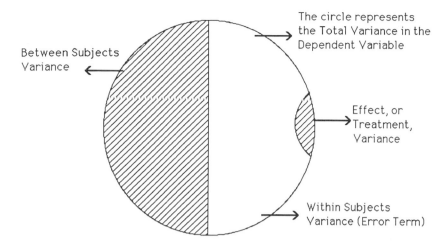

FIGURE 12-13. Schematic representation of within-subjects (repeated-measures) ANOVA. Note that because a substantial portion of the variance in most research designs is attributable to between-subjects differences, by using a within-subjects approach the error term can be reduced. That is, the effect variance is compared only to error variance purged of between-subjects variance, thus increasing the sensitivity of the comparison. In this schematic, half of the variance of interest is due to between-subjects differences, so when it is partialed out, the remaining error variance is reduced substantially.

they were two different dependent variables; after all, the pressure measurements were made at two different times and while wearing two different sockets. If socket-A-pressure and socket-B-pressure represent the patellar tendon pressures while wearing sockets A and B respectively, the multivariate GLM would be

socket-A-pressure, socket-B-pressure = error

In other words, we are contrasting the variance between the means of the two dependent variables to the error variance. The error term is the within-subjects, or within-groups, variance, because the groups in this case are identical across sockets except that in one instance the subjects wear one socket and in another instance, the other socket. If you find this MANOVA approach confusing, do not despair. Only within the late 1980s have computer programs begun to conform to this MANOVA approach to repeated-measures designs. It is slightly less powerful than the univariate approach, but the MANOVA approach does not require the stringent assumptions described previously to be met.

More Complex Examples

It should be clear that just as in conventional ANOVA, to investigate more complex designs, more terms can be added to the within-subjects GLM. For example, we could have the amputees walk with each socket at three different speeds. As a result, we could examine the within-subjects walking speed effect, as well as the interaction of walking speed and socket type.

Between-subjects effects can also be added to the model. For example, half the subjects could be given special instructions runs prior to data collection, and data from the other half could be collected without prior instructions. In this case, the between-subjects effects are again inextricably linked to the instructions conditions—they cannot be treated as within-subjects effects because only half were exposed to each condition. In other words, between-subjects effects in repeated-measures designs generate very complex models that, unless analyzed with a GLM, generally require so many assumptions to be satisfied that the resulting statistics are often meaningless. In addition, sample size requirements increase when between-subjects factors are examined in a within-subjects design.

Significance Testing

The *F* test is used, as in all ANOVA applications, to determine whether mean differences are likely or unlikely to be due to chance. As in other ANOVA models, the *F* test compares MS_{effect} to MS_{error}.

Significance tests for univariate repeated-measures ANOVAs may seem confusing, but they are the essence of simplicity. In general, the error term—the denominator of the *F* ratio—is the interaction between the effect you are testing and the subject term. Thus the significance test in our example would compare the *MS* for socket to the *MS* for the socket × subject interaction. If the experiment also involved walking speed, the *F* test for the walking speed effect would compare the *MS* for walking speed to the walking speed × subject interaction. To test the interaction of walking speed by socket type, compare its *MS* to the *MS* for the three-way interaction walking speed × socket × subject.

The significance tests for the MANOVA approach to repeated-measures statistical analysis are calculated similarly. In this case, the significance test amounts to comparing the difference between the means of the two dependent variables to zero. If the difference between the two mean pressure values is close to zero, the test will be insignificant. If this testing procedure sounds like a *t*-test, it is. This multiple dependent variable generalization of the familiar *t*-test is called *Hotelling's T-test*. It is one of many multivariate techniques.

Multivariate Analysis: Univariate Generalizations

Having covered at some length the univariate or one-dependent-variable designs, we should now consider their multivariate or multiple-dependent-variable generalizations. These multivariate analyses are, or should be, calculated using the least-squares or multiple regression approach, but they are divided into *named families* for the sake of clarity. The families again are distinguished by the nature of the independent variable; continuous IVs have the word *regression* in their name, and categorical IVs have some variant of *analysis of variance* in their name. Because of their calculation complexity and the limited space available, only brief comments are offered here.

The multivariate extension, or generalization, of multiple correlation/regression is canonical correlation/regression. Whereas multiple correlation/regression typically examines the effect of a set of (usually) continuous variables on a single, continuous dependent variable, canonical correlation/regression examines the effect of a set of (usually) continuous independent variables on a set of continuous variables. Note that in both cases the dependent variables must be continuous variates. Strictly speaking, canonical correlation does not distinguish mathematically between independent and dependent variables. The goal of canonical correlation is to generate linear combinations of the two sets of variables that are maximally related to one another. In so doing, canonical correlation determines the relationship between two sets of variables. For example, we may wish to determine the relationship between (1) age, height, weight, and years following diagnosis to (2) activities of daily living (ADL) status, walking speed, and muscle power. Canonical correlation would not only determine the effect size (an R^2 value) but also a significance test that looks and is interpreted like the univariate analogue as determined in multiple correlation/regression analysis. In effect, the canonical R is the Pearson correlation between the weighted average of the IVs and the weighted average of the DVs.

The multivariate generalization of ANOVA is MANOVA. As touched upon previously when discussing repeated measures, MANOVA generates F values to determine whether a set of categorical IVs are significantly related to two or more DVs (the DVs being measured as continuous variates, just as in the univariate case, ANOVA). As in canonical correlation, the multivariate generalization consists of a special method of averaging the IVs and DVs and performs a variance test on these averages.* A MANOVA tests the overall effect of the IVs on the DVs taken as a whole. For example, MANOVA would be used to test the overall of the IVs gender and treatment on two DVs, such as ROM and muscle power. The GLM statement would be

ROM, muscle power = gender + treatment + gender $\times$ treatment + error

Lastly, you should be aware of such techniques as discriminate analysis and factor analysis. The references listed at the end of this chapter cover these techniques in some detail.†

The important conceptual point to remember is that virtually all multivariate techniques are more conservative than their univariate counterparts. Thus they are less likely to find significance among a set of variables than if the same data are examined with several multivariate techniques. The practical problem is that multivariate analysis compels more degrees of freedom and thus generally requires

---

*The student familiar with matrix algebra should conduct the formal proof of this statement. In other words, matrix operators degenerate into scalars in the 1×1 matrices of univariate statistics. Thus the operational difference between univariate and multivariate approaches to data analysis is the requirement of matrix algebra in the latter.

†It is sufficient here to point out that discriminate analysis uses a set of measured or dependent variables to discriminate among group membership (for example, using muscle power and integrated EMG activity to discriminate patients with or without neuropathy). Factor analysis is a statistical technique that generates a smaller number of dimensions, or factors, from a set of variables. Factor analysis assumes that a small number of latent variables underlies or causes the variability in the measured variables and attempts to identify these latent causes by calculating the variance each measured variable shares with the variance unique to each.

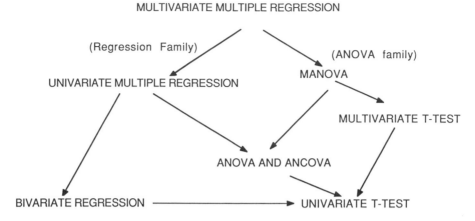

MULTIVARIATE MULTIPLE REGRESSION

(Regression Family)

(ANOVA family)

MANOVA

UNIVARIATE MULTIPLE REGRESSION

MULTIVARIATE T-TEST

ANOVA AND ANCOVA

BIVARIATE REGRESSION   UNIVARIATE T-TEST

FIGURE 12-14. Genealogy of and interrelationships among the named statistical tests. Note that position of tests is important: those below and connected by a line to another are special cases of the test named above. For example, the *t*-test is a special case of ANOVA, which in turn is a special case of multiple regression and MANOVA.

larger sample sizes. This power penalty for not knowing the one best DV to examine increases directly with the number of DVs in the model.

Conclusion: Relationships Among the Named Statistical Tests

Given that variance is the common element in all inferential statistical comparisons, it follows that the various statistical tests should be related in a structured way. The "family tree" depicted in Figure 12-14 shows that the named statistical procedures we learn in introductory statistical courses are simply special cases of the GLM. Each in turn has its progeny and its parent statistical procedure.

Perhaps the most important example is that analysis of variance (ANOVA) is really a special case of multiple regression. As shown in Figure 12-14, one can analyze any data using multiple regression that could be analyzed with ANOVA, but not the converse. In fact, ANCOVA has virtually always been calculated with a least squares or multiple regression approach, rather than the traditional sums of squares ANOVA method. The important message is simply that the researcher obtains precisely the same results regardless of whether such a problem is addressed with an ANOVA approach or a multiple regression approach.

The most important feature of the GLM approach is that it preserves the experimentwise alpha or p values. For example, the literature will occasionally include articles reporting both univariate *t*-tests and ANOVAs. Apparently the authors believe that this approach does not violate the proscription against multiple comparisons. Recognizing that the *t*-test is simply a special case of ANOVA, it becomes perfectly obvious that multiple ANOVAs are just as likely to violate the nominal alpha levels as are multiple *t*-tests.

It is also important, however, to recognize the hierarchical relationship among the various statistical tests. The hierarchical relationships depicted in Figure 12-14 indicate the statistically prudent approach to legitimate post hoc or multiple comparison tests. Just as Sheffé's t-test is applied only if a significant overall F value is obtained in an ANOVA, so may univariate categorical relationships be explored with ANOVA only if a significant MANOVA F result is found. In other words, if the overall test is not significant, one should not go "data snooping" to try to find particular combinations of IVs and DVs that are significant. Such an approach violates the assumptions of the probabilities associated with the various statistical tests. If, however, a particular combination of IVs and DVs or a particular pair of means is hypothesized a priori to have a specified relationship independent of the overall test outcome, such tests may not violate the nominal p values. In short, although the GLM relieves the researcher of many of the calculation and mathematical drudgeries often associated with statistical analysis, it does nothing to relieve the requirements of research design and interpretation responsibility and integrity.

In summary, the GLM is the most general and least limited statistical approach among those depicted in Figure 12-14. It is not, however, applicable to all situations, particularly if the data being analyzed are not homoscedastic and normal (e.g., skewed or kurtotic); for such data, an entirely new, computer-intensive approach is required.

The Structural Equations Approach: Our Robust Future

Although this chapter has focused on the GLM approach to data analysis, the general linear model—as its name implies—assumes a linear relationship among variables. If the distribution of data to be analyzed is unknown, or is known to depart significantly from the assumptions of GLM approaches, the GLM may yield incorrect results. The structural equations approach (SEA) to data analysis is even more general than the GLM; it uses a generalized least squares approach to provide solutions without making assumptions concerning the underlying relationships. Furthermore, the SEA accommodates latent variables and path analysis in a bit less cumbersome way than does GLM.*

Such extensive computations and the complex mathematics that underlie the computations were not realistic until recent events made computer power available to the mass market for statistics. Although we may not see SEA applications in the physical therapy literature for several years, I would not be surprised if by the end of this century, SEA was the accepted statistical standard.

SUMMARY

This chapter presents the GLM as a means of analyzing experimental and quasi-experimental results. The assumptions of the general variance test (the F

*See, e.g., Bentler, P.M. and Weeks, D.G., Linear structural equations with latent variables, *Psychometrika* 45: 289–308, 1980.

test) are described and the conceptual procedures for determining inferential statistics are presented. No attempt is made to outline the calculation procedures, because this chapter assumes that the analyses will be performed by computer programs. However, just as a calculator does not relieve the accountant from the responsibilities of ensuring that the credit and debits balance, computer programs cannot replace the statistician's functions of sound research and statistical design and interpretation of the results. Therefore this chapter focuses on conceptual interpretation of the statistical procedures.

Readers stimulated to obtain further information on the material presented in this chapter should consult the publications in the reference list.

BIBLIOGRAPHY

Bock, R.D. *Multivariate statistical methods in behavioral research.* New York: McGraw-Hill, 1975.

Cohen, J. and Cohen P. *Applied multiple regression/correlation analysis for the behavioral sciences.* Philadelphia: Lawrence Erlbaum Associates, 1975; New York: John Wiley and Sons, 1975.

Harris, R.J. *A primer of multivariate statistics.* New York: Academic Press, 1975.

Kerlinger, F.N. and Pedhazur, E.J. *Multiple regression in behavioral research.* New York: Holt, Rinehart and Winston, 1973.

Morrison, D.F. *Multivariate statistical methods,* 2nd ed. New York: McGraw-Hill, 1976.

Overall, J.E. and Klett, C.J. *Applied multivariate analysis.* New York: McGraw-Hill, 1972; reprint, Malabar, FL: Robert E. Krieger, 1983.

Runyon, R.P. and Haber, A. *Fundamentals of behavioral statistics,* 5th ed. Reading, MA: Addison-Wesley, 1984.

Winer, B.J. *Statistical principles in experimental design,* 2nd ed. New York: McGraw-Hill, 1971.

PART IV

ORGANIZING RESEARCH AND WRITING FOR PUBLICATION

13

THE RESEARCH PROPOSAL

Christopher E. Bork

THE RATIONALE FOR PREPARING A RESEARCH PROPOSAL

THE RESEARCH PROPOSAL PROCESS

THE STRUCTURE OF THE RESEARCH PROPOSAL
The Title
The Introduction
Introducing the Content Area of the Proposed Study
The Problem Statement or Research Question
The Purpose and the Significance
The Research and A Priori Hypotheses
The Plan for Further Literature Review
The Method
The Sample
The Procedure
The Design of the Study
Operational Definitions
Instrumentation
Location of the Study
The Protocol for Data Collection
The Limitations
The Data Analysis
Advisors and Consultants
Timeline
Human or Animal Subjects Protection Documents

SUMMARY

Generating a research proposal is the most useful exercise for ensuring that one's research efforts result in a quality report. A well-prepared research proposal communicates in a clear and concise fashion the intent of the research, why it is important, and how the research will be accomplished. My objective in this chapter is to enable you to prepare such a research proposal. By chapter's end, you will (1) understand the rationale for preparing a research proposal; (2) be able to identify the major sections in a research proposal; and (3) understand the information contained in each section of the proposal.

THE RATIONALE FOR PREPARING A RESEARCH PROPOSAL

A sailor who decides to embark upon a voyage does not hoist anchor and leave port immediately but, rather, plans the voyage, taking key elements into consideration—determining the destination, consulting navigational charts, plotting the ship's course, checking supplies, provisions, and equipment, and preparing the vessel for the voyage. The sailor may seek advice from others who have made similar voyages. By this careful preparation, the sailor attempts to avoid problems that could ruin the voyage or result in disaster.

Likewise, the researcher never embarks upon a research project without a well-thought-out plan. The research proposal is the researcher's plan for an investigation. The researcher first decides what specific question will be addressed by the investigation. Then he or she sets a course by determining the approach and method necessary to obtain and analyze relevant data that will help answer the question. Next the researcher decides what equipment and supplies are needed to conduct the research. Input from others is sought in order to improve the proposed research and avoid problems. Optimally, the result will be the successful achievement of the research goals with a minimum of problems along the way.

Research is often done to satisfy educational requirements, in which case the project must be approved. The proposal should explain what is to be done and allow research advisors to determine the extent to which the intended study meets requirements. A clearly written proposal that identifies what the researcher wants to investigate and how the research will be performed will serve as a vehicle for obtaining expert advice on how to improve the project. If human or animal subjects are used in the research, the proposal will be reviewed by the Institutional Review Board (IRB) to determine whether the subjects are sufficiently informed and protected from harm or hazards related to participation in the study. When a researcher seeks outside funding, the research proposal serves to identify why support is needed, how much support is necessary, and whether the study will meet the objectives of the funding agency. Research proposals for funding by agencies or foundations include information specific to the agency providing the support and are beyond the scope of this chapter.

A carefully prepared research proposal can help the researcher avoid mistakes that may result in frustration and disaster. During the proposal stage, the researcher should logically explore the consequences of each step of the project, asking questions such as, What do I intend to accomplish? What will happen if I do this? and, What alternatives are available? In a real sense, the research proposal serves as a proving ground for the research to be undertaken.

The completed research proposal serves as the researcher's guide for the collection and analysis of data. No prudent sailor or researcher depends on memory to guide her or him to the goal. Just as the sailor follows a plotted course to reach a harbor, the researcher follows a proposal to answer a particular question. In this way, each avoids the temptation to stray into interesting but irrelevant explorations, and, as a result, the chances for success are enhanced.

THE RESEARCH PROPOSAL PROCESS

Before discussing the major sections of the proposal, some advice about the process of fashioning a proposal is in order. The first step for the researcher is to identify a topic that he or she is very interested in or has already learned a great deal about. I stipulate "very interested" because a researcher will invest a considerable amount of time learning about the topic. If one is only casually interested in the topic, it will grow old very quickly, and, as it does, the likelihood that the proposal will be completed will diminish proportionately.

Long before a researcher begins to craft a proposal, a considerable amount of time must be spent in the library reading about the topic. A researcher must be fully cognizant of what is known about the topic, especially studies that are similar to or lead to what the researcher wants to investigate. The goals of library research are to (1) identify and critically analyze the literature related to the topic; (2) ascertain that there is a gap in knowledge that the proposed study will address (i.e., that the question the researcher is asking has not already been answered and there is a need for further investigation); (3) identify studies that have developed valid and reliable procedures to measure the variables or phenomena of interest and gather the necessary data; and (4) become aware of any major problems and limitations that are peculiar to the topic.

The generation and development of a well-written research proposal involves revision, refinement, and at least several drafts. It is not uncommon to discover that decisions made in one section of the proposal lead to alteration and revision of other sections. That is, one works back and forth between the various proposal sections and components of sections until there is a useful and logical "fit" of all the sections. While many find the decision-revision aspect of proposal writing frustrating and tedious, it is essential. It is the process all researchers use to hone their ideas into viable research projects.

Another essential element in proposal development is obtaining feedback and constructive advice. Because the proposal writer is so involved with the research topic he or she may inadvertently overlook some elements or fail to recognize potential problems that are immediately apparent to another reviewer. Therefore, it is wise to circulate drafts of the proposal to individuals knowledgeable about the topic or the methods of the proposed study. Their comments and suggestions should be carefully considered.

The remainder of this chapter is devoted to the sections of a research proposal. I present what I consider a generic proposal format. Academic institutions, clinical facilities, and funding agencies may include somewhat different sections to meet their specific needs. For example, a funding agency may have a very complex format for an estimated budget, while an academic institution may require no budget section for a research proposal prepared for a master's thesis. My intent here is to provide general information about proposal sections and components with the understanding that these sections can be adjusted or modified to suit specific needs.

THE STRUCTURE OF THE RESEARCH PROPOSAL

There are six basic sections contained in a generic research proposal: (1) the title, (2) the introduction, (3) the method, (4) the advisors and consultants, (5) the timeline, and (6) the human or animal subjects protocol. Specific information concerning the use and protection of human and animal subjects appears in chapter 3.

An outline overview for proposal development used by the Department of Physical Therapy at Temple University and an actual proposal written by Irene Naughton, M.S., P.T., appear at the end of this chapter (Appendixes 13-A and 13-B). Ms. Naughton has allowed the use of her proposal to provide concrete examples of the various proposal sections and components.* In the following discussion, I shall refer to the individual who is writing the proposal as the "writer" and the individual who is reading and approving the proposal as the "reviewer."

The Title

The title of the proposal should be the same as the title of the intended research. It is rare for a writer to sit down with a blank piece of paper and write a definitive title for a research proposal. Instead, the content of the title, even the working title, is derived from the research question or the statement of the problem. The title should be concise—descriptive but not overly wordy.

The Introduction

This section introduces the topic and educates the reviewer about the proposed study. It begins from a broad perspective and then progressively becomes more specific. It usually includes a brief discussion of the need for the study, a

---

*Several sections have been omitted from Naughton's proposal. The advisors (section 4) were Katherine Shepard and myself. A timeline (section 5) was not required in this proposal. Because Naughton's work did not directly involve human or animal subjects, it was exempt from review by the Temple University Institutional Review Board.

review and synthesis of the most relevant literature, a statement of the problem or research question the study will address, the purpose and significance of the study, the research and a priori hypotheses, and (in some cases) a plan for an in-depth review of the literature the writer has not already reviewed. The following sections describe in more detail the components of the introduction section.

Introducing the Content Area of the Proposed Study

The initial paragraphs of the proposal should introduce the reviewer to the topic of the study in a clear and interesting manner. The researcher's aim is to whet the curiosity of the reviewer. In the sample proposal (Appendix 13-B), the researcher is interested in studying the incidence of denials of Medicare payment to physical therapy providers. She introduces the reviewer to the topic by identifying billing procedures and incorporating an example from her clinical experience: a total joint arthroplasty. By explaining how and why denials occur and the fiscal consequences of the denials, she incorporates and synthesizes the relevant literature and begins to convince the reviewer that the topic warrants study. Specifically she states: "It is incumbent upon the physical therapy profession to improve the quality of documentation in order to merit coverage under these new regulations."

When summarizing the literature that applies to a topic, the writer presents the most recent and relevant literature in a manner that informs the reviewer, focuses on the issue, and logically convinces the reviewer that a gap in knowledge exists. The writer should not attempt to impress the reviewer by including everything she or he has read because, in most cases, a substantial portion of the literature may not be *directly* relevant to the proposed research. For this reason, the sample proposal does not include the development of Medicare or the diagnostic related guidelines (DRGs).

The Problem Statement or Research Question

The problem statement is a sentence that identifies the major area the intended research will address and declares that there is a lack of literature or consensus in the literature related to the proposed study. In Appendix 13-B, the proposal clearly identifies and states that the problem is a gap in the literature: "At this point in history there is little known about the types of denials received." Some individuals prefer to pose a research question or questions instead of or in addition to a problem statement. A research question or questions provide focus for the intended research. In Appendix 13-B, several research questions are posed: "Are there a greater number [of denials] given for one reason than another? Is one type of diagnosis more prone to denials than another? Is one type of facility's (acute vs rehabilitation) documentation such that it is prone to one type of denial over any other?" What should be clear to the reviewer is that both the problem statement and the research questions are succinct yet allow the writer considerable latitude in choosing exactly how the study will be framed and conducted.

The Purpose and the Significance

The purpose identifies what will be studied by performing the proposed research. One sentence is generally sufficient to describe the purpose of a study. In Appendix 13-B, the purpose is evident: "The purpose of this descriptive study is to examine the incidence of outpatient physical therapy denials across six categories of denials listed by the fiscal intermediary. . . ." The reviewer should note how specific and focused the purpose is; it tells the reviewer in more detail how the problem identified in the problem statement will be addressed.

The significance, on the other hand, informs the reviewer why the study should be undertaken. It should convince the reviewer that there is substantial need for the knowledge the proposed investigation will yield. The significance in the sample proposal is succinct: "By obtaining fewer denials, physical therapy services can be viewed as necessary, timely and unique to third-party payers." While the pursuit of knowledge for the sake of knowing is noble and, indeed, at times justifiable, a writer is well advised to justify the need for the proposed research in terms of disciplinary, professional, or societal needs.

The Research and A Priori Hypotheses

Near the end of the first section of the proposal, the writer should present the hypotheses that further focus the reviewer and provide the basis for the methods employed to gather and analyze data. It is suggested that the writer present both the research hypothesis/hypotheses and the statistical, or a priori, hypothesis/ hypotheses which may be stated as null, alternative, or directional hypotheses. The research hypothesis is what the writer believes will happen, that is, his or her hunch or best guess. On the other hand, a statistical hypothesis, referred to by some researchers as the a priori hypothesis, is framed so that an objective analysis of the data can be performed. The statistical hypothesis should always identify the level of probability for statistical significance. Descriptive research proposals, such as appears in Appendix 13-B, which do not involve hypothesis testing, do not include research or a priori hypotheses.

The Plan for Further Literature Review

This section is optional and is included in thesis and dissertation proposals only if called for by the policies of the reviewers or their institutions. In some institutions, the writer must have completed an intensive literature review prior to generating the proposal. In other institutions, the writer may be allowed to generate a proposal after reviewing the most important literature in the content areas relevant to the proposed investigation. In the latter case, the writer is expected to include in the proposal a plan for further review of the literature in all content areas germane to the proposed investigation. In Irene Naughton's case, she reviewed all the available literature. If, however, there had been reason to believe that the U.S. Congress or the third-party payers were about to change the laws or protocols regarding outpatient coverage, then she would have had to include a section describing the sources she would review.

The Method

The method section specifies how data will be collected and analyzed to validate or refute the statistical hypotheses or, in the case of descriptive or qualitative research, to describe the phenomenon being studied. There are three essential components of the method section: the sample, the procedure, and the data analysis.

The Sample

A detailed description of the sample that will be used in the proposed study is provided for the reviewer. This section identifies the number of subjects and the procedure for obtaining them. The proposal also should clearly state the type of sampling procedure that will be employed. The sample proposal in Appendix 13-B states that the sample will be obtained through a cluster method from a telephone directory.

The *inclusion criteria*, that is, the criteria for eligibility in the study, are specified in detail. In Appendix 13-B, each of the subjects is a hospital, and the inclusion criteria are "all acute care hospitals and rehabilitation hospitals within an eight-mile radius of Glenside, Pennsylvania." *Exclusion criteria*, which disqualify a subject from participation in a proposed study, are also described in detail. For the sample proposal, the exclusion criteria "include facilities not treating Medicare patients or those whose Medicare fiscal intermediary is not Blue Cross/Blue Shield." Although the sample proposal presents the inclusion and exclusion criteria in the narrative, they may be presented as a list.

The last element included in the sample section, if applicable, is a description of how subjects are assigned to groups. If the subjects will be assigned to groups randomly, the writer must describe in detail how the randomization is accomplished. If the subjects are matched and assigned to groups, the characteristics that are used for matching must be described in detail.

The Procedure

The procedure describes in detail how the data will be collected. A well-written procedure will allow another individual to replicate the study. The elements of this section include (1) the design of the study; (2) instrumentation for data collection; (3) a protocol for data collection; and (4) limitations, or the expected difficulties in collecting the data.

The Design of the Study

The writer should state the type of research design for the proposed study—descriptive, preexperimental, experimental, quasi-experimental, and so forth. Chapters 5-8 describe various types of research design. By identifying the design used, the writer establishes a framework for justifying decisions concerning equipment, data collection instruments, location, protocol, and the limitations of the study. In the sample proposal, Irene Naughton states that she will be performing descriptive research.

Operational Definitions

Next, the variables are described in such a manner that they can be measured, or operationally defined. In the sample proposal: "Acute care outpatient departments are defined as those hospitals providing acute care or acute care plus rehabilitation beds. Rehabilitation outpatient departments are defined as those facilities providing primarily rehabilitation beds."* Because the denials for payment were the letters received, there was no need to further define them. In proposals which examine phenomena which can be measured in different ways, the operational definition informs the reviewer precisely how the data will be measured for that particular study; for example, outcome measures such as strength or pain relief can be measured in several ways. The operational definition also allows the reviewer to ascertain if appropriate statistical measurements and tests will be employed later on in the data analysis.

Instrumentation

This subsection provides information on exactly what tools will be used to measure the variables which are operationally defined. The writer should justify the use of any instrument in terms of its validity and should also report its reliability. All equipment used should be described, including the model, the manufacturer, and the manufacturer's address. Often a picture or photograph of a specialized piece of equipment is included as an appendix. If other instruments, such as questionnaires, are used, the writer should report their source, or, if they were developed by the writer, the development protocol should be described. "Pen and paper instruments" such as questionnaires should always be included in an appendix.

Location of the Study

This element is a description of the location where the data will be collected: the physical facilities and any special place or other location requirements. If the description of the space requirements is complex, a schematic drawing may be included.

The Protocol for Data Collection

The protocol for data collection provides the directions for gathering the data. Included in the protocol are the detailed plans for (1) designating who will

---

*Notice that in Appendix 13-B the operational definitions are in the sample section of the proposal. The proposal's advisors preferred the definitions there. Similarly the research design is not identified in the procedure section. Recall that the research design was identified in the purpose. As explained, the format for the proposal presented in this chapter is not meant to be construed as rigid; indeed, logic and clarity should never be sacrificed to adherence to a particular format. On the other hand, the format provides a convenient means of ensuring that all the essential sections, components, and elements germane to a study are addressed.

administer treatment if applicable, and who will collect the data; (2) establishing intrarater and interrater reliability (if necessary for the study); (3) instructions to participants and subjects; (4) data collection forms; (5) the time required to collect data from subjects; (6) informed consent from subjects (if appropriate); and (7) the step-by-step process for data collection. Whether or not all these elements are included in the proposal depends on the nature of the study. When planning research and the generation of a research proposal, the writer should consider the elements and answer certain questions within the protocol. Some questions the proposal writer may wish to address when developing the protocol are presented below. Although these questions are neither exhaustive nor content specific, they are helpful in emphasizing the need for the proposal writer to scrutinize every aspect of the protocol for data collection.

Designating personnel. Ordinarily the researcher, in this case the proposal writer, collects the data. However some studies may require that the researcher be "blind," that is, not know which subjects were exposed to a specific treatment. In the case of a blinded study, who are the personnel to administer the treatment? In any study, the person(s) who will collect the data must be clearly identified.

Establishing reliability. If more than one individual is gathering data, is there a need to establish interrater reliability? If there is the need, how will interrater reliability be established and how will it be statistically assessed? When will the equipment be calibrated and by whom?

Instructions. Do participants or subjects require instructions? If so, what will the instructions be? How will the instructions be conveyed?

Data collection forms. Will data collection forms be necessary and, if so, what must be recorded? Are the forms organized for logical and sequential recording of data?

Time required. How much time will it take to gather the data from one subject? How long will the entire data collection take? Is the time allotted realistic, and, if not, where should the modifications take place?

Informed consent. Is informed consent required and, if so, when will it be obtained and by whom?

The actual data collection. Exactly what steps must be taken to actually collect the data? If multiple measurements will be made, what is the sequence? When will each measurement be recorded? Are there special tasks that must be completed by a certain date? If so, the times for initiation and completion of the tasks should be stated. For example, if a mail questionnaire is used, when will follow-up letters and post cards be sent?

These questions and others that are specific to the content area of a proposal must be asked and answered to ensure that critical steps in the protocol are not overlooked. The objective is to develop a protocol that limits as many threats to reliability and validity as possible. Two of the best pieces of advice concerning protocols are (1) have knowledgeable individuals read and critique the protocol; and (2) pilot-test the protocol on a small number of subjects. Any flaws or oversights should become readily, if not embarrassingly, apparent. An additional benefit of a pilot-test is that the researcher is able to ascertain if the data collected are what was anticipated.

In Appendix 13-B, the sample proposal describes the instructions to the subject hospitals and the assurance of anonymity. She identifies that she wants the directors to assemble the denial letters and states when she will visit to actually collect the data. She then describes, step-by-step, exactly how she will collect and record the data. She even describes how she would categorize the diagnosis. After reading this protocol or, for that matter, any carefully planned protocol, another researcher should be able to replicate the study.

The Limitations

Here, the writer identifies anticipated difficulties in obtaining the data. These difficulties are assumed to be beyond the control of the investigator. Nonetheless the expected difficulties, which can be sources of error, must be identified, and, if possible, their effects upon the outcome of the proposed study must be estimated. Simply including sources of error that can be controlled through design or procedural care in the limitations does not excuse the investigator for a poorly conceived investigation. The sample proposal identifies potential problems with compliance and multiple problems affecting the classification of the patients' diagnoses.

The Data Analysis

This component of the method section describes how the proposal writer will analyze and present the data collected in the investigation. The plan for data analysis is essential, for all too often beginning researchers and graduate students, who have worked diligently to collect data, become literally lost in their data. Without a clear understanding and a plan for analyzing the data there is the potential to over-analyze or incorrectly analyze the data. Remember, the power and ease with which computers can manipulate data is seductive. Often the investigator ends up with reams of printouts when only one or two tests would have been sufficient for the analysis. Thus it is in the proposal writer's best interest to include a plan for the data analysis in the proposal.

The data analysis should consist of identifying (1) plans for the descriptive statistics and (2) the analytical or hypothesis-testing statistical tests that will be used to analyze the data. Descriptive statistics always precede hypothesis testing, because the procedure is always to describe the sample and, in many instances, the data before analyses and comparisons are made. The inferential or hypothesis-testing statistical tests are always presented in the same order as the hypotheses are presented in the introduction section of the proposal. In order to be sure that the descriptive and inferential statistical tests are appropriate for the data that will be collected, the writer is encouraged to include dummy data presentation in the proposal. This allows both the reviewer and the writer to develop an appreciation for the quality of the data and the best way to present the results.

Advisors and Consultants

This section of the proposal indicates who the writer will use as advisors and consultants while performing the investigation. The writer should obtain consent from these individuals to serve as advisors or consultants prior to including their names in the proposal. One additional item that the investigator should discuss with the advisors and consultants concerns the authorship of any publications that will result from the research. In order to avert problems in the future, a form such as shown in Appendix 13-C may prove helpful. All parties who contribute to the research should know what their role in the authorship of publications entails and how they will be recognized for their contributions.

Timeline

Including a timeline for the completion of the investigation helps the reviewer gain a better overall understanding of the proposed research. A timeline also helps the writer develop a sense of the time commitment that the project will involve and allows for planning. Finally, the timeline sets objectives and milestones for the researcher when the investigation is undertaken.

Human or Animal Subjects Protection Documents

The final section of the proposal is the inclusion of the materials which must be sent to the Institutional Review Board (IRB) for approval. These documents vary among institutions and must be submitted and approved before the investigation is initiated. The writer should contact the IRB at her or his institution in order to obtain the appropriate forms.

SUMMARY

The preparation of a research proposal is an essential first step when one decides to begin an investigation. A carefully prepared research proposal helps the investigator to avoid pitfalls and serves as a guide while the research is conducted.

The purposes of the research project are to (1) convey the researcher's reasons and methods for engaging in the research; (2) gather input and advice from research advisors and other experts; (3) identify the resources required to conduct the proposed research; (4) identify potential problems so that they can be averted; and (5) serve as a guide while the project is conducted.

The preparation of a research proposal is not an academic exercise but a necessary precursor to any research project. Because research represents an investment of substantial time, effort, and resources, it is essential that a research proposal optimize one's ability to complete an investigation.

SUGGESTED READING

Francis, J.B., Bork, C.E., and Carstens, S. *The proposal cookbook*, 3rd ed. Naples, FL.: ARA Press, 1986.

Krathwohl, D.R. *How to prepare a research proposal*, 2nd ed. (1977). Available from the Syracuse University Bookstore, Syracuse, NY.

APPENDIX 13-A
The Temple University Department of Physical Therapy
Proposal Outline

Research Proposal Format

I. Title

The title should be formed out of the research question

II. Introduction
   A. Why the study is needed
      1. Statement of the problem
   B. Review and synthesis of the literature
   C. Purpose and significance of the study
   D. Hypotheses
      1. Research hypothesis—what you expect to find
      2. Statistical or a priori hypothesis/hypotheses

III. Method
   A. Sample
      1. Subjects
         a. Number of subjects
         b. Source of subjects
         c. Inclusion criteria
         d. Exclusion criteria
      2. Method of selecting and, if applicable, assigning subjects
   B. Procedure
      1. Design of the study
      2. Instrumentation for data collection
         a. Operational definitions of the variables
         b. Equipment
         c. Other data collection instruments such as surveys, attitudinal scales, functional indices, etc.
         d. Location
            (1) Space and facilities
      3. Protocol for data collection
         a. Participants—who will collect data
            (1) Establishment and assessment of reliability
         b. Instructions to participants and subjects
         c. Data collection forms
         d. Estimate of time needed for data collection
         e. Plan for obtaining informed consent from subjects
         f. Step-by-step process for collecting data
      4. Limitations (expected difficulties)
   C. Data analysis (using simulated data)
      1. Descriptive statistics
         a. Graphs, tables, charts

      2. Inferential or analytical statistics
         a. Display of outcome of appropriate test(s)
            (1) Presented in order of hypothesis(es)
  IV. Names of advisors and consultants
   V. Timeline
 VI. Human subjects or animal subjects protocol for institutional review board
     (if applicable)

APPENDIX 13-B
A Sample Proposal

The Incidence of Outpatient Physical Therapy Medicare Denials Across the Six Categories Listed by Fiscal-Intermediary Blue Cross/Blue Shield

Irene Naughton, P.T.

On November 11, 1988, the Health Care Financing Administration (HCFA) established new billing procedures for Medicare Part B Outpatient Physical Therapy (OPT) Services.[1] These new procedures included an edit system whereby each medical diagnosis is assigned a specific number of physical therapy visits and/or a specific duration of time during which physical therapy services rendered would be reimbursed. An example of one such edit is that given for a total joint arthroplasty. The number of allowable visits is 18, along with a duration of 2 months, whichever comes first. If physical therapy services exceed the parameters of the edits, a medical review of these services will be conducted.

Medical Information Form (MIF) was created by HCFA to expedite the review process. [In this proposal an actual MIF was included as an appendix.] This form is to be completed monthly by a physical therapist for each patient covered by Medicare, and forwarded with the claim. Each claim is subject to review when the quantity of treatments provided exceeds the edit criteria.

If it is found upon review that the physical therapy services did not meet the Medicare guidelines for being "reasonable" and "necessary" or, if the MIF was incorrectly completed, the claim for payment is denied. Physical therapy providers who receive a 5% or greater denial rate in any one quarter are placed on 100% pre-pay medical review in the following quarter.[1] Once put on 100% review, all MIFs submitted with claims are read thoroughly. Reviewers are looking for documentation justifying that the services rendered were necessary and required the skills of a qualified physical therapist. This in-depth review takes more time, thus withholding reimbursement for a longer time as well as increasing the likelihood for further denials. In addition to a 5% denial rate review, a random review of all claims which meet the edit criteria are performed.

The fiscal intermediary Blue Cross/Blue Shield issues the reasons for denials as the following:

1. The diagnosis/service provided on the claim was too vague.
2. The diagnosis provided on claim does not justify the services provided.
3. The services provided were at a maintenance level of care.
4. The services provided do not require a skilled therapist.
5. Documentation does not support improvement in the patient's status or does not specify functional changes in measurable terms.
6. Date of evaluation, date of onset not given.[2]

This new Outpatient Physical Therapy (OPT) payment system is similar to the prospective payment system introduced by Medicare in October, 1983.[3] The prospective payment system established diagnostic related groups (DRG) which established the amount of reimbursements for all services rendered by acute care hospitals according to diagnostic group. Similarly, the OPT edits are categorized by diagnosis and provide an average length of treatment per diagnosis. The goals of the DRG system were to decrease hospital length of stay and to decrease the use of in-patient ancillary services, thereby forcing hospitals to become more cost-efficient.[3,4] A result of this increased efficiency was an increase in outpatient services, including physical therapy.[5] Daniel Dore noted a significant increase in utilization of outpatient physical therapy services in the post-DRG period of 1983-85.[6]

With this increase in utilization of outpatient services comes an increase in the claims against Medicare Part B funds. An HCFA study described an increase in Medicare Part B benefit payments of 18.3% in fiscal year 1986.[7] This author speculates that the development of the edit system is an attempt at cost containment in these Part B expenditures.

The new edit system demands increased efficiency from the providers of physical therapy services. Medicare guidelines state that the treatment must be:

Reasonable: A 50% probability that the patient will attain significant improvement as a result of therapy.

Within a predictable amount of time: The duration/frequency of treatment sessions established by the therapist are an estimate of how long it will take to achieve goals based upon diagnosis and prognosis.[8]

It is incumbent upon the physical therapy profession to improve the quality of documentation in order to merit coverage under these new regulations. By obtaining fewer denials, physical therapy services can be viewed as necessary, timely, and unique by third-party payers. At this point in history there is little known about the types of denials received. Are there a greater number given for one reason than another? Is one type of diagnosis more prone to denials than another? Is one type of facility's (acute vs rehabilitation) documentation such that it is prone to one type of denial over any other? The more that is known about these denials the better able the profession of physical therapy will be to avoid denials by improving its own efficiency. The purpose of this descriptive study is to examine the incidence of outpatient physical therapy denials across the 6 categories of denial listed by the fiscal intermediary Blue Cross/Blue Shield. Also to be examined will be the incidence of denial as it relates to the type of facility reviewed (acute care vs rehabilitation), and the diagnostic group reviewed (orthopedic vs neurologic vs other).

Method

Sample

A cluster sample of all acute care hospitals and rehabilitation hospitals within an eight-mile radius of Glenside, Pennsylvania, will be taken from the telephone directory listings. Exclusion criteria for this sample include facilities not treating

Medicare patients or those whose Medicare fiscal intermediary is not Blue Cross/ Blue Shield. Acute care outpatient departments are defined as those hospitals providing acute care or acute care plus rehabilitation beds. Rehabilitation outpatient departments are defined as those facilities providing primarily rehabilitation beds.

Protocol

Upon selection of the sample, physical therapy directors will be requested to collect all outpatient Medicare denial letters for a three-month period of time [the proposal included a sample denial letter in an appendix]. They will be instructed to document the primary diagnosis of the patient whose payment for physical therapy services is denied. These diagnoses are to be listed as orthopedic, neurologic, or other (any diagnosis not being orthopedic or neurologic). Also to be noted on the letter will be the type of facility (acute care or rehabilitation) receiving it. The researcher will explain to participants that she will visit the facility at the end of each of the next three months to obtain the denial letters collected. No patient name or facility name will appear on the letter. Clinicians will be informed that all denial letters received in their offices during the three-month period are to be collected, regardless of the payment period for which these denials were applicable.

The researcher's procedure for obtaining data will be as follows: A telephone call will be placed to each clinic one week prior to the researcher's arrival to ensure that all data will be ready for collection. Upon arrival at a facility, each letter will be inspected for its content. If portions of the data are not present, the clinician will be asked to supply the missing information. No denial letter will be removed from a clinic if complete information is not contained within it.

Limitations

One limitation of this study may be the ability to obtain full compliance from physical therapy directors/private practice owners when gathering letters and documenting diagnosis and facility type. Also limiting may be the information obtained comparing diagnostic group to denial rate. Since all patients whose physical therapy services are denied for reimbursement will be receiving Medicare and generally will be over 65 years old, there is a likelihood that more than one diagnosis may be present. These additional diagnoses could impede progress in remediation of the primary diagnosis, thus causing the denial.

Data Analysis

A single-sample chi-square test for homogeneity will be performed between the category of denial and the facility type. Another chi-square test will be performed between categories of denial and diagnostic type. This type of testing allows any relationship present between independent variables to be visualized.

Once data are collected, the researcher will tally the number of denials given for categories 1 through 6 on the denial letter. These data will be converted to percentages of denial per category. The number of denial letters for each facility will be counted along with the percentage of denial per facility. Lastly, the number of denial letters per diagnostic type will be tabulated.

APPENDIX REFERENCES

1. Department of Health and Human Services, Health Care Financing Administration, Medicare Hospital Manual, Section 515, Revised Material: Billing for Part B, Outpatient Physical Therapy Services, Revised 8/88.

2. Independence Blue Cross, Health Care Financing Administration fiscal intermediary for Medicare, "Dear Administrator" letter, see Appendix II.

3. Guterman, S., Dobson, A. Impact of the Medicare prospective payment system for hospitals. Health Care Financing Review, Vol. 7, No. 3, p. 97–114, Spring 1986.

4. Weiner, S., Maxwell, J., Sapolsky, H., Dunn, D., Hsiao, W. Economic incentives and organizational realities: managing hospitals under DRG's. The Milbank Memorial Fund, Health and Society, Vol. 65, No. 4, p. 463–487, 1987.

5. Helbing, C., Latta, V. Use and cost of hospital outpatient services under Medicare, 1985. Health Care Financing Review, Vol. 9, No. 4, p. 113–125, Summer 1988.

6. Dore, D. Effect of the Medicare prospective payment system on the utilization of physical therapy. Physical Therapy, Vol. 67, no. 6, p. 964–966, June 1987.

7. Guterman, S., Eggers, P., Riley, G., Greene, T., Terrell, S. The first three years of Medicare prospective payment: An overview. Health Care Financing Review, Vol. 9, No. 3, p. 67–77, Spring 1988.

8. Bernstein, F., Eguchi, K., Messer, S., Dugawson, R., Elkhousy, N., Komorowski, D., Rubenstein, B. Documentation for outpatient physical therapy. Clinical Management in Physical Therapy, Vol. 7, No. 2, p. 28–30, March-April 1987.

(Used with permission of Irene Naughton, Glenside, PA.)

APPENDIX 13-C
A Sample Agreement for Authorship

Note: This agreement may be adapted for research leading to a degree when the wording within the parentheses is retained.

Agreement on Authorship

The guidelines for authorship on any publication or oral presentation resulting from the research project entitled:

_____ and carried out for fulfillment of

requirements for the _____ degree are as follows.

The investigator (graduate student), _____, will retain first authorship on all written or oral presentations.

Second authorship is reserved for the major advisor. Second authorship indicates that the major advisor made significant contributions to one or more of the following: conception of the idea and design of the project; analysis and interpretation of the data; and writing of the manuscript for publication.

Third authorship and so forth are normally reserved for other advisors and consultants depending upon their contributions to the research and the manuscript.

(The graduate student has the professional responsibility to submit a manuscript for publication which will contribute to the physical therapy body of knowledge. If the student does not submit the manuscript for publication or present the findings of the research at the national level within one year of the completion of the study, and the major advisor deems the research to be of merit, the major advisor has the prerogative to submit the manuscript with the student listed as first author.)

_____
Investigator (graduate student)

_____
Major advisor

_____
Advisor

_____
Date

14

WRITING
RESEARCH REPORTS

Marilyn J. Lister

PREPARING FOR PUBLICATION

COMPONENTS
    Title
    Abstract
    Introduction
        Defining the Problem
        Providing Supportive Rationale
        Stating the Purpose
        Identifying the Type of Study
        Stating the Hypothesis or Expected Results
        Justifying the Need for Descriptive Study
    Method
        Subjects
        Procedures
        Data Analysis
    Results
    Discussion
    Conclusion
    References
    Figures
    Appendixes
    Acknowledgments
    Title Page

PREPARATION AND SUBMISSION OF MANUSCRIPTS

RECOMMENDATIONS FOR WRITING
Reviewing the Rules
Selecting Style and Syntax

SUMMARY

Research is not complete until a report of it is published. Assuming that your research is valid and that you have valuable information to contribute to the physical therapy literature, you now can start on one of the most rewarding, albeit frustrating, experiences—writing.

As you start writing, diminish your negative anticipation by keeping in mind what you already know about learning new technical skills: start with small steps; review the parts you already know; see how others do it; get feedback as you go along; and practice.

Writing a report on your research can be done more easily if you follow certain steps. First, learn and follow the style and organization advocated for a scientific paper. Once you learn the basic content required, subsequent manuscripts are easier to write, and your decisions about organizing your next research project are more effective. Second, use appropriate language. This skill, however, does not come without study and experience. To help you publish your research report, this chapter provides general guidelines on preparing yourself for publication, presents the components of a research report, identifies what to consider when preparing a manuscript, and provides a review of common rules of English and a few suggestions on word usage.

PREPARING FOR PUBLICATION

Before you begin the writing phase, you must decide to which journal you will submit your manuscript. Ask yourself questions such as, Who is my intended audience? What readership does the journal have? Does it matter that my manuscript is peer-reviewed? Does the journal have a reputable review process? Do I have to pay to get my manuscript published? Does the journal have highly regarded standards for style and editorial policy? and, Does the journal provide editorial assistance should I need help? You may decide, for example, that you want to submit your basic research paper for consideration to a journal not related to physical therapy because your findings would be of greater interest to basic scientists than to physical therapists. You may decide to submit your paper to a specialty journal within your own profession because of your intended audience and the specificity of the subject matter. You even may consider submitting it to an international journal if the topic is more suitable for that journal's readership.

Next, gather the specific guidelines and instructions for submitting manuscripts to the intended journal. These guidelines and instructions are set forth, generally, by scientific experts and, specifically, by authorities who represent the journal. Generally, for example, most scientific communities advocate using the International System of Units (SI) for all physical measurements, but, specifically, some authorities differ in their preferred format for citing and presenting references. The rules are intended to enhance clarity by providing uniform conversion of manuscripts written in many styles to published articles in one consistent style. This consistency prevents a variety of forms from distracting the readers and promotes a universal understanding of the content. The key point to remember is that you must use the style and format called for by your intended publication. You should forget the style and format of your university compositions and your thesis or dissertation and become familiar with the requirements for a publishable manuscript.

Instructions to authors are published by most journals in almost every issue. The differences in guidelines among journals usually exist because of traditional or common usage of style and language in a particular discipline. The instructions usually include information about (1) the types of articles considered for review; (2) the specific requirements for such factors as title page, abstract, length of text, use of footnotes, citation of references, double spacing, tables, and figures; and (3) the submission procedures, permission to reprint regulations, and copyright transmittal requirements. Most journals will not accept a manuscript for review unless it is submitted according to their instructions and is accompanied by a copyright release statement. Become familiar with the instructions in your intended journal to ensure that your manuscript will at least be considered for review. Your attention to the details of these instructions reflects your interest in and commitment to publishing your study.

Also become knowledgeable about the technical writing style required by your intended journal. To ensure that you are understood by the scientific community you wish to address, you must pay attention to its vocabulary and style of presentation. It is not enough just to complete your study. Conducting research requires not only that you publish your results, but that you write about your study in a particular manner for publication. Some associations have their own style manuals. They vary in specificity, but each contains specific material related to preparing manuscripts and presenting technical data and language for a particular journal. Despite differences, the basic content of some manuals can be used by specialists in other disciplines as well because the language is similar. Physical therapists have many language uses similar to those found in the manuals of the American Psychological Association (APA),[1] the American Medical Association (AMA),[2] and the Council of Biology Editors (CBE),[3] because the physical therapy vocabulary derived from a combination of knowledge of many fields. The American Physical Therapy Association currently advocates use of the AMA style manual when writing for *Physical Therapy,* the journal of the APTA.

If the journal you choose does not have a style manual, look at recent issues of that journal for examples of style and format. You also may find that the journal's instructions follow an established style manual such as the AMA or APA manual. In any case, it is essential that you make yourself familiar with a journal's style, format, and published appearance.

Finally, prepare yourself psychologically for the task at hand. Take heed of the advice given by experts to overcome, reduce, or at least channel writing anxiety. Shilling, for example, summarized 20 valuable tips for conquering writing anxiety that included familiar ideas such as making sure you have a deadline; setting aside a work area; arranging for regular, short writing sessions; breaking the project into small steps; starting whether you are in the mood or not; and giving up on perfectionism.[4] Her other practical ideas included using tape recorders to document a flow of ideas, posing questions to yourself to get ideas on what to include, reading outside your field for ideas on language use and style, and seeking feedback about your writing from reliable sources. Do not assume you already know or use efficient or effective practices. Review these concepts and consider the advice when beginning your professional writing so you can (1) prevent bad habits from forming and (2) correct inefficient practices.

Maybe you also need to determine if you are hindered by misunderstanding the writing process. Do you think your writing has to be perfect the first time? Do you have to know what you are going to say before you start? Do you believe there is one best way to approach a writing project? Shilling also dispelled 10 such myths about professional writing, while providing sound principles that could apply to other writing tasks, such as grant proposals, budget justifications, and even poetry.[5]

Because professional writing is so important, take the time to develop a good understanding of the writing process and of yourself as a writer. Your professional career can depend on the success of your efforts to be effective in written communication.

COMPONENTS

Even before you begin writing, you have already completed the hardest part of your research project: designing and conducting the study. The writing component of your research essentially is nothing more than putting down on paper the thought and actions that went into your work, the findings from the analysis of your data, and your observations regarding your results. If you have not done so already, learn to collect and organize these bits and pieces about your project according to the sections you will be using in your paper: introduction, method, results, discussion, conclusion, references, tables, and figures. You can complete the title and abstract later.

Some researchers use file folders labeled with the manuscript headings as places to collect information or ideas to include when writing. This way, you can collect the thoughts you get while away from the project and put them on note cards or in note form for filing.

You many also want to consider writing about your study while it is in progress. This can enhance the clarity of your detail because the procedures are fresh in your mind. If you have co-authors, you can also resolve more readily any critical issues about the content of the paper or inconsistencies in the procedures.

Title

The title of your paper should be concise, specific, and clear. Choose your words with great care because the title is used not only by indexing and abstracting services to reach intended audiences but also by readers who wish to locate relevant material without reading the entire article.

Write your final title after you have completed your paper. By then you will have established more clearly the key words and phrases of your content and the precise wording of your purpose. In the meantime, select a working title that focuses on your purpose and will keep you from getting sidetracked.

Keep your title short; a title longer than two lines is usually unacceptable. Use specific words and avoid meaningless generalities. Compare the following: (1) "The Results of Comparing Two Different Treatment Techniques Used for Increasing the Strength and Range of Motion in the Knees of Patients on the Neuromedical Rehabilitation Ward" and (2) "Comparison of Methods to Increase Knee Strength and Range of Motion in Patients with Hemiplegia." In the latter, note the precision and succinctness.

Be sure to omit all extraneous words and phrases at the beginning of titles, such as "the," "a," "use of," "report of," and "treatment using." Because the title is not a complete sentence, you can remove verbs and arrange the subject, verb, and object in a nonroutine fashion. It is important, however, to watch for errors in syntax when you choose your word order, because your efforts to be precise can lead to humor at your expense. Consider the errors in this title: "An Interesting Review of the History of the Development and Use of Electricity in the Treatment of Pain Dating Back Long Before Man."

Use subtitles sparingly. They can clarify generalities or give a frame of reference for the content, but they should not duplicate the title.

Be sure to follow the particular journal's style requirements for capitalization, abbreviations, and footnotes. Attention to such details can signify to the reviewers and editor a serious interest in publishing with their journal.

Abstract

An abstract is a brief summary of the manuscript that enables readers to identify the essential facts of the study. It should be a single paragraph of about 150 words that discloses the problem and the solution discussed in the manuscript. Clearly, you must finish writing your manuscript before trying to summarize it. A well-written abstract permits readers to identify quickly and accurately the content of your report and thus to decide whether to read it. Your abstract should permit readers to save time and to understand clearly what you dealt with in your study. Abstracts are often reproduced without change in secondary sources as a service to readers. Think of what you have or have not found useful in the abstracts you reviewed when preparing for your research.

Abstracts of studies should contain statements of purpose, method, results (including significance levels), conclusions, and clinical relevance. For examples of acceptable abstracts, review those in your intended journal. Especially note in the method portion how authors condense information about their subjects, study design, and procedures and instrumentation. You also will find that the order of presentation of the different statements follows the order of the text. This order should help you when you write your abstract after completing the final editing on your paper.

Do not include information that is not stated in the text or is not related to your findings. For accuracy and consistency, double-check your numerical values, word choices and descriptive phrases, and conclusions. It is preferable to use consistent terminology throughout your report and to use the same sequence that is in the text when describing a series of events or results. Finally, check the style preference of the journal about the use of abbreviations or acronyms in abstracts.

Introduction

The introduction should (1) define clearly the problem or question of the study; (2) provide supportive rationale for the importance of the problem by including material that is relevant and of appropriate quality; (3) clarify the purpose of the study; (4) clarify or imply the type of study being reported; (5) include a statement of the null hypothesis or a statement of the expected results if the study is experimental or correlational; and (6) include the need for collecting data or reporting findings if the study is descriptive.

Defining the Problem

When defining the problem, focus on the nature and the scope of the problem. If possible, relate your concerns in a tangible way to the clinical need for the answer to the question or the solution to the problem. Ask yourself specific questions to help refine the issue, such as, What specific dilemma needs resolving? Is it important to mention how the problem came into being? Who sees the problem as worthy of being solved? How does this problem relate to the solution of another problem? and, What are the advantages to having the study question answered? Get feedback from knowledgeable colleagues about your preliminary wording to make sure you are inclusive but succinct. Think of this section of your manuscript as setting the stage, making readers anxious to learn if you solved the problem.

Providing Supportive Rationale

When providing supportive rationale from the literature, use only those essential primary references that specifically deal with your topic. Use this section of the introduction to relate your work to the work of others or to previous work of your own. Weeding out references may take considerable effort, especially if you are converting a thesis or dissertation into manuscript format, because the requirements are different. It is best to avoid using secondary references unless the original source is unavailable or unknown. If you use a secondary source, be sure to check on the journal's style for noting in the reference list such quotations or referrals. To save space, also think of using key sources that refer to the valuable references you would include if you had the space. And remember to follow the style required for citing references by the intended journal.

Stating the Purpose

State the purpose of your study clearly and succinctly. Remember that later, when you do the final writing, your title and abstract must be consistent with your purpose. If you have an extensive literature review section, place your purpose in the first paragraphs of your introduction. This placement enables readers to know immediately your intent, and you can let the rationale follow with a subheading entitled "Literature Review." If your review section is minimal, place your purpose in the paragraph preceding the method section. Your decision should be based on how you can best help inform readers about the logic of your thinking and the intent of your research.

Identifying the Type of Study

Use the introduction to inform readers of the type of study done to solve the problem. For an experimental design, for example, you can state the type either directly (e.g., "The purpose of this experimental study was to . . .") or indirectly (e.g., immediately after the purpose, state, "The null hypothesis for this study was . . . ," which implies an experimental design was used).

Stating the Hypothesis or Expected Results

For any experimental or correlational study, you must include a statement of the null hypothesis or a statement of your expected results (your research hypothesis). If you will be using a one-tailed statistical test, you should indicate here the expected direction of the result and the reason why. You could, for example, say, "I expected to find that age was a greater factor in achieving a high salary level than . . . because . . ." If you will be using a two-tailed statistical test, you should indicate here the expected result (do not include the direction) and the reason why. Be sure to clarify if your hypotheses or expectations are based on the works of others.

Why are this precision and trouble necessary? The information is critical in enabling readers to be sure you collected the appropriate data, presented the data appropriately, analyzed the data correctly, and made legitimate statements about your findings. You, in turn, can look for the same clues when critiquing the work of others.

Justifying the Need for Descriptive Study

For descriptive studies, you must justify the need for collecting the data or reporting your results. This clarification is done easily in your discussion of the importance of the problem. When elaborating on the value of your work, avoid making the common error of including material that is not pertinent to your research problem, purpose, or type of study.

If you need to elaborate on your reasons for selecting a particular test or procedure for part of your study, clarify your rationale in the introduction. If several tests are applicable for measuring what you want, and if you chose one of the methods for a specific reason, then justify your selection. Also clarify what the tests you will be using actually measure if that is not common knowledge. This information is essential; it allows readers not only to understand your thinking but also to replicate your study. You may need to provide this background information by reporting here (or in the method section) on a pilot study you did in preparing for your research.

Subheadings will help readers grasp the flow of your ideas. They can delineate an extensive literature review and also separate remarks about different issues that require distinct presentation of rationale. For example, subheadings could precede the discussion of (1) the ramifications of the pathological condition and (2) the tests used to measure improvement in muscle performance.

In summary, the introduction prepares readers for things to come, enables them to understand why you wanted to do the study, convinces them that you have a solid and logical approach to solving the problem, demonstrates that you know legitimate methods of obtaining answers, and encourages them to read further. The section also allows you to keep the lengthy and complex background material out of the method section, where it interferes with the clarity of your process and flow of ideas.

Method

It is a good idea to write the method section in subsections that represent such divisions as subjects, procedures, instrumentation, special conditions, and statistical analysis of data. The subheadings should match these divisions. In this section you should provide enough detail to enable an experienced person to replicate your study. If some of your procedures are common knowledge and you have followed the steps exactly, cite the primary source for the precise steps.

Subjects

When describing your subjects, clarify such relevant details as numbers, ages (including means and standard deviations), characteristics, and methods of selecting and assigning them to groups. If you developed a special test or measurement, for example, one for screening candidates for your sample, you also may provide the detail in this subsection. Be precise so that another researcher can match your sample with a similar sample. Use tables or figures to consolidate the details if possible.

Your inclusion of pertinent details in this section demonstrates your knowledge of the critical factors about the subjects that might influence their response to your protocol. If you developed any special terminology to describe your subjects, you may give your lengthy or complex operational definitions and explanations in the Introduction section and your brief definitions here. For extremely long lists of definitions, consider using an appendix. Use your judgment about how much to interrupt the flow of your material.

Procedures

The procedures subsection should follow the chronological order of your protocol as much as possible. Use your judgment as to the need to vary the organization of this subsection. Consider the complexity of steps or the advantage of keeping like data together. Give precise detail for all the steps you identify, and provide operational definitions for uncommon or controversial terms. Provide references that give detail whenever possible. Because this part of the paper can contain much complicated detail that often is awkward to present, review how other reports present this material, and determine your own strategies. Some helpful hints are to (1) use lists with a common lead-in sentence; (2) use the active voice; (3) start all sentences in the list with the same kind of word (e.g., a verb or noun); and (4) turn a lengthy and complex procedure into an appendix.

Because the procedures subsection usually contains much technical information, pay particular attention to your need to use footnotes for equipment and materials. Check your style manual for guidelines on what to include; which symbols to use; and the preferred way to present abbreviations, numbers, notations for figures and legends, and subheadings.

Once you have established the order in which to present a study with several parts to your question, keep the subject matter in the same order when you prepare the data analysis, results, discussion, and abstract. If you, for example, first looked at Position A, then Position B, and then Position C, keep that order in mind throughout the rest of the paper. Follow this guideline for all types of material, whether concepts or facts.

Most journals require that you provide evidence in your text that informed consent was obtained or that your study protocol was approved. This statement should be made in the procedures subsection, but you may add it in the subjects subsection if you deem this more appropriate or less awkward.

Data Analysis

The data analysis subsection describes the statistical method(s) used to analyze your data, if applicable. If you believe you used common statistical methods, do not cite a reference. Provide explanations and definitions in the text or cite references for all advanced or unusual methods. Keep in mind the order in which you present your information and maintain the sequence in the rest of the paper. If you have used several analyses, for example, present them in the same order in the results section. In a multipart paper, this ordering should also be coordinated. Also be sure to check your style manual for use of statistical terminology and symbols and advice on how to present equations.

Authors often commit common errors when writing about their data analysis. They provide excessive and erudite explanations of common, simple tests but fail to provide help with the unknown; they do not include the correct name of the test or misspell proper names; they include abbreviations for statistical terms when the words should have been spelled out; they do not mention all the tests reported in the results section; and they include the data analysis information in the results section. As I noted, these are observations about writing errors and not assessments of the overall appropriateness of the analysis for the particular type of study and design, for testing the expectations of null hypotheses, or for the kind of data collected. Those concerns are addressed in the review process.

For descriptive studies, you do not always need a data analysis subsection. Instead, you can state briefly how you compiled or arranged your data if such information is not obvious from your procedures.

Results

The results section requires discrimination in selecting and compiling your data and precision and clarity in preparing and displaying your findings. Your first challenge is to find ways to present data that represent rather than repeat all your raw data. Then you must plan for the most appropriate type and number of tabular or visual presentations that will display your data adequately.

General guidelines to follow include the following:

1. If only a few data are for presentation, add them descriptively in the text.
2. If repetitive data are needed, give them in tables or figures, but include a complementary summary statement in the text.
3. If the data were analyzed for statistical significance, include in the text the relevant critical values (e.g., t, r, F, X), degrees of freedom, and obtained p values.
4. If data are qualitative, include in the text the means and standard deviations or median and range.

The results section, therefore, may be the shortest section of your paper. If you have prepared your readers well in the method section, the results should need little explanation. It is not enough, however, to say merely, "The results are found in the Table."

There are some common errors to avoid: Do not include in this section material that belongs in the procedures or data analysis subsections. Do not present results that are not related to your purpose of the study. And do not discuss the results as you present them.

Some general rules apply when writing about your results. Remember to consider organizing your data according to the procedures and data analysis subsections. Use appropriate subheadings as necessary to enhance the clarity of your organization. Double-check your numbers in the text, and compare them with those in the tables, figures, and abstract. Use the same descriptive words here that you used throughout the rest of the paper.

Discussion

Write the discussion succinctly and in the same order in which you presented your procedures and results. By following the same sequence, you and your readers will not be sidetracked, and you will be sure to cover all the essential material.

Avoid adding "nice to know" information as afterthoughts. If an idea is not factual or does not relate directly to an aspect of the procedures or results, leave it out. Do not repeat the results in this section except in a general sense. If, as a result of your findings, you did an additional statistical test to analyze your findings further, include the test rationale, the test, and the findings in this section.

If your study involved testing a hypothesis, clarify early in this section whether (1) the hypothesis was accepted or rejected or (2) the results were as expected. If you used a one-tailed statistical test and your results did not occur in the expected direction stated in the introduction section, then you cannot give an explanation here other than that the reasons originally put forth were not confirmed. If your results occurred in the expected direction, you can expand here on the reasons for your expectations as stated in the introduction section. If you used a two-tailed statistical test and your expected results occurred, you can expand here on the reasons for your expectations stated in the introduction. If your expected results did not occur, you cannot give an explanation here other than that the reasons originally put forth were not confirmed. This means that with a two-tailed statistical test, you cannot discuss the apparent direction of your result.

Next, proceed with the discussion by relating your comments to such considerations as (1) the importance of the findings (as pertains to what was done in and obtained from the study); (2) the problem, importance of the problem, purpose of the study, and either the expectations and reasons for them (if an experimental or correlational study) or the need for the data (if a descriptive study); and (3) the work done by others.

Unless your research was theoretical, summarize the clinical relevance of your findings and make practical suggestions for the clinical application of your results. If the research was theoretical, discuss where you think your results might lead. If applicable, consider using a separate subheading entitled "Clinical Implications." And, finally, be sure to discuss the limitations of your findings and include suggestions for further research or additional research questions raised by your study results.

Conclusion

Close your paper with a brief conclusion based on your findings and the implications of your results. Use this section to highlight the major thoughts you have about your findings so readers know your final perspective and considerations. Do not create a summary for this section as in an abstract, which includes your purpose and method, and do not draw conclusions unless they are based on fact.

References

References are often the most problematic part of the manuscript for authors and editors. There are two reasons for this. First, authors frequently do not obtain adequate information for a complete citation. Second, journals have different styles. To avoid having inadequate information, develop a system of collecting all the information you might need for most journals of your interest. The confusion that results from various journal styles is remedied by becoming familiar with the preferred style of the journals for which you choose to write. Most scientific journals have enough common rules so your task should not be impossible. As I noted earlier, the rules are easy to find in the journal's instructions or manuals and are easy to observe by example. Although authors are accountable for the accuracy of their references, the editorial staff of some journals will assist authors with completeness and accuracy by asking pertinent questions.

As I mentioned in the introduction section, select only important primary sources, especially those containing related references. For the journal *Physical Therapy*, limit the number of references to 15 to 20 for a manuscript of 15 pages. Avoid using nonscientific publications, such as newsletters or magazines, unless they are exceptionally critical to your purpose; such references reflect poorly on your credibility. Do not include a suggested reading list.

Cite the references in the text and make a reference list according to the system advocated by your intended journal. Each system has its own advantages and disadvantages. The journal *Physical Therapy*, for example, uses the *citation order system* that calls for numbering the references consecutively as they appear in the text and listing them in that numerical order. This system minimizes interruptions to the flow of reading because the citation numbers are set in small type and placed as superscripts. The other systems are *name and year* (placed in parentheses within a sentence in the text) and *alphabet-number* (the list is alphabetized and numbered, and the numbers are used in the text as superscripts). When listing references for *Physical Therapy*, pay attention to special instructions such as double spacing your list, using only certain abbreviations for journal names, and not including unpublished data on the list.

Figures

Use figures, or illustrations, to complement the text, support your conclusions, or demonstrate your results and concepts. Figures include all types of illustrations, such as line drawings, graphs, photographs, photographs of roentgenograms, and recorded graph tracings. It is important to be very selective in your choice of figures. Every figure should have a definite purpose. In this way, you cut down on your own preparation costs and on the journal's production and publication costs.

Each type of figure has specifications that must be followed. You will save time and money by finding out in advance each journal's requirements not only for content but also for such factors as format, number of copies, labeling, size of lettering, preparation of ink line drawings, legend sheets, abbreviations, protection of photographs, and photograph-release statements.

Use figures only for a specific purpose that is not duplicated in the text, for example, to show results; reveal trends and relationships; show actual records; or demonstrate ideas, equipment, positions, and activities. Also remember that because your figure will be reduced in size when printed, much of the detail and wording may be lost. The final product will be only as good as the original art work.

Appendixes

You may be permitted to use an appendix in certain journals, but the option is rare because of space constraints. *Physical Therapy* allows appendixes because they help prevent the text from being cluttered with details that (1) are not critical for readers to know immediately and (2) would impede the flow of thought. However, such material must also be unsuitable for a table or a figure.

Acknowledgments

Write acknowledgments sparingly and succinctly. The two general categories of acknowledgments are the personal type and those for equipment or supplies. Use this opportunity to express appreciation for such considerations as important ideas, supplies, equipment, consultation, or assistance. Check your intended journal for examples and placement. Avoid flowery or superfluous language.

Title Page

When you are ready to type your manuscript, check the journal's instructions or the style manual for what to include on the title page. Most journals require basic content such as authors and affiliations. You will find, however, a variety of preferences for the presentation of other information, including degrees, corresponding author, previous presentation, and acknowledgment of financial support.

In the case of co-authors, the first person listed usually is considered the primary or senior author and the one responsible for handling all correspondence and making revisions. If you and your co-authors agree to a different plan, be sure to make that clear to the editor. The list of authors should include only those who actively made an important contribution to designing or conducting the research protocol. Furthermore, the list should be in the order of the authors' importance to the experiment. These decisions are not always easy to make but are important because the primary author usually gets the recognition for having done most of the work (the recognition may be in the form of an award).

Decide early in your professional writing career how you will present your name, and be consistent thereafter. Cumulative author indexes for most journals have separate notations for a name presented with and without a middle initial. If you are inconsistent, you may not have all of your work recognized.

PREPARATION AND SUBMISSION OF MANUSCRIPTS

Before you make the final copy of your manuscript, someone else should read and edit your work. You undoubtedly will have had consultants look at the content as you have gone along, but you need a critique of your final draft to ensure that your manuscript is the best that it can be. Consider having different people check your work for various purposes, for example, one who knows the material as well as you do, another whose knowledge is at the level of the readers you want to reach, and someone else who is an accomplished writer or editor but is not in your field. Be specific in your requests to each person so you can take advantage of their expertise.

As noted before, you must remember to prepare and submit your manuscript according to the instructions and style preferred by your journal. You are account-able not only for the content of your manuscript but also for the detail and accuracy of the presentation. This means you may have to oversee the typist if the person is unfamiliar with your journal specifications. Be sure that the person who types your revision is just as familiar with your preferences, or the individual inadvertently may undo your acceptable presentation, which could call for an additional revision on your part. Learn the basic style yourself so that you can instruct and oversee the typist.

Submit your manuscript according to the instructions for your intended journal. Be sure to comply with all the requirements: numbers of copies, duplicates of figures, copyright release statement, photograph-release forms, and permission-to-reprint statements.

RECOMMENDATIONS FOR WRITING

Writing scientific and scholarly reports calls for applying the same basic lan-guage rules required for all communication. Problems can arise in applying the rules, however, because these common rules are not a primary professional interest and also because the current literature frequently contains examples of misused and incorrect language. Despite these obstacles, you must learn to achieve a practi-cal application of basic rules if you intend to write professionally.

Writing for scientific literature also calls for establishing and demonstrating a style of writing that can be understood by your peers and is acceptable to your scientific community. As stated before, achieving this writing skill takes study and practice. If you are successful in developing your writing skills using a simple, basic style that is understood easily and quickly, you may never need or want to become an eclectic author who writes more with literary flair than with clarity. The unique-ness of your individual writing style will still be evident, even with a simple style of writing.

You must pay attention to your writing skill if you are to be successful in reporting your research or documenting your practice. Numerous books are avail-able that give detailed descriptions and examples, so here I will provide only highlights based on my observations of beginning authors' needs.[6–8]

Reviewing the Rules

Find, review, and keep on hand reliable sources that will help you remember the rules or solve the problems about usage. Do not try to keep all the complex requirements in your head, but learn to use and rely on your resources. Be cautious about turning to the current literature you read for good examples of syntax or grammar, even if you believe the publication is reputable. Review and use English rules from such sources as *Words Into Type*[9] and the *Harbrace College Handbook*[10] so that you do not propagate common errors and poor writing. Refresh your memory about such grammatical rules as avoiding split infinitives and split predicates and the common rules for punctuation. As you become more experienced in writing and more knowledgeable about the basic rules, you will become wise about detecting problems in the writing of others and about knowing which authors to emulate.

When reviewing the rules for using English, pay particular attention to guidelines on subject-verb agreement, consistent syntax, consistent and accurate tenses, dangling participles, ambiguous and unnecessary ramblers, and singular and plural word forms. The following examples, which represent the more common types of errors found in my experience, clarify the above concerns.

Subject-verb agreement. Keep agreement of a verb with its subject and a pronoun with its antecedent. You would need to say, for example, "The *assessment* for shoulders, hips, and knees *is* completed . . ." rather than ". . .*are* completed."

Syntax. Keep syntax consistent by using the same construction to present similar material in a sentence. Start each phrase of a series in a sentence with the same type of construction, such as a verb, a noun, or a complete sentence. For example, a construction using verbs would be, "The author's first manuscript was submitted, revised, and accepted because she had developed good professional writing skills." A cumbersome construction would be, "The author's first manuscript was submitted, the requests for revisions were acted on, and the paper met with acceptance."

Tenses. Keep tenses straight and accurate in the different sections of your paper. It is permissible to move between the past and present tenses. In general, use the past tense when preparing your abstract, writing parts of the literature review, describing your methods, presenting your results, and elaborating in parts of your discussion. Use the present tense when presenting the purpose of your paper in the abstract and introduction: "The purpose of this article *is* to . . ." In parts of the literature review, use the past tense to demonstrate that someone's work was done in the past, but use the present tense to describe their results: "Morra showed that the position of the upper extremity inhibits the action of the wrist flexors.[21]" Refer to your results in the past tense until after your article is published. In those parts of the discussion where you compare your findings with those of previously published work, use the past tense for your findings and the present tense for the findings of others. For further examples, consult various journals.

Dangling participles. Avoid dangling participles. Double-check to see that sentences beginning with "-ing" word forms have the modifier placed immediately following the introductory phrase in the sentence. You would not want to say, for example, "Lying directly under the electrode, you will be able to find many small blisters" because this means that "you" are under the electrode. You could improve this by saying, "Lying directly under the electrode, many small blisters will be found." Best of all, however, avoid the problem by converting the sentence to the active voice: "You will find many small blisters directly under the electrode."

Ramblers. Avoid ambiguous ramblers and meaningless phrases, such as "there are" and "it is," by rewording your sentences. Use the active voice to identify the subject of the sentence and to clarify your intent. Instead of saying, "There are three important reasons for learning the rules of grammar . . . ," say "Three important reasons exist for learning grammatical rules . . ." or "The three reasons for learning grammatical rules are. . . ."

Singular vs plural. Prevent problems with singular and plural word forms by double-checking in a dictionary the word forms, for example, criterion/criteria, datum/data, and curriculum/curricula. You will then know whether to use a singular or plural verb form.

Selecting Style and Syntax

Develop and use a simple writing style. Your ability to write simple declarative statements not only will enable readers to understand you better but will enable you to avoid most of the common grammatical problems. Writing short, simple sentences also will enhance the clarity and preciseness of your sentences. Some of the elements of simple writing are as follows:

- Use the active voice if at all possible. Most scientific journals currently advocate the use of active voice and personal pronouns to enhance the author's accuracy and the readers' understanding. The old style of scientific writing that mandated only using the passive voice and avoiding personal pronouns no longer is advocated because it could result in lack of clarity and preciseness. It is permissible to mix the active and passive voices. And, in some cases, it still is more appropriate to use the passive voice, such as when the object is more important than the subject. If using the passive voice, be careful to avoid ambiguity. When the option of voice is yours, however, using the active voice will facilitate the ease of your writing.
- Keep verbs close to the subject, especially when you have a sentence with multiple and long phrases. Writing several sentences instead of one sometimes helps solve this problem.
- Watch for misplaced modifiers that could destroy your intent. Can you believe the following description? "The therapist used a posture training device at a state facility for staff members who slouched." Was it really the staff members who slouched?
- Use fewer or shorter words, for example, (1) use the verb form of a word instead of the noun pattern (say "planning" instead of "the planning of," and "analyzes" instead of "presents an analysis of"); (2) eliminate long-winded expressions by using short substitutions (say "can" instead of "are capable of,"

and "motor skills" instead of "skills in the motor area"); and (3) delete redundant words (say "few" not "few in number," and "outcome" not "final outcome"). Refer to a style manual for lists of other suggestions.

Another important consideration in writing clearly is choosing words carefully. The accuracy of your word choice is critical to the universal understanding of your ideas. The misuse of many words has become so common that some authors resist editorial corrections and fight to maintain errors because they find published examples to support them. The mistakes involve not only misusing technical words such as "parameter," "interface," and "valgus/varus," but also creating imprecise meanings by using "since" for "because," "while" for "although," "which" for "that," and "presently" for "currently." Keep in mind not to accept what you read in every journal as being the best example to copy. Use your dictionary constantly to keep your language accurate and precise. Also remember that the use of superlatives is not indicated when reporting scientific data.

Clear writing also demands knowledge about word usage and placement. Some words must be used in conjunction with other words to complete a thought. For example, you must use "either–or," "greater–than," "neither–nor," and "not only–but" in the same sentence. These pairs are important to remember particularly when you present your results by saying one factor had greater response than another factor. To avoid making a comparative statement, you may be able to reword your sentence and use such words as "increased" and "decreased" for larger and smaller. You also might use words like "most," "biggest," and "smallest."

Other words must be placed in a specific order in a sentence. Adverbs, for example, such as "however" and "also," must be placed within the sentence as close as possible to the words they modify. This means that the words "however" and "also" rarely can begin a sentence. There are exceptions, of course.

Finally, avoid jargon and sexist language. The coined phrases or clinical slang used during the working day or in the laboratory are generally not acceptable in a professional journal but may be used if you introduce them in quotation marks and provide your operational definitions. Become familiar with acceptable terms by reading the most current textbooks and medical dictionaries. Be selective if you consider using journals for help in determining what is jargon. Contemporary literature supports the use of nonsexist language. Refer to the available style manuals for suggestions on rewording and substitutions for gender-specific language.

SUMMARY

One of the most rewarding professional experiences is to complete a research project and have your report published. The steps leading to publication call for commitment, perseverance, and patience in writing. A few aspects of the writing tasks, however, are relatively simple because a format and organization exist for you to follow and examples abound for you to emulate. Because the more difficult aspects of professional writing are not mastered without concentrated effort and study, you need to take steps to do the following: prepare yourself with the tools and guidelines to use when writing, learn the basic content and organization required for an acceptable research report, and review commonly used rules of English and writing techniques so you can practice exemplary writing skills.

While you diligently practice applying the basic rules and recommended guidelines, remember that you are not alone in your anxieties and frustrations. As you gain experience, you probably will find that most readers, editors, and other authors have more empathy and support for you than you originally thought. We commend you for undertaking and enduring your professional writing career.

REFERENCES

1. *Publication manual of the American psychological association,* 3rd ed. Washington, DC: American Psychological Association, 1983.

2. Barclay, W.R., Southgate, M.T., and Mayo, R.W., eds. *Manual for authors and editors: Editorial style and manuscript preparation,* 7th ed. Los Altos, CA: Lange Medical Publications, 1981.

3. *CBE style manual,* rev. 5th ed. Bethesda, MD: Council of Biology Editors, 1983.

4. Shilling, L.M. Twenty tips for conquering writing anxiety: Writing tips. *Physical Therapy* 65:1113–1115, 1985.

5. Shilling, L.M. Ten myths about professional writing: Writing tips. *Physical Therapy* 64:1417–1423, 1984.

6. Day, R.A. *How to write and publish a scientific paper,* 2nd ed. Philadelphia, PA: ISI Press, 1983.

7. DeBakey, L. *The scientific journal: Editorial policies and practices—guidelines for editors, reviewers, and authors.* St. Louis, MO: C. V. Mosby, 1976.

8. Strunk, W. and White, E.B. *The elements of style,* 2nd ed. New York: Macmillan, 1972.

9. Skillen, M. and Gay, R. *Words into type,* 3rd ed. Englewood Cliffs, NJ: Prentice Hall, 1974.

10. Hodges, J.C. and Whitten, M.E. *Harbrace college handbook,* 9th ed. New York: Harcourt Brace Jovanovich, 1982.

INDEX

Numbers followed by an *f* indicate a figure; *t* following a page number indicates tabular material.

ISBN 0-397-54803-6

90000

9 780397 548033